T0259481

Sleep Hypoventilation: A State-of-the-Art Overview

Editor

BABAK MOKHLESI

SLEEP MEDICINE CLINICS

www.sleep.theclinics.com

Consulting Editor
TEOFILO LEE-CHIONG Jr

September 2014 • Volume 9 • Number 3

ELSEVIER

1600 John F. Kennedy Boulevard • Suite 1800 • Philadelphia, Pennsylvania, 19103-2899

http://www.theclinics.com

SLEEP MEDICINE CLINICS Volume 9, Number 3
September 2014, ISSN 1556-407X, ISBN-13: 978-0-323-32680-3

Editor: Patrick Manley
Developmental Editor: Donald Mumford

© **2014 Elsevier Inc. All rights reserved.**

This periodical and the individual contributions contained in it are protected under copyright by Elsevier, and the following terms and conditions apply to their use:

Photocopying
Single photocopies of single articles may be made for personal use as allowed by national copyright laws. Permission of the Publisher and payment of a fee is required for all other photocopying, including multiple or systematic copying, copying for advertising or promotional purposes, resale, and all forms of document delivery. Special rates are available for educational institutions that wish to make photocopies for non-profit educational classroom use. For information on how to seek permission visit www.elsevier.com/permissions or call: (+44) 1865 843830 (UK)/(+1) 215 239 3804 (USA).

Derivative Works
Subscribers may reproduce tables of contents or prepare lists of articles including abstracts for internal circulation within their institutions. Permission of the Publisher is required for resale or distribution outside the institution. Permission of the Publisher is required for all other derivative works, including compilations and translations (please consult www.elsevier.com/permissions).

Electronic Storage or Usage
Permission of the Publisher is required to store or use electronically any material contained in this periodical, including any article or part of an article (please consult www.elsevier.com/permissions). Except as outlined above, no part of this publication may be reproduced, stored in a retrieval system or transmitted in any form or by any means, electronic, mechanical, photocopying, recording or otherwise, without prior written permission of the Publisher.

Notice
No responsibility is assumed by the Publisher for any injury and/or damage to persons or property as a matter of products liability, negligence or otherwise, or from any use or operation of any methods, products, instructions or ideas contained in the material herein. Because of rapid advances in the medical sciences, in particular, independent verification of diagnoses and drug dosages should be made. Although all advertising material is expected to conform to ethical (medical) standards, inclusion in this publication does not constitute a guarantee or endorsement of the quality or value of such product or of the claims made of it by its manufacturer.

Sleep Medicine Clinics (ISSN 1556-407X) is published quarterly by Elsevier Inc., 360 Park Avenue South, New York, NY 10010-1710. Months of issue are March, June, September and December. Business and Editorial Offices: 1600 John F. Kennedy Blvd., Ste. 1800, Philadelphia, PA 19103-2899. Customer Service Office: 3251 Riverport Lane, Maryland Heights, MO 63043. Periodicals postage paid at New York, NY and additional mailing offices. Subscription prices are $195.00 per year (US individuals), $95.00 (US residents), $406.00 (US institutions), $230.00 (Canadian individuals), $235.00 (foreign individuals), $135.00 (Canadian and foreign residents) and $452.00 (Canadian and foreign institutions). Foreign air speed delivery is included in all *Clinics* subscription prices. All prices are subject to change without notice. **POSTMASTER:** Send change of address to *Sleep Medicine Clinics*, Elsevier Health Sciences Division, Subscription Customer Service, 3251 Riverport Lane, Maryland Heights, MO 63043. Customer Service: **Tel: 1-800-654-2452 (U.S. and Canada); 314-447-8871 (outside U.S. and Canada). Fax: 314-447-8029. E-mail: journalscustomerservice-usa@elsevier.com (for print support); journalsonlinesupport-usa@elsevier.com (for online support)**.

Reprints. For copies of 100 or more of articles in this publication, please contact the Commercial Reprints Department, Elsevier Inc., 360 Park Avenue South, New York, NY 10010-1710. Tel.: 212-633-3874; Fax: 212-633-3820; E-mail: reprints@elsevier.com.

PROGRAM OBJECTIVE
The goal of *Sleep Clinics of North America* is to keep practicing physicians up to date with current clinical practice by providing timely articles reviewing the state of the art in patient care.

TARGET AUDIENCE
All practicing physicians and other healthcare professionals.

LEARNING OBJECTIVES
Upon completion of this activity, participants will be able to:
1. Review hypoventilation syndromes of infancy, childhood, and adulthood.
2. Discuss advances in PAP treatment modalities for hypoventilation syndromes.
3. Recognize diagnostic consideration and technological limitations related to sleep hypoventilation.

ACCREDITATION
The Elsevier Office of Continuing Medical Education (EOCME) is accredited by the Accreditation Council for Continuing Medical Education (ACCME) to provide continuing medical education for physicians.

The EOCME designates this enduring material for a maximum of 15 *AMA PRA Category 1 Credit*(s)™. Physicians should claim only the credit commensurate with the extent of their participation in the activity.

All other health care professionals requesting continuing education credit for this enduring material will be issued a certificate of participation.

DISCLOSURE OF CONFLICTS OF INTEREST
The EOCME assesses conflict of interest with its instructors, faculty, planners, and other individuals who are in a position to control the content of CME activities. All relevant conflicts of interest that are identified are thoroughly vetted by EOCME for fair balance, scientific objectivity, and patient care recommendations. EOCME is committed to providing its learners with CME activities that promote improvements or quality in healthcare and not a specific proprietary business or a commercial interest.

The planning committee, staff, authors and editors listed below have identified no financial relationships or relationships to products or devices they or their spouse/life partner have with commercial interest related to the content of this CME activity:

Loutfi S. Aboussouan, MD; Dan Adler, MD; Maged Argalious, MD, MBA; Nevin Arora, MD; Indu A. Ayappa, PhD; Jay S. Balachandran, MD; Kenneth I. Berger, MD; Rakesh Bhattacharjee, MD; Michelle Cao, MD; Michael S. Carroll, PhD; Frances Chung, MBBS; Daniel Combs, MD; Olivier Contal, PhD; Katherine A. Dudley, MD; Marieke Leontine Duiverman, MD, PhD; Roberta M. Goldring, MD; Jésus Gonzalez-Bermejo; David Gozal, MD; Nicholas Hart, FRCP, PhD; Kristen Helm; Brynne Hunter; Jean-Paul Janssens, MD; Roop Kaw, MD; Sandy Lavery; Stephen W. Littleton, MD; Atul Malhotra, MD; Patrick Manley; Juan Fernando Masa, MD, PhD; Jill McNair; Babak Mokhlesi, MD, MSc; Gökhan M. Mutlu, MD; Mahalakshmi Narayanan; Pallavi P. Patwari, MD; Jean-Louis Pepin, MD, PhD; Claudio Rabec, MD; Casey M. Rand, BS; David M. Rapoport, MD; Rehan Saiyed, BS; Safal Shetty, MD; Aiman Tulaimat, MD; Debra E. Weese-Mayer, MD; Lisa F. Wolfe, MD.

The planning committee, staff, authors and editors listed below have identified financial relationships or relationships to products or devices they or their spouse/life partner have with commercial interest related to the content of this CME activity:

Jean-Christian Borel, PhD has an employment affiliation with AGIR a Dom; has a research grant and is a consultant/advisor for Koninklijke Philips N.V.

Shahrokh Javaheri, MD is on speakers bureau and has research grant from Respironics; is on speakers bureau for ResMed; and is a consultant/advisor for Respicordia.

Teofilo Lee-Chiong, Jr., MD has stock ownership, a research grant and an employment affiliation with Koninklijke Philips N.V. is a consultant/advisor for CareCore National and Elsevier; and has royalties/patents with Elsevier, Lippincott, Wiley, Oxford University and CreateSpace.

Patrick B. Murphy, MRCP, PhD is on speakers bureau for Koninklijke Philips N.V.; has research grant from Koninklijke Philips N.V.; and ResMed.

Robert L. Owens, MD is a consultant/advisor for Koninklijke Philips N.V.

Sairam Parthasarathy, MD has royalties/patents with Up-To-Date, Inc.; is on speakers bureau for Koninklijke Philips N.V.; and has research grants from Younes Sleep Technologies and Koninklijke Philips N.V.

Amanda J. Piper, BAppSc, MEd, PhD is a consultant/advisor for ResMed and Koninklijke Philips N.V., and has a research grant from the ResMed Foundation.

Renaud Tamisier, MD, PhD has research grants from Resmed Foundation and AGIR a Dom is on speakers bureau for AstraZeneca.

Peter Jan Wijkstra, MD, PhD is on speakers bureau and has research grants from Vivisol, Resmed and Koninklijke Philips N.V.; also has research grants from Medicq TEFA and Emdamed.

UNAPPROVED/OFF-LABEL USE DISCLOSURE
The EOCME requires CME faculty to disclose to the participants:
1. When products or procedures being discussed are off-label, unlabelled, experimental, and/or investigational (not US Food and Drug Administration (FDA) approved); and

2. Any limitations on the information presented, such as data that are preliminary or that represent ongoing research, interim analyses, and/or unsupported opinions. Faculty may discuss information about pharmaceutical agents that is outside of FDA-approved labelling. This information is intended solely for CME and is not intended to promote off-label use of these medications. If you have any questions, contact the medical affairs department of the manufacturer for the most recent prescribing information.

TO ENROLL

To enroll in the Sleep Medicines Clinic Continuing Medical Education program, call customer service at 1-800-654-2452 or sign up online at http://www.theclinics.com/home/cme. The CME program is available to subscribers for an additional annual fee of USD $126.

METHOD OF PARTICIPATION

In order to claim credit, participants must complete the following:
1. Complete enrolment as indicated above.
2. Read the activity.
3. Complete the CME Test and Evaluation. Participants must achieve a score of 70% on the test. All CME Tests and Evaluations must be completed online.

CME INQUIRIES/SPECIAL NEEDS

For all CME inquiries or special needs, please contact elsevierCME@elsevier.com.

SLEEP MEDICINE CLINICS

ISSUES OF RELATED INTEREST

Sleep Medicine Clinics, Vol. 9, No.1 (March 2014)
Central Sleep Apnea
Peter Gay, MD, *Editor*

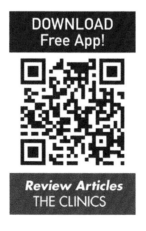

**DOWNLOAD
Free App!**

Review Articles
THE CLINICS

NOW AVAILABLE FOR YOUR iPhone and iPad

Contributors

CONSULTING EDITOR

TEOFILO LEE-CHIONG Jr, MD
Professor of Medicine, Division of Pulmonary,
Critical Care and Sleep Medicine, Department
of Medicine, National Jewish Health, University
of Colorado, Denver, Colorado; Chief Medical
Liaison, Philips Respironics, Pennsylvania

EDITOR

BABAK MOKHLESI, MD, MSc
Professor of Medicine, Section of Pulmonary
and Critical Care, Department of Medicine,
Director, Sleep Disorders Center and Sleep
Fellowship Program, University of Chicago,
Chicago, Illinois

AUTHORS

LOUTFI S. ABOUSSOUAN, MD
Cleveland Clinic, Cleveland, Ohio

DAN ADLER, MD
Division of Pulmonary Diseases, Geneva
University Hospitals, Geneva, Switzerland

MAGED ARGALIOUS, MD, MBA
Cleveland Clinic, Cleveland, Ohio

NEVIN ARORA, MD
Stanford Sleep Medicine, Stanford University,
Redwood City, California

INDU AYAPPA, PhD
Associate Professor of Medicine, Division of
Pulmonary, Critical Care and Sleep Medicine,
Department of Medicine, New York University
School of Medicine; André Cournand
Pulmonary Physiology Laboratory, Bellevue
Hospital, New York, New York

JAY S. BALACHANDRAN, MD
Section of Pulmonary and Critical Care,
Department of Medicine, Sleep Disorders
Center, University of Chicago, Chicago, Illinois

KENNETH I. BERGER, MD
Associate Professor of Medicine, Physiology
and Neuroscience, Division of Pulmonary,
Critical Care and Sleep Medicine, Department
of Medicine, New York University School of
Medicine; André Cournand Pulmonary
Physiology Laboratory, Bellevue Hospital,
New York, New York

RAKESH BHATTACHARJEE, MD
Sections of Pediatric Sleep Medicine
and Pediatric Pulmonology, Department
of Pediatrics, Comer Children's Hospital,
Pritzker School of Medicine, The
University of Chicago, Chicago, Illinois

JEAN-CHRISTIAN BOREL, PhD
Research and Development Department,
AGIR à dom, Meylan, France

MICHELLE CAO, MD
Stanford Sleep Medicine, Stanford University,
Redwood City, California

MICHAEL S. CARROLL, PhD
Center for Autonomic Medicine in Pediatrics (CAMP), Ann & Robert H. Lurie Children's Hospital of Chicago; Northwestern University Feinberg School of Medicine, Chicago, Illinois

FRANCES CHUNG, MBBS
Department of Anesthesia, Toronto Western Hospital, University Health Network, University of Toronto, Toronto, Ontario, Canada

DANIEL COMBS, MD
Department of Pediatrics, Arizona Respiratory Center, University of Arizona; Division of Pulmonary, Critical Care, Allergy and Sleep Medicine, Department of Medicine, Arizona Respiratory Center, University of Arizona, Tucson, Arizona

OLIVIER CONTAL, PhD
Department of Physiotherapy, HESAV School of Health Sciences, University of Applied Sciences Western Switzerland, Lausanne, Switzerland

KATHERINE A. DUDLEY, MD
Research and Clinical Fellow, Harvard Combined Program of Pulmonary and Critical Care and Division of Sleep and Circadian Disorders at Brigham and Women's Hospital, Boston, Massachusetts

MARIEKE LEONTINE DUIVERMAN, MD, PhD
Department of Pulmonary Diseases/Home Mechanical Ventilation, University Medical Centre Groningen, Groningen, The Netherlands

ROBERTA M. GOLDRING, MD
Professor of Medicine, Division of Pulmonary, Critical Care and Sleep Medicine, Department of Medicine, New York University School of Medicine; André Cournand Pulmonary Physiology Laboratory, Bellevue Hospital, New York, New York

JÉSUS GONZALEZ-BERMEJO, MD, PhD
Department of Respiratory and Critical Care Medicine, Groupe Hospitalier Pitié-Salpêtrière, Assistance Publique-Hôpitaux de Paris; Neurophysiologie Respiratoire Expérimentale et Clinique, INSERM, Hôpital de la Pitié-Salpêtriére, Paris, France

DAVID GOZAL, MD
Sections of Pediatric Sleep Medicine and Pediatric Pulmonology, Department of Pediatrics, Comer Children's Hospital, Pritzker School of Medicine, The University of Chicago, Chicago, Illinois

NICHOLAS HART, FRCP, PhD
Lane Fox Clinical Respiratory Physiology Research Centre, Guy's & St Thomas' NHS Foundation Trust; Division of Asthma, Allergy and Lung Biology, King's College London; Lane Fox Respiratory Unit, Guy's & St Thomas' NHS Foundation Trust, London, United Kingdom

JEAN-PAUL JANSSENS, MD
Division of Pulmonary Diseases, Hôpital Cantonal, Geneva University Hospitals, Geneva, Switzerland

SHAHROKH JAVAHERI, MD
Professor Emeritus, Division of Pulmonary, Critical Care & Sleep Medicine, University of Cincinnati, Cincinnati, Ohio

ROOP KAW, MD
Associate Professor, Cleveland Clinic Lerner College of Medicine; Departments of Hospital Medicine and Outcomes Research Anesthesia; Cleveland Clinic, Cleveland, Ohio

STEPHEN W. LITTLETON, MD
Assistant Professor, Rush University Medical Center; Pulmonary, Critical Care and Sleep Medicine, John H. Stroger Hospital of Cook County, Chicago, Illinois

ATUL MALHOTRA, MD
Kenneth M. Moser Professor of Medicine, Chief of Pulmonary and Critical Care Medicine, Director of Sleep Medicine, University of California San Diego, San Diego, California

JUAN FERNANDO MASA, MD, PhD
Pulmonary Division, San Pedro de Alcantara Hospital, Caceres; CIBERES National Research Network, Madrid, Spain

BABAK MOKHLESI, MD, MSc
Professor of Medicine, Section of Pulmonary and Critical Care, Department of Medicine, Director, Sleep Disorders Center and Sleep Fellowship Program, University of Chicago, Chicago, Illinois

PATRICK B. MURPHY, MRCP, PhD
Lane Fox Clinical Respiratory Physiology
Research Centre, Guy's & St Thomas' NHS
Foundation Trust; Division of Asthma, Allergy
and Lung Biology, King's College London,
London, United Kingdom

GÖKHAN M. MUTLU, MD
Professor of Medicine, Section of Pulmonary
and Critical Care Medicine, University of
Chicago, Chicago, Illinois

ROBERT L. OWENS, MD
Assistant Professor of Medicine, Divisions of
Pulmonary and Critical Care and Sleep and
Circadian Disorders, Brigham and Women's
Hospital, Boston, Massachusetts

SAIRAM PARTHASARATHY, MD
Division of Pulmonary, Critical Care, Allergy
and Sleep Medicine, Associate Professor of
Medicine, Department of Medicine, Arizona
Respiratory Center, University of Arizona,
Tucson, Arizona

PALLAVI P. PATWARI, MD
Assistant Professor of Pediatrics, Sleep
Medicine Center, Department of Pediatrics,
Ann & Robert H. Lurie Children's Hospital of
Chicago, Chicago, Illinois

JEAN-LOUIS PEPIN, MD, PhD
INSERM U 1042, Sleep Laboratory, Grenoble
University Hospital, CHU de Grenoble,
Grenoble, France

AMANDA J. PIPER, BAppSc, MEd, PhD
Department of Respiratory and Sleep
Medicine, Royal Prince Alfred Hospital,
Camperdown; Sleep and Circadian Group,
Woolcock Institute of Medical Research,
Glebe, New South Wales, Australia

CLAUDIO RABEC, MD
Service de Pneumologie et Réanimation
Respiratoire, Centre Hospitalier et Universitaire
de Dijon, Dijon, France

CASEY M. RAND, BS
Center for Autonomic Medicine in Pediatrics
(CAMP), Ann & Robert H. Lurie Children's
Hospital of Chicago, Chicago, Illinois

DAVID M. RAPOPORT, MD
Professor of Medicine, Division of Pulmonary,
Critical Care and Sleep Medicine, Department
of Medicine, New York University School of
Medicine; André Cournand Pulmonary
Physiology Laboratory, Bellevue Hospital,
New York, New York

REHAN SAIYED, BS
Center for Autonomic Medicine in Pediatrics
(CAMP), Ann & Robert H. Lurie Children's
Hospital of Chicago, Chicago, Illinois

SAFAL SHETTY, MD
Division of Pulmonary, Critical Care, Allergy
and Sleep Medicine, Department of Medicine,
Arizona Respiratory Center, University of
Arizona, Tucson, Arizona

RENAUD TAMISIER, MD, PhD
INSERM U 1042, Sleep Laboratory, Grenoble
University Hospital, CHU de Grenoble,
Grenoble, France

AIMAN TULAIMAT, MD
Assistant Professor, Rush University Medical
Center; Pulmonary, Critical Care and Sleep
Medicine, John H. Stroger Hospital of Cook
County, Chicago, Illinois

DEBRA E. WEESE-MAYER, MD
Chief, Center for Autonomic Medicine
in Pediatrics (CAMP), Ann & Robert H.
Lurie Children's Hospital of Chicago;
Professor of Pediatrics, Northwestern
University Feinberg School of Medicine,
Chicago, Illinois

PETER JAN WIJKSTRA, MD, PhD
Department of Pulmonary Diseases/Home
Mechanical Ventilation, University Medical
Centre Groningen, Groningen, The
Netherlands

LISA F. WOLFE, MD
Associate Professor of Medicine and
Neurology, Pulmonary and Critical Care
Medicine, Northwestern University Feinberg
School of Medicine, Chicago, Illinois

Contents

of breathing while maintaining breathing comfort. Although such devices are increasingly used in clinical practice, supporting clinical evidence—specifically comparative-effectiveness studies in real-life conditions—needs to be gathered. There is opportunity to refine these devices, including the ability of the device to monitor gas exchange and sleep-wakefulness state, and for reducing variability in device efficacy owing to provider-selected device settings.

of sleep, daytime arterial blood gases, and survival. NIV does not treat the underlying cause of obesity hypoventilation syndrome (ie, obesity). Furthermore, NIV is poorly tolerated in a subset of patients, may fail because of poor adherence, and may not reduce significantly the comorbidities associated with obesity. Exploring alternative or complementary options to NIV is important. Among these options, the contribution of exercise, surgical or nonsurgical weight reduction, tracheostomy, respiratory stimulants, and oxygen are discussed in this article.

Overlap syndrome refers to the coexistence of chronic lung disease and obstructive sleep apnea (OSA) in the same patient. To date, overlap syndromes have been poorly studied for a variety of reasons. One difficulty is that each of the underlying disorders in an overlap syndrome occurs along a spectrum of disease severity. Thus, patients with an overlap syndrome are heterogeneous, and the goals of therapy may differ in different patients. However, the importance of overlap syndromes is highlighted by recent data demonstrating increased morbidity and mortality in patients with the overlap of both chronic obstructive pulmonary disease (COPD) and OSA compared with either underlying disorder alone. Unrecognized OSA may also contribute to symptoms of sleepiness/fatigue in patients with chronic lung disease. Clinicians should be mindful of the possibility of overlap syndromes in these patients.

Until now, there has been no conclusive evidence that noninvasive ventilation (NIV) should be provided routinely to stable patients with chronic obstructive pulmonary disease. Nevertheless, patients who are clearly hypercapnic, who receive confirmed effective ventilation by applying higher inspiratory pressures, and have a better compliance, might show clinical benefits. The combination of rehabilitation and nocturnal ventilatory support seems to provide more benefits than rehabilitation alone, so this might be a situation in which chronic NIV is effective.

The emphasis on improved pain control and the focus on treating chronic pain syndromes have led to a large increase in the number of patients on chronic opioid medications. The use of opioids chronically is associated with a variety of breathing disorders and potential for fatal outcomes. Understanding the mechanisms underlying control of respiration and opioid-mediated respiratory depression is essential in applying treatment options and providing new directions for management without sacrificing adequate pain control.

Obesity hypoventilation syndrome represents an embedded epidemic within the larger epidemic of obesity and sleep apnea. It's prevalence is largely unknown but seems much lower than that of obstructive sleep apnea. Preoperative identification is key because most patients are largely undiagnosed at the time of surgery.

Perioperative challenges include difficult intubation, failed airway, rapid oxygen desaturation predisposing to anoxic/hypoxic injury, associated comorbidities like heart failure and pulmonary hypertension, and higher chances of opioid-induced ventilatory failure. Special preparedness is required on the part of the anesthesiologist, and most of the management strategies are empiric.

Preface

Sleep Hypoventilation: A State-of-the-Art Overview

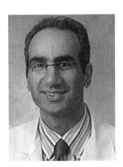

Babak Mokhlesi, MD, MSc
Editor

The association between obesity and hypoventilation has long been recognized. Of historical interest, obesity hypoventilation syndrome was described well before obstructive sleep apnea was recognized in 1969. Since then, we have made great strides to advance our understanding of sleep hypoventilation syndromes. Sleep hypoventilation, particularly obesity hypoventilation syndrome, should no longer be considered a rare condition in the current global epidemic of obesity. Despite the increased recognition of this condition by health care providers, a significant proportion of the population afflicted by sleep hypoventilation remains undiagnosed and untreated, and the potential societal, health-related, and economic consequences remain poorly defined. It therefore gives me great pleasure to see the outstanding contributions from a cast of highly qualified experts and researchers who discuss in great detail the recent advances in epidemiology, pathophysiology, diagnosis, and treatment of adult and pediatric sleep hypoventilation syndromes.

While extensive research spanning several decades has increased our understanding of sleep hypoventilation syndromes, the specific purpose of this issue of *Sleep Medicine Clinics* is to provide a forum that allows a group of internationally recognized experts in the field to thoroughly and critically review the current state of knowledge and to provide insight and guidance on important questions that require further investigation. My

most fervent hope is that the state-of-the-art discussions in this issue will stimulate the readership and provide a focused assessment of the current state of knowledge on sleep hypoventilation. I am confident that the outstanding contributions by my colleagues will help current and future investigators and clinicians to formulate many probing questions waiting to be asked and help us find the answers in this exciting and important area of respiratory and sleep medicine.

The issue begins with an article providing a historical perspective on sleep hypoventilation syndromes. The following article provides an overview of the pathophysiology of sleep hypoventilation and how it can progress from hypoventilation during sleep to hypoventilation during wakefulness. This is followed by an in-depth discussion regarding diagnostic considerations and technological limitations related to capnometry. The next article provides an update of advances in various modalities of positive airway pressure therapy. Scoring respiratory events during noninvasive ventilation can be challenging, and a systematic description of these events has been summarized in the following article. The next three articles provide a detailed and up-to-date summary of diagnosis, epidemiology, and treatment of obesity hypoventilation syndrome. These three articles are followed by a series of outstanding reviews covering the spectrum of hypoventilation,

Sleep Med Clin 9 (2014) xv–xvi
http://dx.doi.org/10.1016/j.jsmc.2014.07.001
1556-407X/14/$ – see front matter © 2014 Elsevier Inc. All rights reserved.

such as the overlap syndrome, neuromuscular disorders, hypoventilation due to opioids and sedatives, as well as the interaction between anesthesia and sleep hypoventilation syndromes. The last two articles provide a comprehensive review of pediatric hypoventilation syndrome and treatment with noninvasive ventilation in children.

I am indebted to my colleagues who graciously accepted my invitation to make exceptional contributions to this issue of *Sleep Medicine Clinics*. I am also grateful to Dr Teofilo Lee-Chiong for providing a forum that allows an in-depth analysis and discussion of the topic. I hope you will enjoy reading these outstanding articles.

Babak Mokhlesi, MD, MSc
Section of Pulmonary and Critical Care
Sleep Disorders Center and Sleep Fellowship
Program
University of Chicago
5841 S. Maryland Avenue
MC6076/Room M630
Chicago, IL 60637, USA

E-mail address:
bmokhles@medicine.bsd.uchicago.edu

The History of Hypoventilation Syndromes

Stephen W. Littleton, MD*, Aiman Tulaimat, MD

KEYWORDS

• Sleep hypoventilation • History • Obesity • Sleep apnea

KEY POINTS

- An understanding of sleep hypoventilation requires some basic advancements in chemistry, physics, and physiology.
- It could not be studied until scientific discoveries led to tools that could measure sleep and ventilation.
- Before that, there were only impressive descriptions by observant historians, physicians, and novelists of the look and behavior of patients who hypoventilated during sleep.

FROM DIONYSIUS TO SERVETIUS

Although obstructive sleep apnea syndrome and obesity-hypoventilation syndrome were not discovered until the 1950s, striking descriptions of individuals likely to have had either are ancient. The oldest known is an account of Dionysius of Hereclea, a tyrant and:

> I am informed that Dionysius the Heraclote, son of Clearchus the tyrant, through daily gluttony and intemperance, increased to an extraordinary degree of Corpulency and Fatness, by reason whereof he had much adoe to take breath.[1]

> The voluptuous life he led made him grow so fat, that he did little but sleep, and his drowsiness was so great, that they could hardly awake him by running long needles into his flesh.[2]

> The physicians who attended Dionysius, the son of Clearchus, who lived in continual fear of suffocation from fat, adopted a very curious mode of keeping him awake: they appointed a person to prick his sides with very long and sharp needles, whenever he fell into a profound sleep, which was not interrupted by the operation, till the needle having passed through the fat, arrived at the sensible parts beneath.[3]

Such drastic measures to keep a man awake strongly imply his physicians were afraid he would be suffocated by fat in his sleep. He died at 55, perhaps later than one would expect.[2]

Other accounts in the ancient literature are mainly limited to the association of obesity with dyspnea. Caelius Aurelianus and Soranus noted that an obese person, after walking just a few steps, sweat, become short of breath, and "feel suffocated by his own body and cannot endure even light clothing."[4] Hippocrates noted an association between obesity, excessive daytime sleepiness, and sleep quality. He stated:

> Others, when their diet bears too great a proportion to their exercise, not only sleep well at

Disclosures: None.
Pulmonary, Critical Care and Sleep Medicine, John H. Stroger Hospital of Cook County, 14th Floor, Administration Building, 1900 West Polk, Chicago, IL 60612, USA
* Corresponding author.
E-mail address: slittleton@cookcountyhhs.org

Sleep Med Clin 9 (2014) 281–288
http://dx.doi.org/10.1016/j.jsmc.2014.05.011
1556-407X/14/$ – see front matter © 2014 Elsevier Inc. All rights reserved.

night, but are likewise drowsy in the day; the repletion still increases, and their nights begin to grow restless...[5]

Galen (**Fig. 1**), a Greek physician practicing in Rome around 150 AD and considered to be Hippocrates' successor, described a condition he called polysarkos, from poli (many) and sarka (flesh). He noted that in such patients, "the body deviates toward obesity to such a point that person cannot walk without sweating, cannot reach (when seated at) the table because of the mass of his stomach, cannot breath easily..."[6]

The Greeks, who readily recognized asthma, bronchitis, and pneumonia, also described hypoventilation from kyphoscoliosis. It was a Hippocratic aphorism that those with such "hump back" deformities die young.[7] He recognized that the mechanism was hypoventilation:

And in those cases where the gibbosity is above the diaphragm, the ribs do not expand properly in width, but forward, and the chest becomes sharp-pointed and not broad, and they become affected with difficulty of breathing and hoarseness; for the cavities

which inspire and expire the breath do not attain their proper capacity.[8]

Hippocrates' and Galen's hypotheses on breathing and circulation remained unchallenged until the early 13th century. Ibn al-Nafis observed that there is no direct passage for blood between the right and left ventricles, as Galen had thought, that the substance of the heart is not porous, and that blood flowed from the right ventricle through the lung to reach the left ventricle.[9]

Around 1550, Vesalius revived the practice of cadaveric dissection. He also questioned Galen's idea of blood flow. Inspired by Vesalius, Servetus published a description of the true flow of blood, for which he and his books were burned at the stake[10]:

However, this communication is made not through the middle wall of the heart, as is commonly believed, but by a very ingenious arrangement, the refined blood is urged forward from the right ventricle of the heart over a long course through the lungs; it is treated by the lungs, becomes reddish-yellow, and is poured from the pulmonary artery to the pulmonary vein.

ΓΑΛΗΝΟΣ   "The target (skopos) of medical science is
GALEN   health, its end (telos) is the achievement of it"

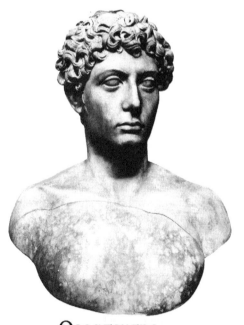
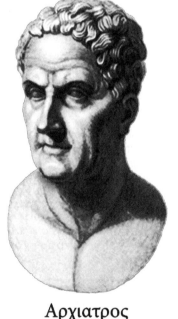

Θεραπευτης
Medical student

Αρχιατρος
Senior Roman court physician

Fig. 1. Galen father of modern medicine. (*From* Pasipoularides A. Galen, father of systematic medicine. An essay on the evolution of modern medicine and cardiology. Int J Cardiol 2014;172:48; with permission.)

William Harvey fully described the circulatory path of blood, and reiterated the idea that waste vapors were carried by the blood and eliminated through the lungs. This inspired chemists to determine what these waste vapors were, and what the pneuma zotikon, or vital spirit, of air was.

CHEMISTS AND CLINICIANS: NE'ER THE TWO SHALL MEET

In the late 16th century, Boyle discovered that a flame in a bell jar will eventually extinguish. An animal in such a jar will eventually die; another animal placed into the jar with the dead animal will die much sooner than the first. From this, he concluded that air must be a mixture of different substances. The description of air pressure by Galileo led to the invention of the vacuum pump, which Boyle used to show that blood contained gas. Hales invented a device that could distinguish between a gas dissolved in air from a gas dissolved in liquid (a pneumatic trough); measurement of gases in blood soon followed.

Although the chemists were making great headway in understanding the composition of air, this knowledge was not much used by the clinicians of the day. This did not stop them from making astute observations, such as the description by Christianus Helwich in 1722 of a patient with kyphoscoliosis and perhaps obesity hypoventilation syndrome. In it, he described the final days of a patient on whom he was called to attend, and may have described sleep-disordered breathing:

During her lifetime, a certain fat and hunchbacked woman had rather severe difficulty in breathing during bodily movement... toward the close of her mortal lifetime the distress in her chest was greatly increased. Moreover, having called me three days before her death, she indicated, in words frequently interrupted, that the symptoms which she now suffered seemed to her to be of a different kind from those which she had been afflicted since early life and which were caused by bad conformation of her chest and by conspicuous obesity... most of all the symptoms disturbed her at the time of the first sleep, when the most urgent danger of suffocation threatened [her]...these attacks of strangulation she so greatly dreaded that she had spent many sleepless nights...Thus far my guiding star in the recognition of pectoral dropsy [heart failure] had been the difficulty and frequency in breathing which afflicts the patient in the first period of sleep.[11]

The next likely description of obesity hypoventilation syndrome did not come until 1781. John

Fothergill, in his *A Complete Collection of the Medical and Philosophic Works*, related a case:

A country tradesman, aged about thirty of a short stature, and naturally of a fresh, sanguine complexion, and very fat... complained of perpetual drowsiness and inactivity. His countenance was almost livid, and such a degree of somnolency attended him, that he could scarce keep awake whilst he described his situation.[12]

Kryger interpreted the "sanguine complexion" as possibly polycythemia,[1] and the "livid" (meaning purplish) appearance could have described cyanosis.

Fothergill's accounts were revisited in 1818, and others added, including Surgeon Extraordinary to the King William Wadd, in *Cursory Remarks on Corpulence, or Obesity Considered as a Disease: With a Critical Examination of Ancient and Modern Opinions Relative to its Causes and Cure*. In it, he noted that obese patients tend to be sleepy. He described 1 patient he had treated:

Mr. W.W. Whitehaven, at about 30 years of age weighted twenty-three stone (146 kg)... He became at length so lethargic, that he frequently fell asleep in the act of eating, even in company.

He attempted bloodletting on a 44 year-old woman weighing 23 stone (146 kg) because of her severe drowsiness, but could not find a vein. In addition to sleepiness, he noted that obese patients tend to have respiratory difficulty.

A preternatureal accumulation of fat in (the chest), cannot fail to impede the free exercise of the animal functions. Respiration is performed imperfectly, or with difficulty... suffocation and death from corpulency be not uncommon.

By the time Wadd and Fothergill published their accounts, understanding of gases and blood had advanced. Around 1754, Joseph Black discovered carbon dioxide when he noticed that limestone lost weight after it was heated to produce caustic lime. He called the gas liberated by this process "fixed air". He found that fixed air was also produced by fermentation. He later discovered that fixed air was produced by respiration when he noticed that chalk precipitated on lime soaked rags that he stuffed into the air ducts of a crowded church before a 10-hour service.

In the 1770s, oxygen was discovered by Priestly and Steele by heating mercuric oxide. The gas, which they called "pure air," allowed a flame to burn brighter and a mouse to live longer in an airtight container. They described their findings to Lavosier (the father of modern chemistry), who later concluded that air had a nonrespirable component, and a respirable component that was responsible for combustion. He and others concluded that combustion must then occur in living things. His work came to an abrupt halt upon his beheading during the French Revolution in May 1794. In 1797, Davie measured oxygen and carbon dioxide in blood, and this was repeated, and more widely disseminated, by Magnus in 1837.[10] The groundwork for blood gas analysis had been laid.

Around the same time of Magnus' publication, the most famous obese, sleepy patient (Joe, the "fat boy") was described by Charles Dickens in *The Posthumous Papers of the Pickwick Club*. Dickens was known as the most astute parliamentary reporter in England, and his keen observational skills were put to good use in describing Joe (**Fig. 2**). The fat boy was the servant of Mr. Wardle, and was so prone to falling asleep, that Mr. Wardle had to give him very particular instructions to ensure that they were actually carried out:

A most violent and startling knocking was heard at the door; it was not an ordinary double knock, but a constant and uninterrupted succession of the loudest single raps, as if the knocker were endowed with the perpetual motion, or the person outside had forgotten to leave off.

Mr. Lowten hurried to the door... the object that presented itself to the eyes of the astonished clerk was a boy—a wonderfully fat boy—habited as a serving lad, standing

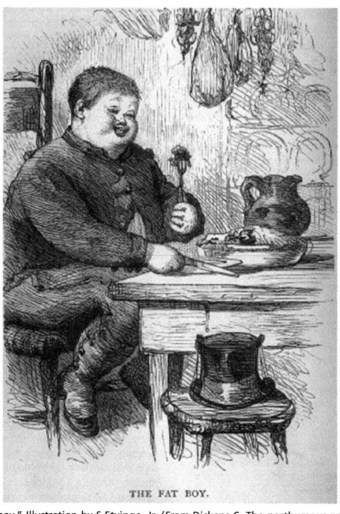

THE FAT BOY.

Fig. 2. Joe the "fat boy." Illustration by S Etyinge, Jr. (*From* Dickens C. The posthumous papers of the Pickwick Club. Boston: Ticknor and Fields: Boston; 1867.)

upright on the mat, with his eyes closed as if in sleep.

'What's the matter?' inquired the clerk.

The extraordinary boy replied not a word, but he nodded once, and seemed, to the clerk's imagination, to snore feebly.

'What in the devil do you knock that way for?' inquired the clerk, angrily.

…'Because master said I wasn't to leave off knocking till they opened the door, for fear I should go to sleep,' said the boy.[13]

Other passages describe Joe has having "young dropsy" (ie, edema associated with congestive heart failure), and red-faced, which could again be polycythemia, and decreased attentiveness "the fat boy's perception being slow".[14] Kryger went on to say, "Despite a brilliant, accurate description in 1836, a clear understanding of the strange disorder of the fat boy did not emerge for a very long time."

Almost 30 years later, the chemists' work was making its way into the clinical realm. In 1866, *BMJ* published what was likely the first case of death from obesity hypoventilation syndrome where hypoxemia and hypercapnia were suspected. James Russell wrote:

In the case which I am about to relate a condition of complete cyanosis was established sometime before death, evidently by very gradual stages. Venous blood had been evidently circulating through the vessels for a considerable length of time, and the patient died poisoned by carbonaceous matter. This state of cyanosis seems attributable to want of pulmonary capacity, sufficient to meet the increased demand for oxygen created by the highly carbonized state of the blood. The disproportion between the size of the lungs and that of the entire body… was most striking after death.

He went on to describe a woman who had become both increasingly obese and increasingly short of breath over the last 3 years of her life, and suffered from such terrible somnolence that "as an out-patient, she requested to be dismissed speedily, lest she should fall asleep in the hall."[15] Russell's description is familiar to those who treat such patients on a regular basis, and his description of the pathophysiology was not inaccurate, even by today's standards.

A little more than 20 years later, the *BMJ* published a remarkably accurate description of a

patient with obstructive sleep apnea, and possibly obesity hypoventilation syndrome, although there was no reference to Russell's case. Caton described what he called "a remarkable case of narcolepsy":

The patient was a man, aged 37. He would fall asleep while standing, when selling articles in his shop, or even when walking the streets. If he attempted to read or sit in a chair he invariably fell asleep for a moment. During sleep a spasmodic closure of the glottis always took place, lasting nearly a minute. Violent contraction of the diaphragm and other respiratory muscles would come on, increasing in force, and the patient would get more and more cyanosed, until at length the violence of the inspiratory efforts partially roused him, and the spasm of the glottis yielded. Loud noisy respirations would now come on, and the cyanosis would disappear, to be followed by deep sleep and the same round of symptoms.[16]

Interestingly, Caton would go on to be the first person to record the electrical signals from an animal brain. He gave this account at a meeting of the Clinical Society of London. The president of the society, Christopher Heath, remarked that the patient reminded him of Joe the fat boy, and the term Pickwickian syndrome was born, or at least hinted at.[17] Not long after, in the seventh edition of his seminal work *On the Principles and Practice of Medicine*, Osler made a similar comparison:

An extraordinary phenomenon in excessively fat persons is an uncontrollable tendency to sleep—like the fat boy in Pickwick. I have seen one instance of it. Caton has reported a case.[18]

Even President Taft made the comparison, although, frighteningly, he was referring to himself. Referring to recent weight loss, he wrote, "I have lost that tendency to sleepiness which made me think of the fat boy in Pickwick. My color is very much better and my ability to work is greater."[19]

Around the same time, an American physician, Silas Weir Mitchell, described pure sleep hypoventilation. In 1890, he described an entity he named "respiratory failure in sleep":

Where for some reason, the respiratory centers are diseased or disordered, a man may possess enough gangionic energy to carry on breathing well, while the will can supplement that automatic activity of the lower centers. But in sleep, these being not quite competent, and the volition off guard, there ensues a gradual failure of respiration, and the man awakes with a sense of impending suffocation.

He drew a distinction between this disorder and Cheyne-Stokes respiration, attributing this condition to "a failure of the chest and diaphragmatic movements."[20]

PARTIAL PRESSURES, POLIO, AND POLYSOMNOGRAPHY

After the descriptions by Osler and Heath, there were a few case reports that trickled into the literature, but most cases were likely mislabeled narcolepsy and dismissed as untreatable.[20] One case report stands out. Entitled *Polycythemia in the Course of Neuropsychiatric Conditions*, it (unwittingly) chronicled patients with both sleep hypoventilation and obesity hypoventilation syndrome. The former was the case of a 38-year-old man, who,

In April 1934… began having generalized headaches… He further complained of… excessive salivation for many years; a tremor of the extremities for about the same period of time; somnolence dating back to 1920…

Exam showed a (body mass index) BMI of 31 and generalized hyperreflexia. Laboratory studies showed polycythemia, and "arterial blood obtained under oil in afternoon, carbonic acid content 62.1 vol. per cent (normal 45–54 vol. per cent)."

It is notable that measurement of arterial blood gases was not routine clinical practice at the time. This patient likely had sleep hypoventilation secondary to bulbar amylotropic lateral sclerosis. His headaches were likely secondary to the hypoventilation and hypercapnia, and the polycythemia secondary to nocturnal hypoxemia. The excess salivation was probably mistaken for an inability to handle his own saliva. The authors then discussed 3 other case reports in which polycythemia was accompanied by narcolepsy, including one:

In 1929, Gunther described a case of what he termed cerebral polyglobulia in a patient with narcolepsy, obesity, cyanosis, and polyuria.[21]

The authors failed to realize the significance of their findings, probably because they were inexperienced in interpreting arterial blood gases. This is understandable, because the routine measurement and interpretation of arterial blood gases were 2 decades away.

Four years before that case report, the first commercial pH electrode was produced. It received little attention until a huge number of respiratory complications arose in a 1951 Danish polio epidemic, where it would change the course of respiratory medicine. The pH probe was used to analyze the blood of patients dying of respiratory failure. Their high CO_2 levels were initially interpreted as metabolic alkalosis, but an anesthesiologist, Ibsen, thought it was respiratory in origin. He performed a tracheostomy in a girl and attempted bag ventilation. He was unable to ventilate her until he paralyzed her. Then, she immediately improved. Many other patients were saved using this technique, the first widespread application of positive pressure ventilation.

In 1954 the CO_2 electrode was invented, and Ibsen no longer had to guess whether the elevated CO_2 content was metabolic or respiratory.[10,22] The oxygen partial pressure (PO_2), carbon dioxide partial pressure (PCO_2) and pH monitors were incorporated into a single device in 1958, and finally hypoventilation could be routinely identified and quantified. Around the same time, rapid eye movement (REM) sleep was discovered by Aserinsky and Kleitman (**Fig. 3**), but drew little attention.[23]

With the availability of tools to measure sleep, blood gases, and lung function, sleep hypoventilation was about to be formally recognized. There was interest in respiratory physiology during sleep, in both normal subjects and those with narcolepsy.[24,25] In 1956, Bickelmann and Burwell published *Extreme Obesity Associated with Alveolar Hypoventilation: a Pickwickian Syndrome*, but

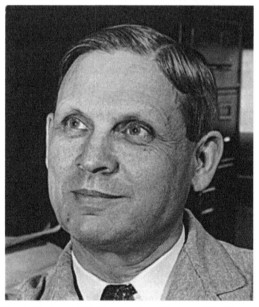

Fig. 3. Nathaniel Kleitman. (*From* Dement WC. History of sleep physiology and medicine. In: Kryger MH, Roth T, Dement WC, editors. Principles and practice of sleep medicine. 5th edition. St Louis (MO): Elsevier; 2011. p. 7.)

they too failed to recognize the presence of sleep-disordered breathing. Two years later, Robin and colleagues[24] elegantly described how ventilation decreases during sleep in normal subjects. In 1965, European neurologists interested in sleep gave the first description of obstructive sleep apnea.[26,27] It took at least 15 years for the medical community to recognize the importance of the report.

Although cardiopulmonary complications of kyphoscoliosis and neuromuscular disorders were described decades before obstructive sleep apnea was,[8,21] the understanding of sleep apnea led to the study of breathing during sleep in other conditions. The first case report of sleep hypoventilation in patients with amyotrophic lateral sclerosis was published in 1979,[28] and the first case report in kyphoscoliotic patients (with an analogy to the dim-witted Quasimodo) was published in 1981.[29] Technology had finally caught up with history and fiction.

The history of sleep hypoventilation syndromes is 1 example of the usual progress of medicine; careful observation is the first step in discovery. Recognition of an abnormality is the first step in its study. In this case, the recognition of the condition preceded the technology by which to explain it by hundreds, if not thousands, of years. This only leaves one to wonder: what is it that is recognized today but has not the technology to explain it? Will medical descendants look back at this era with wonder and appreciation, as has been done here?

REFERENCES

1. Kryger MH. Sleep apnea. From the needles of Dionysius to continuous positive airway pressure. Arch Intern Med 1983;143(12):2301–3.
2. Bayle P, Maizeaux PD, Gaudin A, et al. The dictionary historical and critical of Mr. Peter Bayle. Printed for J.J. and P. Knapton et al, London, 1735.
3. Wadd W. Cursory remarks on corpulence; or obesity considered as a disease. 3rd edition. London: Callow Medical Bookseller; 1816.
4. Papavramidou N, Christopoulou-Aletra H. Management of obesity in the writings of Soranus of Ephesus and Caelius Aurelianus. Obes Surg 2008;18(6):763–5. http://dx.doi.org/10.1007/s11695-007-9362-1.
5. Haslam D. Obesity: a medical history. Obes Rev 2007;8(Suppl 1):31–6. http://dx.doi.org/10.1111/j.1467-789X.2007.00314.x.
6. Papavramidou NS, Papavramidis ST, Christopoulou-Aletra H. Galen on obesity: etiology, effects, and treatment. World J Surg 2004;28(6):631–5.
7. Hippocrates. The genuine works of Hippocrates. Translated by Adams F. New York: William Wood and Company; 1886.
8. Bergofsky EH, Turino GM, Fishman AP. Cardiorespiratory failure in kyphoscoliosis. Medicine (Baltimore) 1959;38:263–317.
9. West JB. Ibn al-Nafis, the pulmonary circulation, and the Islamic golden age. J Appl Physiol (1985) 2008;105(6):1877–80. http://dx.doi.org/10.1152/japplphysiol.91171.2008.
10. Colice G. Historical perspective on the development of mechanical ventilation. In: Tobin M, editor. Principles and practice of mechanical ventilation. 2nd edition. Chicago: McGraw-Hill Medical Pub. Division; 2006. p. 1–36.
11. Jarcho S. Christianus Helwich on difficulty of respiration (Augsburg, 1722). Bull N Y Acad Med 1970; 46(1):34–8.
12. Elliott J. A complete collection of the medical and philosophical works of John Fothergill. London: Printed for John Walker; 1781.
13. Dickens CJ. The posthumous papers of the Pickwick Club: containing a faithful record of the perambulations, perils, travels, adventures, and sporting transactions of the corresponding members. Leipzig: Tauchnitz; 1842.
14. Kryger MH. Fat, sleep, and Charles Dickens: literary and medical contributions to the understanding of sleep apnea. Clin Chest Med 1985;6(4):555–62.
15. Russell J. A case of polysarka, in which death resulted from deficient arterialisation of the blood. 1866. Obes Res 1994;2(4):384–5.
16. Caton R. Reports of societies, "a case of narcolepsy". Br Med J 1889;357(1):358.
17. Lavie P. Who was the first to use the term Pickwickian in connection with sleepy patients? History of sleep apnoea syndrome. Sleep Med Rev 2008; 12(1):5–17. http://dx.doi.org/10.1016/j.smrv.2007.07.008.
18. Osler SW. The principles and practice of medicine: designed for the use of practitioners and students of medicine. New York: D. Appleton; 1910.
19. Sotos JG. Taft and Pickwick: sleep apnea in the White House. Chest 2003;124(3):1133–42.
20. Lavie P. Nothing new under the moon. Historical accounts of sleep apnea syndrome. Arch Intern Med 1984;144(10):2025–8.
21. Ferraro A, Sherwood WD. Polycythemia in the course of neuropsychiatric conditions. Psychiatr Q 1937; 11(1):21–33. http://dx.doi.org/10.1007/BF01563882.
22. Colice G. A historical perspective on intensive care monitoring. In: Tobin M, editor. Principles and practice of intensive care monitoring. St Louis (MO): McGraw-Hill Health Professions Division; 1998. p. 1–31.
23. Dement W. History of sleep physiology and medicine. In: Kryger M, Roth T, Dement W, editors. Principles and practice of sleep medicine. 5th edition. St Louis (MO): Elsevier Science Health Science div; 2011. p. 3–15.

24. Robin ED, Whaley RD, Crump CH, et al. Alveolar gas tensions, pulmonary ventilation and blood pH during physiologic sleep in normal subjects. J Clin Invest 1958;37(7):981–9. http://dx.doi.org/10.1172/JCI103694.

25. Birchfield RI, Sieker HO, Heyman A. Alterations in blood gases during natural sleep and narcolepsy; a correlation with the electroencephalographic stages of sleep. Neurology 1958;8(2):107–12.

26. Gastaut H, Tassinari CA, Duron B. Polygraphic study of the episodic diurnal and nocturnal (hypnic and respiratory) manifestations of the Pickwick syndrome. Brain Res 1966;1(2):167–86.

27. Jung R, Kuhlo W. Neurophysiological studies of abnormal night sleep and the Pickwickian syndrome. Prog Brain Res 1965;18:140–59.

28. Minz M, Autret A, Laffont F, et al. A study on sleep in amyotrophic lateral sclerosis. Biomedicine 1979;30(1):40–6.

29. Guilleminault C, Kurland G, Winkle R, et al. Severe kyphoscoliosis, breathing, and sleep: the "Quasimodo" syndrome during sleep. Chest 1981;79(6):626–30.

Pathophysiology of Hypoventilation During Sleep

Kenneth I. Berger, MD[a,b,*], David M. Rapoport, MD[a,b],
Indu Ayappa, PhD[a,b], Roberta M. Goldring, MD[a,b]

KEYWORDS

- Carbon dioxide • Hypercapnia • Hypoventilation • Pathogenesis • Sleep
- Sleep-disordered breathing

KEY POINTS

- Alveolar hypoventilation is determined by more than the level of minute ventilation and is defined by an increase in arterial PCO_2.
- Sleep hypoventilation occurs in a variety of disease states with potential carryover to the daytime manifesting as chronic hypercapnia during wakefulness.
- Maintenance of eucapnia during wakefulness requires adequate compensatory mechanisms. Elevation of blood bicarbonate concentration, while appropriate to defend blood pH, provides a mechanism for perpetuation of chronic hypercapnia.

INTRODUCTION

In healthy individuals, the arterial blood gas tensions and pH remain constant within a remarkably narrow range over a spectrum of activities. This stability is maintained by the precise adjustment of alveolar ventilation to metabolic rate. Reduction in alveolar ventilation (ie, hypoventilation) produces an immediate increase in arterial partial pressure of carbon dioxide (P_aCO_2), with a corresponding reduction in arterial partial pressure of oxygen (P_aO_2). For clinical purposes, monitoring of P_aCO_2 is the parameter used to monitor alveolar ventilation; values higher than 45 mm Hg at sea level have been used to define presence of alveolar hypoventilation.[1]

It has been well established that metabolic rate falls during sleep in healthy subjects, with a concomitant reduction in minute ventilation.[2-6]

However, in some individuals, an elevation in P_aCO_2 can be detected, defining a state of alveolar hypoventilation.[5,7] The etiology of alveolar hypoventilation can be ascribed to 2 major categories. Alveolar ventilation may fall either because of a reduction in the overall level of ventilation or because of a maldistribution of ventilation with respect to pulmonary capillary perfusion (ie, an increase in anatomic and/or physiologic dead space). This latter mechanism of increase dead space is independent of overall (total) level of ventilation and may occur even in circumstances in which the total ventilation is at an elevated level.

In many disease states, the initial manifestation of alveolar hypoventilation occurs during sleep before development of chronic hypercapnia during wakefulness. Sleep-related hypoventilation events range from short transient to longer sustained events. Regardless of etiology or duration of event,

Disclosure statement: The authors have no disclosures that are relevant to the content of this article.
[a] Division of Pulmonary, Critical Care and Sleep Medicine, Department of Medicine, New York University School of Medicine, New York, NY, USA; [b] André Cournand Pulmonary Physiology Laboratory, Bellevue Hospital, New York, NY, USA
* Corresponding author. André Cournand Pulmonary Physiology Laboratory, Bellevue Hospital, 240 East 38th Street, Room M-15, New York, NY 10016.
E-mail address: Kenneth.berger@nyumc.org

1556-407X/14/$ – see front matter © 2014 Elsevier Inc. All rights reserved.

maintenance of eucapnia during wakefulness requires adequate compensatory mechanisms. Compensatory mechanisms require an intact integration between respiratory control and acid-base regulatory systems. Because this issue of the journal includes articles for each disease state associated with sleep hypoventilation, this review characterizes the disease states based on pathophysiologic derangements and focuses on the compensatory regulatory mechanisms that would be common to all disorders.

NORMAL SLEEP PHYSIOLOGY AND RELATIONSHIP TO SLEEP STAGE

There are a variety of changes in respiratory mechanics and in the respiratory control system that occur during sleep that predispose subjects to development of reduced minute ventilation. Although a modest degree of hypoventilation with increased P_aCO_2 may occur in healthy subjects,[5,7] this respiratory phenomenon is accentuated in patients with sleep hypoventilation disorders. Regardless of etiology, the severity of resultant hypoventilation and associated CO_2 retention imposes a burden for the CO_2 excretion that is required on awakening to prevent development of chronic hypercapnia during wakefulness.

Respiratory Drive

Alterations in respiratory control during sleep have been well established and may predispose to alveolar hypoventilation. Numerous studies have documented blunted responsiveness to CO_2 during sleep attributable to both an increase in the set point for CO_2 and to a decrease in the ventilatory response slope to increasing PCO_2.[7-11] The precise mechanism for the reduced ventilatory response slope is unclear, and may relate to decreased chemosensitivity, decreased ventilatory output from skeletal muscle hypotonia and/or increased upper airway resistance,[12,13] and to local phenomena in chemosensitive areas.[10,11,14,15] For example, regional PCO_2 at the site of the central chemoreceptors may fall independent of the arterial level when blood flow to the chemoreceptors increases relative to the local metabolic rate.[15] Regardless of the mechanisms involved, the cumulative effect is a modest reduction in CO_2 responsiveness that is most evident during rapid eye movement (REM) sleep. In addition to CO_2 responsiveness, the ventilatory response to hypoxemia also is affected by sleep. Decreased hypoxic response has been demonstrated in both men and women during REM sleep and in men during non-REM (NREM) sleep.[16] Last, sleep has been shown to alter the pattern of breathing; ataxic

breathing is commonly observed during phasic portions of REM sleep.[17-19] Although the foregoing alterations are modest in NREM sleep, more profound changes occur during REM, potentially explaining the increased propensity for alveolar hypoventilation to initially manifest during REM in many disease states.

Respiratory Mechanics

Changes in body position may impact gas exchange and respiratory muscle function during sleep. In particular, the supine position is associated with reduction in functional residual capacity (FRC) in all subjects[20,21]; this effect is magnified in obesity due to mass loading on the chest cage. Further reduction in FRC occurs during REM sleep due to hypotonia of the chest wall and accessory muscles.[14] In selected circumstances, the reduction in FRC may decrease resting lung volume to values below the closing volume. For example, in obesity, reduction of FRC is already apparent in the upright position and is exacerbated when patients are supine.[22-26] Alternatively, even in subjects with normal FRC, resting lung volume may fall below closing volume, when the latter is increased due to the presence of underlying diseases (eg, chronic obstructive pulmonary disease [COPD]).[27-29] In either case, persistence of blood flow to regions with airway closure produces shuntlike behavior with resultant hypoxemia. In addition, even in the absence of hypoxemia, reduction in lung volume may predispose patients to develop alveolar hypoventilation due to the increased load on inspiratory muscles in the supine position (eg, obesity).[24,25]

With the onset of sleep, multiple changes occur in the upper airway that ultimately result in an increased resistance to airflow.[13,30-32] First, in the supine position, posterior movement of tongue and soft palate increases upper airway resistance and collapsibility.[33-36] These changes may be responsible for the observation that snoring is generally more prominent in the supine position. Upper airway resistance may be further increased as a result of the reduction in resting lung volume, as reduction in FRC may reduce axial forces along the trachea, thereby reducing that stabilize the pharyngeal airway.[37-40] Second, sleep may be associated with reduced activation of upper airway muscles.[41-48] This effect has been shown to be associated with transient increases in upper airway resistance with a corresponding reduction in ventilation.[32,49] Third, the potential for altered chemical responsiveness of the upper airway has been suggested. Decreased responsiveness of the genioglossus muscle to rising PCO_2 has been demonstrated during NREM sleep.[47] Although not studied, similar effects during REM sleep appear likely. Last, sleep is associated with reduced responsiveness to airway loading as compared with wakefulness. Whereas addition of a mechanical load to the upper airway during wakefulness results in an increase in respiratory drive, this response is either absent or greatly attenuated during sleep.[31,48,50] Although this perturbation would not produce hypoventilation per se, it would impair the response of a given patient to other factors that increase the load on the respiratory system during sleep.

Respiratory muscle function also is altered during sleep, predisposing selected individuals to development of alveolar hypoventilation. REM sleep is accompanied by generalized skeletal muscle hypotonia.[14] Although the diaphragm is spared, the accessory muscles of respiration are not. Thus, subjects who are dependent on the accessory muscles to maintain ventilation at the eupneic level are at risk for development of hypoventilation during REM sleep (eg, patients with COPD and hyperinflation and subjects with neuromuscular diseases that involve the diaphragm).

Sleep Stage

The magnitude of the perviously described perturbations in respiratory control and respiratory mechanics are in large part dependent on the stage of sleep. REM sleep in particular is associated with the greatest stress, as it involves changes throughout the respiratory system from the central controller to upper airway and respiratory mechanics, as well as to gas exchange. Changes in chemosensitivity, resting lung volume, neuromuscular control of the upper airway, and hypotonia are at maximal levels during REM sleep.[11,14,16,32,51] The cumulative effects explain the additional increase in P_aCO_2 observed in healthy subjects during REM sleep. Furthermore, these considerations explain occurrence of hypoventilation during REM sleep before NREM sleep and before wakefulness.[51–54]

Minute Ventilation

All of the foregoing discussion leads to a decrease in minute ventilation during sleep even in healthy adults. The magnitude of the decreased ventilation is disproportionate when related to the simultaneous decline in metabolic rate. As a result, a modest increase in P_aCO_2 may be observed during sleep even in healthy subjects (up to 4–6 mm Hg).[5] Although this CO_2 load is readily excreted on awakening in the morning, patients with disease may manifest greater degrees of CO_2 retention during

the night with the potential for carryover throughout wakefulness, producing a chronic state of alveolar hypoventilation with associated chronic hypercapnia. Potential mechanisms for this carryover effect in the daytime are discussed in later sections of this review.

MECHANISMS FOR SLEEP HYPOVENTILATION

There are a multitude of diseases associated with alveolar hypoventilation during sleep (either due to decreased minute ventilation or increased dead space). Diseases discussed in the following sections were chosen either based on relative frequency with which they are encountered in the clinical setting or to exemplify a given pathophysiology. Although the list is not comprehensive, additional diseases can be readily added to this framework based on the underlying abnormalities. Moreover, a pathophysiologic approach is helpful in deciding optimal therapy for individual patients based on the balance between the underlying derangements that are manifest or uncovered during routine clinical evaluation and during polysomnography.

Upper Airway Diseases

Numerous diseases are associated with abnormalities in the upper airway structure and control that predispose patients to airway obstruction during sleep. Obstructive sleep apnea (OSA) is a common disorder characterized by short apneic or hypopneic events due to total or partial collapse of the upper airway.[55–57] Abnormalities in upper airway and central respiratory control coupled with functional and structural abnormalities in the airway may contribute to pathogenesis of OSA.[37,58–67] The short apneic/hypopneic events reflect transient reduction in ventilation that is occasionally associated with chronic sustained hypercapnia during wakefulness.[68–73] In addition, longer episodes of hypoventilation due to partial upper airway obstruction have been described in the spectrum of this disease.[74] Whereas OSA likely occurs as a consequence of an interaction between structural airway abnormalities and abnormalities in respiratory control, there are a variety of diseases that are predominantly caused by anatomic abnormalities. For example, OSA can be seen in the setting of macroglossia (eg, Down syndrome) or caused by distortion of the upper airway (eg, due to glycosaminoglycan storage in the mucopolysaccharidoses).[75,76] Regardless of etiology, the diagnosis of these disorders is readily obtainable via standard nocturnal polysomnography and the diseases are treatable with continuous positive airway pressure (CPAP), which primarily reverses the obstruction of the upper airway by acting as a pneumatic splint. CPAP also may have other beneficial effects, such as increasing FRC through positive end expiratory pressure (raising tracheal traction) and have effects on dead space that help stabilize oscillations in CO_2 excretion.

Respiratory Muscle Diseases

Weakness of the inspiratory muscles is commonly associated with hypoventilation during sleep.[53,77,78] Common neuromuscular diseases associated with hypoventilation include spinal cord injury, muscular dystrophies, amyotrophic lateral sclerosis, postpolio syndrome, and myasthenia gravis. In addition to hypoventilation from reduced motor output, these diseases are subject to impaired compensation to the increased respiratory impedance that occurs during sleep. Moreover, these subjects may demonstrate impaired excretion of accumulated CO_2 load after awakening, predisposing them to development of chronic hypercapnia during wakefulness.

There are 2 subgroups of patients that are particularly at risk for sleep hypoventilation related to disproportionate weakness in the diaphragm as compared with other inspiratory muscles. Patients with COPD may develop hyperinflation with associated compromise in diaphragmatic function. Although skeletal muscle function may be normal in these subjects, hypoventilation is frequently encountered during sleep. Abnormalities are particularly prominent in REM sleep because of the hypotonia of the accessory muscles of inspiration coupled with the baseline abnormalities in diaphragm function.[51,79–85] An additional group of patients at risk for hypoventilation includes those with neuromuscular diseases that have a predilection for compromising diaphragm strength.[52,53] For example, Pompe disease is a glycogen storage disorder that may affect diaphragm function early in the disease course at time points in which peripheral muscle function is only minimally abnormal. Patients with diaphragm weakness have been shown to be at risk for sleep hypoventilation, particularly during REM sleep.[54] Although Pompe disease is rare in the general clinical population, similar findings may occur in any of the muscular dystrophies.[52,53]

For all of the diseases discussed previously, hypoventilation initially presents during REM sleep, progresses to hypoventilation during all sleep stages, and finally to persistence of hypoventilation during wakefulness.[53] Diagnosis requires full night polysomnography with electroencephalography to monitor for sleep stage–related abnormalities.

Treatment requires ventilatory support, which can be applied either noninvasively (eg, bilevel positive airway pressure) or invasively (eg, via a tracheostomy). The decision to proceed with tracheostomy is a frequent dilemma that requires consideration of the progressive nature of the underlying disease counterbalanced by the associated morbidities related to invasive mechanical ventilation.

Chest Wall Diseases

Diseases of the chest bellows have long been recognized as causes for hypoventilation. Common disorders include kyphoscoliosis, ankylosing spondylitis, and pleural restriction.[86] These disorders may present with concomitant hypoxemia from either atelectasis and/or from ventilation-perfusion (V/Q) mismatch. Although obesity is associated with altered chest wall compliance, elevated work of breathing from obesity per se is not a likely cause for chronic daytime hypercapnia, as patients with equivalent degrees of obesity may demonstrate normal blood gases during wakefulness.[87] Nevertheless, obesity, with its associated mass loading and increased work of breathing, would impair respiratory compensation for other disorders (eg, OSA).[25,88] For a patient with hypoventilation caused by chest wall disease, treatment with noninvasive positive-pressure or negative-pressure ventilation has been shown to result in normalization of P_aCO_2 during wakefulness and reduced health care utilization.[86,89]

Abnormal Gas Exchange

Abnormalities in gas exchange related to underlying cardiopulmonary disease have received a great deal of attention as a cause of alveolar hypoventilation. COPD is a well-recognized cause for alveolar hypoventilation. Alveolar ventilation is reduced in some patients with COPD despite normal or high total minute ventilation due to an elevation of the dead space fraction. Chronic daytime hypercapnia caused by COPD generally is manifest only in subjects with severe airflow limitation on standard spirometry. For patients with milder degree of disease, chronic hypercapnia has been associated with concomitant OSA (ie, the overlap syndrome).[90–92] Although the precise contribution of COPD to the chronic hypercapnia not been established in this circumstance, it is clear that elevation of dead space would impair ventilatory compensation for the acute CO_2 retention during obstructive events in these subjects, and thus could potentiate any effect on chronic CO_2 retention.

An additional form of gas exchange abnormality that may contribute to alveolar hypoventilation during sleep occurs whenever cyclical or intermittent reductions in ventilation are present. Temporal dissociation between ventilation and perfusion may occur during any periodic pattern of breathing.[93] The initial description was applied to short apneic episodes in which ongoing perfusion during periods of absent ventilation (ie, shunt) alternates with hyperpnea during arousal with unchanged perfusion (ie, dead space). The consequence of this form of V/Q mismatch is identical to V/Q mismatch from underlying COPD. This form of V/Q mismatch also would occur during a broad range of events, including short hypopneas and prolonged periods of alveolar hypoventilation, as long as ventilation oscillates out of proportion to simultaneous changes in blood flow.

Abnormal Respiratory Control

A variety of abnormalities in respiratory control, both intrinsic and iatrogenic, have been associated with hypoventilation. Ondine's curse, also known as congenital central hypoventilation syndrome, is associated with hypoventilation during sleep in subjects without identifiable pulmonary disease.[94–96] Recently, mutations in the PHOX2b gene have been implicated in this disease.[97] Additional diseases that are associated with impaired respiratory drive and hypoventilation include Arnold-Chiari malformation, brainstem tumors, and vascular malformations.

Perhaps the most frequent etiology for impaired respiratory drive is related to iatrogenic causes. Methadone has been shown to depress ventilatory responsiveness and is a well-established etiology for hypoventilation.[98] Similar concerns are applicable to any medication associated with somnolence and depression of respiratory drive (eg, tricyclic antidepressants, antipsychotics, antihistamines). Particular attention is needed for subjects receiving oxygen or diuretics. These are frequently prescribed either due to misdiagnosis of cardiac disease or to address the obligate hypoxemia that occurs whenever P_aCO_2 is elevated (in accord with the alveolar air equation) or the fluid retention and peripheral edema that is manifest in patients with cor pulmonale; however, oxygen and diuretics do not address the underlying abnormality. In addition, profound effects on respiratory drive may occur either directly (eg, oxygen) or indirectly by producing an increase in serum bicarbonate (eg, furosemide; see discussion later in this article).[99,100]

In addition to the previously mentioned disorders, there is a wide range of normal ventilatory drive that may become manifest in selected circumstances. Variability in both hypoxic and hypercapnic ventilatory responses is identifiable in healthy subjects. Although these abnormities alone would not produce hypoventilation, they may adversely impact an individual subject's ability to compensate for concomitant diseases. For example, a patient with blunted response to CO_2 may maintain normal gas exchange until a disease such as OSA becomes manifest or a respiratory depressant medication is prescribed.

CO_2 LOADING DURING SLEEP

Empiric studies both during sleep and wakefulness allow estimation of the relationship between the volume of CO_2 loaded and the acute change in blood PCO_2.[101,102] The volume of CO_2 load per mm Hg increase in P_aCO_2 ranged from 2 to 7 mL/kg, reflecting differences in baseline P_aCO_2. Importantly, the CO_2 load was directly a function of body weight.[102] For any given change in P_aCO_2, the magnitude of CO_2 loading was greater in obese as compared with thin adults. Because maintenance of eucapnia requires excretion of the CO_2 load, obese subjects require an increase in the compensatory rate of hyperventilation above the level required in thin subjects at similar P_aCO_2. Achievement of the required compensation is further exacerbated by the elevated work of breathing that has been documented in obesity.[23]

CO_2 UNLOADING
Compensatory Mechanisms During Sleep

Maintenance of overall CO_2 homeostasis in the setting of sleep hypoventilation requires a compensatory increase in ventilation during the period between hypoventilation events.[88,101,103] Traditionally, the efficacy of CO_2 unloading has been attributed to the magnitude of CO_2 responsiveness in individual subjects. Recently, breath-by-breath measurements of whole-body CO_2 balance during sleep (**Fig. 1**) has been used to describe the mechanisms for CO_2 responsiveness that are applicable to periods of sleep containing hypoventilatory events.[101] These data demonstrate that CO_2 elimination is ultimately limited by both the duration available and magnitude of ventilation during the compensatory phase between events (eg, between apneas). Thus, when the duration of respiratory events become 3 times longer than the subsequent breathing interval, CO_2 tends to accumulate despite maximal tidal volume because there is insufficient time for adequate hyperventilation between the events. In accord with this observation,

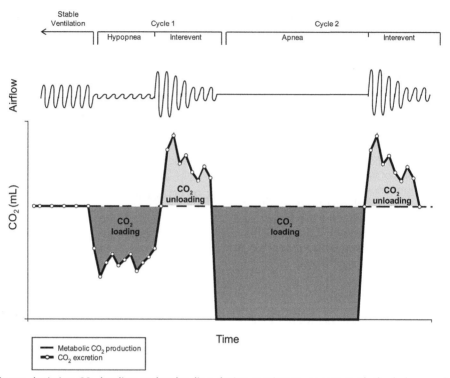

Fig. 1. Schema depicting CO_2 loading and unloading during respiratory events. Dark shaded areas depict CO_2 loading due to reduced CO_2 excretion during events. Light shaded areas depict CO_2 unloading due to compensatory hyperventilation between events. (*Adapted from* Berger KI, Ayappa I, Sorkin IB, et al. CO_2 homeostasis during periodic breathing in obstructive sleep apnea. J Appl Physiol 2000;88(1):259; with permission.)

studies in patients with obstructive sleep apnea demonstrate that hypercapnic subjects have a reduced duration of the interapnea ventilatory period relative to the length of the preceding apnea.[104]

In addition, modeling studies show that full CO_2 unloading during periodic ventilation requires an overall average ventilation that is higher than the average minute ventilation required to maintain P_aCO_2 during steady-state nonperiodic breathing.[93] This further stress imposed by periodic breathing occurs as a consequence of the temporal dissociation between oscillating ventilation and continuous perfusion (temporal V/Q mismatch). It is mathematically similar to the effect of classical V/Q mismatch from spatially nonuniform lung disease.

In most otherwise healthy subjects, full compensation for acute hypercapnia occurs after each episode of hypoventilation and there is no net CO_2 loading with each cycle. The augmented tidal volume that often occurs in the first breath after an apnea in eucapnic patients with obstructive apnea is the most obvious example of this compensation and failure of this augmentation has been demonstrated in patients with chronic hypercapnia.[71]

More detailed experiments demonstrated that the initial ventilation following apnea is directly related to the volume of CO_2 loaded during the preceding respiratory event and thus represents an index of "CO_2 load response."[105] Hypercapnic patients demonstrate reduction of this index of ventilatory responsiveness as compared with eucapnic patients.[105]

At least one study suggests that impaired CO_2 homeostasis after respiratory events (eg, relative shortening of interapnea duration and reduced postevent ventilation) may be mediated by opioids or opioid receptors because endorphin blockade changed this pattern.[106] Increased cerebrospinal fluid (CSF) β-endorphin activity with return to normal values following treatment has also been reported in subjects with sleep apnea.[107] These observations provide a framework for understanding the facilitating effect that opiates (including methadone) may have on the development of hypercapnia in some patients with sleep-disordered breathing.

Whereas the postevent ventilatory response reflects the output of an integrated control system, this ventilatory response to CO_2 load correlates poorly with the traditional ventilatory response to

CO_2 measured during wakefulness.[105] This dissociation suggests that additional inputs to the ventilatory control system may be present during periodic breathing. These could include the fluctuating hyperoxia/hypoxia and the change in ventilatory control that occurs with alternating sleep/wake states.[16] In addition, experimental data suggest that a distinct transiently aroused state characterized by enhanced cardiorespiratory activation may exist immediately on arousal that is distinct from sustained wakefulness.[108] Alterations in all of the foregoing could contribute to the altered magnitude of the postevent ventilatory response in hypercapnic sleep-disordered breathing; however, they have not been studied directly.

The previous observations indicate that there is an integrated ventilatory response to sleep-disordered breathing that controls ventilation between events and appears to respond to the volume of CO_2 loaded during the events. This control system appears to be impaired in patients with established chronic daytime hypercapnia and predisposes susceptible patients to awakening in the morning with an elevated arterial PCO_2 after multiple inadequately compensated acute hypoventilatory events.

Transition to Chronic Hypercapnia During Wakefulness

The previously mentioned considerations explain hypercapnia on awakening after a night of sleep-disordered breathing in the susceptible individual. However, they do not explain why a period of wakefulness free of ventilatory disturbances does not result in normalization of P_aCO_2 before the next period of sleep. Many scientists have postulated that adaption of chemoreceptors may occur in subjects with chronic hypoventilation. Tenney[99] suggested that elevated bicarbonate concentration ([HCO_3]) represents a "compromise adaptation" for hypercapnia. Subsequently, a role for an elevated bicarbonate concentration per se as a mechanism of generating a chronic hypercapnic state was suggested by Goldring and Turino[102] during experimentally induced metabolic alkalosis in healthy subjects. Elevated bicarbonate concentration would blunt the change in hydrogen ion concentration for a given change in P_aCO_2, in accord with the Henderson- Hasselbalch relationship, thereby blunting ventilatory CO_2 drive (**Fig. 2**).

Although the magnitude of the bicarbonate retention after a single night is too small to be measured clinically, modeling studies of whole-body CO_2 kinetics that included a renal bicarbonate controller in addition to a ventilatory controller

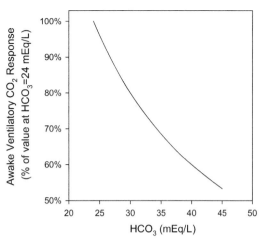

Fig. 2. Awake ventilatory response to CO_2, expressed as a percentage of the value obtained at a HCO_3 concentration of 24 mEq/L, is plotted as a function of increasing blood HCO_3 levels. A hyperbolic relationship between ventilatory response and HCO_3 exists, indicating blunting of the ventilatory response to CO_2 at elevated HCO_3 levels. (*Adapted from* Norman RG, Goldring RM, Clain JM, et al. Transition from acute to chronic hypercapnia in patients with periodic breathing: predictions from a computer model. J Appl Physiol 2006;100(5):1738; with permission.)

suggest that repetitive nights can produce a cumulative effect sufficient to depress ventilatory control (**Fig. 3**).[109] In this study, when ventilatory CO_2 response and renal HCO_3 excretion were normal, PCO_2 and [HCO_3] remained normal (ie, bicarbonate excretion during the day compensated for that retained during the night). However, when CO_2 response was abnormally low, a modest rise in awake PCO_2 and [HCO_3] was seen over multiple days. Similarly, when renal HCO_3 excretion rate was lowered to simulate chloride deficiency, the model demonstrated a modest rise in awake PCO_2 and [HCO_3] over multiple days, even with normal CO_2 response. Significantly, the combination of low CO_2 response and low renal HCO_3 excretion rate produced a synergistic effect on the degree of elevation of PCO_2 during wakefulness. Thus, respiratory-renal interactions may contribute to the development and perpetuation of chronic awake hypercapnia in patients with hypoventilation during sleep.

The foregoing considerations support the concept that a common denominator for the development of chronic hypercapnia during wakefulness is failure of compensation for the acute hypercapnia that occurs during sleep and particularly during sleep-disordered breathing events.[103] Failure of compensation may occur at 2 different points in time. First, immediate ventilatory compensation

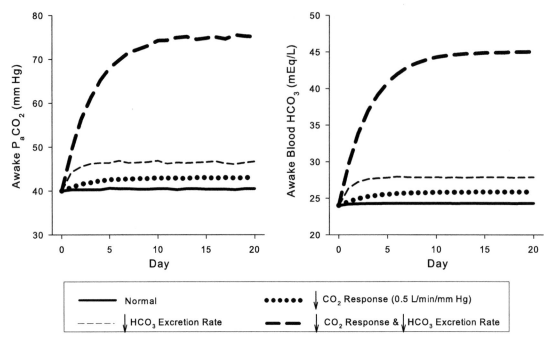

Fig. 3. Results from simulations depicting development of chronic hypercapnia using a model of whole-body CO_2 kinetics. The combination of reduced CO_2 response and reduced renal HCO_3 excretion rate produced a synergistic effect on the degree of elevation of awake PCO_2. (*Adapted from* Norman RG, Goldring RM, Clain JM, et al. Transition from acute to chronic hypercapnia in patients with periodic breathing: predictions from a computer model. J Appl Physiol 2006;100(5):1737; with permission.)

is required after each acute hypercapnic insult (apnea/hypopnea or sustained periods of hypoventilation). Ventilatory compensation may be compromised by either reduced ventilatory drive (eg, reduction in innate ventilator drive or induced by drug or oxygen) or reduced ventilatory efficiency of CO_2 clearance (eg, as in underlying cardiopulmonary disease). Second, adequate renal bicarbonate excretion is required during wakefulness to offset the effects of uncompensated cyclical hypercapnia. Renal compensatory mechanisms may be compromised by diuretic-induced chloride deficiency and/or by increased sodium avidity (eg, congestive heart failure (CHF), hypoxemia, or metabolic syndrome) and contribute to the transition between acute hypercapnia and the chronic hypercapnic state. It must be emphasized that these considerations apply both to short apneic and hypopneic events, as occurs in subjects with OSA and to prolonged central hypoventilation events, as occurs in subjects with sleep hypoventilation syndrome.

SUMMARY

Alveolar hypoventilation defined by an increase in P_aCO_2 occurs due to either reduced minute ventilation and/or increased dead space. Mild alveolar hypoventilation may be observed in healthy subjects during sleep. Sleep hypoventilation is accentuated in disease states with potential carryover to the daytime, producing chronic hypercapnia during wakefulness due to failure of compensation during sleep and/or during wakefulness. Elevation of blood bicarbonate concentration, although appropriate to defend blood pH, provides a mechanism for perpetuation of a chronic hypercapnic state due to blunting of respiratory drive.

REFERENCES

1. Goldring RM, Heinemann HO, Turino GM. Regulation of alveolar ventilation in respiratory failure. Am J Med Sci 1975;269(2):160–70.
2. White DP, Weil JV, Zwillich CW. Metabolic rate and breathing during sleep. J Appl Physiol 1985;59(2):384–91.
3. Kreider MB, Buskirk ER, Bass DE. Oxygen consumption and body temperatures during the night. J Appl Physiol 1958;12(3):361–6.
4. Milan FA, Evonuk E. Oxygen consumption and body temperatures of Eskimos during sleep. J Appl Physiol 1967;22(3):565–7.
5. Robin ED, Whaley RD, Crump CH, et al. Alveolar gas tensions, pulmonary ventilation and blood pH during physiologic sleep in normal subjects. J Clin Invest 1958;37(7):981–9.

6. Brebbia DR, Altshuler KZ. Oxygen consumption rate and electroencephalographic stage of sleep. Science 1965;150(3703):1621–3.
7. Morrell MJ, Harty HR, Adams L, et al. Changes in total pulmonary resistance and PCO_2 between wakefulness and sleep in normal human subjects. J Appl Physiol 1995;78(4):1339–49.
8. Simon PM, Dempsey JA, Landry DM, et al. Effect of sleep on respiratory muscle activity during mechanical ventilation. Am Rev Respir Dis 1993; 147(1):32–7.
9. Worsnop C, Kay A, Pierce R, et al. Activity of respiratory pump and upper airway muscles during sleep onset. J Appl Physiol 1998;85(3):908–20.
10. Berthon-Jones M, Sullivan CE. Ventilation and arousal responses to hypercapnia in normal sleeping humans. J Appl Physiol Respir Environ Exerc Physiol 1984;57(1):59–67.
11. Douglas NJ, White DP, Weil JV, et al. Hypercapnic ventilatory response in sleeping adults. Am Rev Respir Dis 1982;126(5):758–62.
12. Budhiraja R, Parthasarathy S, Drake CL, et al. Early CPAP use identifies subsequent adherence to CPAP therapy. Sleep 2007;30(3):320–4.
13. Ayappa I, Rapoport DM. The upper airway in sleep: physiology of the pharynx. Sleep Med Rev 2003; 7(1):9–33.
14. Johnson MW, Remmers JE. Accessory muscle activity during sleep in chronic obstructive pulmonary disease. J Appl Physiol Respir Environ Exerc Physiol 1984;57(4):1011–7.
15. Krimsky WR, Leiter JC. Physiology of breathing and respiratory control during sleep. Sem Respir Crit Care Med 2005;26(1):5–12.
16. Berthon-Jones M, Sullivan CE. Ventilatory and arousal responses to hypoxia in sleeping humans. Am Rev Respir Dis 1982;125(6):632–9.
17. Gould GA, Gugger M, Molloy J, et al. Breathing pattern and eye movement density during REM sleep in humans. Am Rev Respir Dis 1988;138(4): 874–7.
18. Orem J, Lovering AT, Dunin-Barkowski W, et al. Endogenous excitatory drive to the respiratory system in rapid eye movement sleep in cats. J Physiol 2000;527(Pt 2):365–76.
19. Orem JM, Lovering AT, Vidruk EH. Excitation of medullary respiratory neurons in REM sleep. Sleep 2005;28(7):801–7.
20. Hewlett AM, Hulands GH, Nunn JF, et al. Functional residual capacity during anaesthesia. II. Spontaneous respiration. Br J Anaesth 1974;46(7): 486–94.
21. Watson RA, Pride NB. Postural changes in lung volumes and respiratory resistance in subjects with obesity. J Appl Physiol 2005;98(2):512–7.
22. Jones RL, Nzekwu MM. The effects of body mass index on lung volumes. Chest 2006;130(3):827–33.
23. Rochester DF, Alpert MA, Alexander JK. Obesity and pulmonary function. The heart and lung in obesity. Armonk (NY): Futura Publishing Co; 1998. p. 109–31.
24. Yap JC, Watson RA, Gilbey S, et al. Effects of posture on respiratory mechanics in obesity. J Appl Physiol 1995;79(4):1199–205.
25. Steier J, Lunt A, Hart N, et al. Observational study of the effect of obesity on lung volumes. Thorax 2014. http://dx.doi.org/10.1136/thoraxjnl-2014-205148. [Epub ahead of print].
26. Ferretti A, Giampiccolo P, Cavalli A, et al. Expiratory flow limitation and orthopnea in massively obese subjects. Chest 2001;119(5):1401–8.
27. Cosio M, Ghezzo H, Hogg JC, et al. The relations between structural changes in small airways and pulmonary-function tests. N Engl J Med 1978; 298(23):1277–81.
28. Marco M, Minette A. Lung function changes in smokers with normal conventional spirometry. Am Rev Respir Dis 1976;114(4):723–38.
29. Begin R, Renzetti AD Jr, Bigler AH, et al. Flow and age dependence of airway closure and dynamic compliance. J Appl Physiol 1975;38(2):199–207.
30. Hudgel DW, Martin RJ, Johnson B, et al. Mechanics of the respiratory system and breathing pattern during sleep in normal humans. J Appl Physiol 1984;56(1):133–7.
31. Wiegand L, Zwillich CW, White DP. Collapsibility of the human upper airway during normal sleep. J Appl Physiol 1989;66(4):1800–8.
32. Tangel DJ, Mezzanotte WS, White DP. Influence of sleep on tensor palatini EMG and upper airway resistance in normal men. J Appl Physiol 1991; 70(6):2574–81.
33. Pevernagie DA, Stanson AW, Sheedy PF, et al. Effects of body position on the upper airway of patients with obstructive sleep apnea. Am J Respir Crit Care Med 1995;152(1):179–85.
34. Fouke JM, Strohl KP. Effect of position and lung volume on upper airway geometry. J Appl Physiol 1987;63(1):375–80.
35. Anch AM, Remmers JE, Bunce H. Supraglottic airway resistance in normal subjects and patients with occlusive sleep apnea. J Appl Physiol 1982; 53(5):1158–63.
36. Martin SE, Mathur R, Marshall I, et al. The effect of age, sex, obesity and posture on upper airway size. Eur Respir J 1997;10(9):2087–90.
37. Schwab RJ, Gefter WB, Pack AI, et al. Dynamic imaging of the upper airway during respiration in normal subjects. J Appl Physiol 1993;74(4): 1504–14.
38. Hoffstein V, Zamel N, Phillipson EA. Lung volume dependence of pharyngeal cross-sectional area in patients with obstructive sleep apnea. Am Rev Respir Dis 1984;130(2):175–8.

39. Van de Graaff WB. Thoracic influence on upper airway patency. J Appl Physiol 1988;65(5):2124–31.

40. Breuer J. Die Selbststeuerung der Athmung durch den Nervus vagus. Sitzungsber Akad Wiss Wien 1868;58:909–37.

41. White DP, Lombard RM, Cadieux RJ, et al. Pharyngeal resistance in normal humans: influence of gender, age, and obesity. J Appl Physiol 1985; 58(2):365–71.

42. Fogel RB, Malhotra A, Shea SA, et al. Reduced genioglossal activity with upper airway anesthesia in awake patients with OSA. J Appl Physiol 2000; 88(4):1346–54.

43. Strohl KP, Hensley MJ, Hallett M, et al. Activation of upper airway muscles before onset of inspiration in normal humans. J Appl Physiol 1980;49(4):638–42.

44. Kuna ST, Vanoye CR. Mechanical effects of pharyngeal constrictor activation on pharyngeal airway function. J Appl Physiol 1999;86(1):411–7.

45. Malhotra A, Pillar G, Fogel RB, et al. Genioglossal but not palatal muscle activity relates closely to pharyngeal pressure. Am J Respir Crit Care Med 2000;162(3 Pt 1):1058–62.

46. Tangel DJ, Mezzanotte WS, White DP. Influences of NREM sleep on activity of palatoglossus and levator palatini muscles in normal men. J Appl Physiol 1995;78(2):689–95.

47. Pillar G, Malhotra A, Fogel RB, et al. Upper airway muscle responsiveness to rising PCO(2) during NREM sleep. J Appl Physiol 2000;89(4):1275–82.

48. Wiegand DA, Latz B, Zwillich CW, et al. Upper airway resistance and geniohyoid muscle activity in normal men during wakefulness and sleep. J Appl Physiol 1990;69(4):1252–61.

49. Worsnop C, Kay A, Kim Y, et al. Effect of age on sleep onset-related changes in respiratory pump and upper airway muscle function. J Appl Physiol 2000;88(5):1831–9.

50. Henke KG. Upper airway muscle activity and upper airway resistance in young adults during sleep. J Appl Physiol 1998;84(2):486–91.

51. Becker HF, Piper AJ, Flynn WE, et al. Breathing during sleep in patients with nocturnal desaturation. Am J Respir Crit Care Med 1999;159(1):112–8.

52. White JE, Drinnan MJ, Smithson AJ, et al. Respiratory muscle activity and oxygenation during sleep in patients with muscle weakness. Eur Respir J 1995;8(5):807–14.

53. Ragette R, Mellies U, Schwake C, et al. Patterns and predictors of sleep disordered breathing in primary myopathies. Thorax 2002;57(8):724–8.

54. Mellies U, Ragette R, Schwake C, et al. Sleep-disordered breathing and respiratory failure in acid maltase deficiency. Neurology 2001;57(7): 1290–5.

55. Gastaut H, Tassinari CA, Duron B. Polygraphic study of the episodic diurnal and nocturnal (hypnic and respiratory) manifestations of the Pickwick syndrome. Brain Res 1966;1(2):167–86.

56. Guilleminault C, Eldridge FL, Dement WC. Insomnia with sleep apnea: a new syndrome. Science 1973; 181:856–8.

57. Remmers JE, deGroot WJ, Sauerland EK, et al. Pathogenesis of upper airway occlusion during sleep. J Appl Physiol 1978;44(6):931–8.

58. Longobardo GS, Evangelisti CJ, Cherniack NS. Analysis of the interplay between neurochemical control of respiration and upper airway mechanics producing upper airway obstruction during sleep in humans. Exp Physiol 2008;93(2):271–87.

59. Khoo MC, Gottschalk A, Pack AI. Sleep-induced periodic breathing and apnea: a theoretical study. J Appl Physiol 1991;70(5):2014–24.

60. Khoo MC, Kronauer RE, Strohl KP, et al. Factors inducing periodic breathing in humans: a general model. J Appl Physiol Respir Environ Exerc Physiol 1982;53(3):644–59.

61. Rodenstein DO, Dooms G, Thomas Y, et al. Pharyngeal shape and dimensions in healthy subjects, snorers, and patients with obstructive sleep apnoea. Thorax 1990;45(10):722–7.

62. Haponik EF, Smith PL, Bohlman ME, et al. Computerized tomography in obstructive sleep apnea. Correlation of airway size with physiology during sleep and wakefulness. Am Rev Respir Dis 1983; 127(2):221–6.

63. Schellenberg JB, Maislin G, Schwab RJ. Physical findings and the risk for obstructive sleep apnea. The importance of oropharyngeal structures. Am J Respir Crit Care Med 2000;162(2 Pt 1):740–8.

64. Shelton KE, Woodson H, Gay S, et al. Pharyngeal fat in obstructive sleep apnea. Am Rev Respir Dis 1993;148(2):462–6.

65. Schotland HM, Insko EK, Schwab RJ. Quantitative magnetic resonance imaging demonstrates alterations of the lingual musculature in obstructive sleep apnea. Sleep 1999;22(5):605–13.

66. Sforza E, Bacon W, Weiss T, et al. Upper airway collapsibility and cephalometric variables in patients with obstructive sleep apnea. Am J Respir Crit Care Med 2000;161(2 Pt 1):347–52.

67. Suratt PM, Dee P, Atkinson RL, et al. Fluoroscopic and computed tomographic features of the pharyngeal airway in obstructive sleep apnea. Am Rev Respir Dis 1983;127(4):487–92.

68. Burwell CS, Robin ED, Whaley RD, et al. Extreme obesity associated with alveolar hypoventilation: a pickwickian syndrome. Am J Med 1956;21:811–8.

69. Auchincloss HJ, Cook E, Renzetti AD. Clinical and physiological aspects of a case of obesity, polycythemia, and alveolar hypoventilation. J Clin Invest 1955;35:1537–45.

70. Rapoport DM, Sorkin B, Garay SM, et al. Reversal of the "Pickwickian syndrome" by long-term use

of nocturnal nasal-airway pressure. N Engl J Med 1982;307(15):931–3.

71. Rapoport DM, Garay SM, Epstein H, et al. Hypercapnia in the obstructive sleep apnea syndrome. A reevaluation of the "Pickwickian syndrome." Chest 1986;89(5):627–35.

72. Sullivan CE, Issa FG, Berthon-Jones M, et al. Reversal of obstructive sleep apnoea by continuous positive airway pressure applied through the nares. Lancet 1981;1(8225):862–5.

73. Sullivan CE, Berthon-Jones M, Issa FG. Remission of severe obesity-hypoventilation syndrome after short-term treatment during sleep with nasal continuous positive airway pressure. Am Rev Respir Dis 1983;128(1):177–81.

74. Berger KI, Ayappa I, Chatr-Amontri B, et al. Obesity hypoventilation syndrome as a spectrum of respiratory disturbances during sleep. Chest 2001;120(4): 1231–8.

75. Marcus CL, Keens TG, Bautista DB, et al. Obstructive sleep apnea in children with Down syndrome. Pediatrics 1991;88(1):132–9.

76. John A, Fagondes S, Schwartz I, et al. Sleep abnormalities in untreated patients with mucopolysaccharidosis type VI. Am J Med Genet A 2011; 155(7):1546–51.

77. Mellies U, Dohna-Schwake C, Voit T. Respiratory function assessment and intervention in neuromuscular disorders. Curr Opin Neurol 2005;18(5):543–7.

78. Polkey MI, Lyall RA, Moxham J, et al. Respiratory aspects of neurological disease. J Neurol Neurosurg Psychiatry 1999;66(1):5–15.

79. Barnes PJ. Chronic obstructive pulmonary disease. N Engl J Med 2000;343(4):269–80.

80. Wynne JW, Block AJ, Hemenway J, et al. Disordered breathing and oxygen desaturation during sleep in patients with chronic obstructive pulmonary disease. Chest 1978;73(2 Suppl):301–3.

81. Douglas NJ, Calverley PM, Leggett RJ, et al. Transient hypoxaemia during sleep in chronic bronchitis and emphysema. Lancet 1979;1(8106):1–4.

82. Coccagna G, Lugaresi E. Arterial blood gases and pulmonary and systemic arterial pressure during sleep in chronic obstructive pulmonary disease. Sleep 1978;1(2):117–24.

83. Collop N. Sleep and sleep disorders in chronic obstructive pulmonary disease. Respiration 2010; 80(1):78–86.

84. White JE, Drinnan MJ, Smithson AJ, et al. Respiratory muscle activity during rapid eye movement (REM) sleep in patients with chronic obstructive pulmonary disease. Thorax 1995;50(4):376–82.

85. Hudgel DW, Martin RJ, Capehart M, et al. Contribution of hypoventilation to sleep oxygen desaturation in chronic obstructive pulmonary disease. J Appl Physiol Respir Environ Exerc Physiol 1983;55(3): 669–77.

86. Garay SM, Turino GM, Goldring RM. Sustained reversal of chronic hypercapnia in patients with alveolar hypoventilation syndromes. Long-term maintenance with noninvasive nocturnal mechanical ventilation. Am J Med 1981;70(2):269–74.

87. Rochester DF, Enson Y. Current concepts in the pathogenesis of the obesity hypoventilation syndrome: mechanical and circulatory factors. Am J Med 1974;57:402–20.

88. Javaheri S, Colangelo G, Lacey W, et al. Chronic hypercapnia in obstructive sleep apnea-hypopnea syndrome. Sleep 1994;17(5):416–23.

89. Gonzalez C, Ferris G, Diaz J, et al. Kyphoscoliotic ventilatory insufficiency: effects of long-term intermittent positive-pressure ventilation. Chest 2003; 124(3):857–62.

90. Bradley TD, Rutherford R, Lue F, et al. Role of diffuse airway obstruction in the hypercapnia of obstructive sleep apnea. Am Rev Respir Dis 1986;134(5):920–4.

91. Chaouat A, Weitzenblum E, Krieger J, et al. Association of chronic obstructive pulmonary disease and sleep apnea syndrome. Am J Respir Crit Care Med 1995;151(1):82–6.

92. Flenley DC. Sleep in chronic obstructive lung disease. Clin Chest Med 1985;6(4):651–61.

93. Rapoport DM, Norman RG, Goldring RM. CO_2 homeostasis during periodic breathing: predictions from a computer model. J Appl Physiol 1993;75(5): 2302–9.

94. Severinghaus JW, Mitchell RA. Ondine's curse—failure of respiratory center automaticity while awake. Clin Res 1952;10:122.

95. Mellins RB, Balfour HH Jr, Turino GM, et al. Failure of automatic control of ventilation (Ondine's curse). Report of an infant born with this syndrome and review of the literature. Medicine (Baltimore) 1970; 49(6):487–504.

96. Grigg-Damberger M, Wells A. Central congenital hypoventilation syndrome: changing face of a less mysterious but more complex genetic disorder. Semin Respir Crit Care Med 2009;30(3):262–74.

97. Goridis C, Dubreuil V, Thoby-Brisson M, et al. Phox2b, congenital central hypoventilation syndrome and the control of respiration. Semin Cell Dev Biol 2010;21(8):814–22.

98. Marks CE Jr, Goldring RM. Chronic hypercapnia during methadone maintenance. Am Rev Respir Dis 1973;108(5):1088–93.

99. Tenney SM. Respiratory control in chronic pulmonary emphysema: a compromise adaptation. J Maine Med Assoc 1957;48:375–9.

100. Berger KI, Norman RG, Ayappa I, et al. Potential mechanism for transition between acute hypercapnia during sleep to chronic hypercapnia during wakefulness in obstructive sleep apnea. Adv Exp Med Biol 2008;605:431–6.

101. Berger KI, Ayappa I, Sorkin IB, et al. CO(2) homeostasis during periodic breathing in obstructive sleep apnea. J Appl Physiol 2000;88(1):257–64.

102. Goldring RM, Turino GM. Assessment of respiratory regulation in chronic hypercapnia. Chest 1976;70(1 Suppl):186–91.

103. Berger KI, Goldring RM, Rapoport DM. Obesity hypoventilation syndrome. Semin Respir Crit Care Med 2009;30(3):253–61.

104. Ayappa I, Berger KI, Norman RG, et al. Hypercapnia and ventilatory periodicity in obstructive sleep apnea syndrome. Am J Respir Crit Care Med 2002;166(8):1112–5.

105. Berger KI, Ayappa I, Sorkin IB, et al. Postevent ventilation as a function of CO(2) load during respiratory events in obstructive sleep apnea. J Appl Physiol 2002;93(3):917–24.

106. Greenberg HE, Rapoport DM, Rothenberg SA, et al. Endogenous opiates modulate the postapnea ventilatory response in the obstructive sleep apnea syndrome. Am Rev Respir Dis 1991;143(6):1282–7.

107. Gislason T, Almqvist M, Boman G, et al. Increased CSF opioid activity in sleep apnea syndrome. Regression after successful treatment. Chest 1989;96(2):250–4.

108. Horner RL, Sanford LD, Pack AI, et al. Activation of a distinct arousal state immediately after spontaneous awakening from sleep. Brain Res 1997;778(1):127–34.

109. Norman RG, Goldring RM, Clain JM, et al. Transition from acute to chronic hypercapnia in patients with periodic breathing: predictions from a computer model. J Appl Physiol 2006;100(5):1733–41.

Sleep Hypoventilation
Diagnostic Considerations and Technological Limitations

Amanda J. Piper, BAppSc, MEd, PhD[a,b,*],
Jésus Gonzalez-Bermejo, MD, PhD[c,d],
Jean-Paul Janssens, MD[e]

KEYWORDS

- Nocturnal hypoventilation • Hypercapnia • Blood gas monitoring • Sleep-disordered breathing
- Monitoring

KEY POINTS

- Nocturnal hypoventilation is an early manifestation of progressive hypercapnic respiratory failure in a range of disorders affecting the respiratory system.
- To document and identify nocturnal hypoventilation, some measure of CO_2 level during sleep is required.
- Although widely used, clinical evaluation and daytime measures of respiratory function have limited ability to accurately detect nocturnal hypoventilation.
- End-tidal and transcutaneous CO_2 monitoring allow assessment of CO_2 across the night without disrupting sleep.
- Limitations of these measures need to be appreciated, and results interpreted in the context of other monitoring and clinical findings.

INTRODUCTION

Hypoventilation develops when alveolar ventilation becomes insufficient to meet metabolic demand. As a result of the imbalance between metabolic production and ventilatory elimination of carbon dioxide (CO_2), both alveolar and arterial CO_2 increase. Consequently, assessment of arterial CO_2 is essential for evaluating alveolar ventilation:

$$V_A = k \times V_{CO_2}/Pa_{CO_2}$$

whereby V_A is alveolar ventilation, V_{CO_2} is the rate of metabolic production of carbon dioxide, Pa_{CO_2} is the arterial carbon dioxide tension, and k is a constant. By definition, hypoventilation is present when Pa_{CO_2} rises higher than 45 mm Hg.

Determining whether an individual is hypoventilating is usually achieved by analyzing arterial blood gases during wakefulness with the subject seated. However, such a measurement reflects alveolar ventilation during a single point in the 24-hour period, and may not necessarily reflect changes occurring in alveolar ventilation in circumstances such as lying supine, sleep, or exercise. For many individuals, sleep poses a significant

[a] Department of Respiratory and Sleep Medicine, Royal Prince Alfred Hospital, Missenden Road, Camperdown, New South Wales 2050, Australia; [b] Sleep and Circadian Group, Woolcock Institute of Medical Research, Glebe Point Road, Glebe, New South Wales, Australia; [c] Department of Respiratory and Critical Care Medicine, Groupe Hospitalier Pitié-Salpêtrière Charles Foix, Assistance Publique-Hôpitaux de Paris, 47-83 boulevard de l'Hopital, Paris 75651, Cedex 13, France; [d] Neurophysiologie Respiratoire Expérimentale et Clinique, INSERM, UMR_S 1158, Paris, France; [e] Division of Pulmonary Diseases, Geneva University Hospital, Rue Gabrielle Perret-Gentil 4, 1211, Geneva 14, Switzerland
* Corresponding author. Department of Respiratory and Sleep Medicine, Royal Prince Alfred Hospital, Missenden Road, Camperdown, New South Wales 2050, Australia.
E-mail address: amanda.piper@sydney.edu.au

Sleep Med Clin 9 (2014) 301–313
http://dx.doi.org/10.1016/j.jsmc.2014.05.006
1556-407X/14/$ – see front matter © 2014 Elsevier Inc. All rights reserved.

challenge to ventilation. Not only will it worsen already poor daytime gas exchange, sleep hypoventilation generally precedes the development of daytime hypercapnia in many disorders. Consequently, marked rises in $Paco_2$ may be present during sleep, despite awake $Paco_2$ levels remaining within the normal range. This situation is easily missed if the clinician relies simply on an awake arterial blood sample. Early identification of sleep hypoventilation is desirable to minimize clinically significant ramifications of hypoventilation on daytime function and quality of life.

DEFINING SLEEP HYPOVENTILATION

Fundamental to the issue of monitoring sleep hypoventilation is to define what degree of variance from normal sleep ventilation constitutes hypoventilation. Some degree of hypoventilation is a normal physiologic response to sleep, with an expected decrease in minute ventilation of around 10% to 15% accompanied by increases in $Paco_2$ of up to 7 mm Hg.[1] Various definitions of sleep hypoventilation have been used, with the current American Academy of Sleep Medicine[2] suggesting:

- In adults
  - An increase in $Paco_2$ (or surrogate) greater than 55 mm Hg for 10 minutes or longer, or
  - An increase in $Paco_2$ (or surrogate) of 10 mm Hg or greater during sleep compared with an awake supine value to greater than 50 mm Hg for 10 minutes or longer
- In children
  - Greater than 25% of the total sleep time with $Paco_2$ greater than 50 mm Hg, measured by either arterial Pco_2 or a surrogate

Acceptable surrogates of $Paco_2$ are considered to be end-tidal CO_2 ($P_{ET}co_2$) and transcutaneous CO_2 ($P_{TC}co_2$).[2] However, these are consensus definitions, and various other definitions of sleep hypoventilation have been used.[3,4] Data are also lacking as regards threshold values of nocturnal hypercapnia that are associated with the appearance of specific clinical abnormalities.

CLINICAL EVALUATION AND DAYTIME ASSESSMENT OF AT-RISK INDIVIDUALS

Although it is obvious that monitoring the adequacy of ventilation during sleep is the most direct way of identifying the presence of sleep hypoventilation, it is neither cost-effective nor feasible to carry out such monitoring frequently or over an extended period. Therefore, simpler methods are used to identify the most appropriate time to undertake such monitoring. The first step in this process is to maintain a high level of suspicion in patients with disorders known to be associated with nocturnal hypoventilation (**Box 1**). Patients need to be specifically questioned about sleep quality, breathing, and daytime functioning, and any symptoms suggestive of hypoventilation actively sought (**Box 2**). The major limitation here is that symptoms often develop insidiously or overlap with those related to the primary diagnosis, and there are no signs specific for hypoventilation.

In individuals with neuromuscular disorders, several simple bedside tests are used to monitor respiratory function and identify those likely to have sleep-breathing abnormalities (**Box 3**). Because diaphragmatic function is critical in maintaining adequate ventilation in rapid eye movement (REM) sleep, the pattern of muscle weakness and the extent of diaphragmatic involvement will influence which disorders develop sleep hypoventilation and at what stage in the evolution of the disease this occurs. Although these

---

Box 1
Disorders associated with sleep or daytime and sleep hypoventilation

I. Restrictive lung disorders

　　Chest wall disorders (eg, kyphoscoliosis, pleural disorders)

　　Obesity hypoventilation syndrome

　　Parenchymal disorders (eg, sequelae of tuberculosis, advanced interstitial lung disease)

II. Neuromuscular disorders

　　Central hypoventilation (eg, Ondine's curse, chronic opioid use)

　　Motoneuron disease (eg, amyotrophic lateral sclerosis, poliomyelitis)

　　Disorders of the neuromuscular plaque (eg, myasthenia gravis)

　　Muscular disorders (eg, Duchenne muscular dystrophy, Steinert myotonic dystrophy)

III. Chronic obstructive pulmonary diseases

　　Chronic obstructive pulmonary disease

　　Cystic fibrosis

　　Chronic bronchiolitis

IV. Bronchiectasis

Box 2
Symptoms frequently associated with nocturnal hypoventilation

- Disrupted sleep
- Morning headaches
- Daytime somnolence
- Fatigue
- Insomnia
- Enuresis
- Orthopnea
- Worsening memory or neurocognitive function

daytime tests may correlate poorly with the severity and nature of sleep-disordered breathing, they can flag individuals in whom further screening is warranted (**Fig. 1**).[5] The most useful measure is

the difference between vital capacity while upright versus supine, which when more than 20% to 25% is very specific for diaphragmatic dysfunction,[6] particularly in patients with myotonic dystrophy and amyotrophic lateral sclerosis (ALS).[7,8] When significant bulbar dysfunction is present, daytime lung function and respiratory muscle testing are not informative in detecting possible daytime hypercapnia.[9] The presence of other factors such as obesity, craniofacial abnormalities, chest wall deformity, cardiomyopathy, and upper airway obstruction will place an additional load on an already compromised respiratory system, permitting sleep hypoventilation to occur at more preserved levels of lung function.

Daytime measures of lung function and respiratory muscle strength are not useful for identifying the presence or severity of sleep hypoventilation in obesity or lung disease. Although low vital capacity and a body mass index (BMI) greater than

Box 3
Simple tests suitable for general clinic or bedside use to identify and monitor respiratory muscle weakness and the possibility of sleep hypoventilation in patients with neuromuscular disorders

Measurement	Comments
Vital capacity (VC)	Erect to supine decrease in VC >20% indicating diaphragmatic weakness
	Provides sensitive thresholds for predicting sleep-breathing abnormalities in myopathic diseases[5]
	• VC <60% predicted: onset of sleep-disordered breathing, hypopneas in rapid eye movement sleep
	• VC <40% predicted: hypoventilation >50% of total sleep time
	• VC <20% predicted: daytime hypercapnic respiratory failure
	Is a late predictor of respiratory failure compared with MIP
Maximum mouth inspiratory pressure (MIP)	A value >80 cm H_2O excludes significant inspiratory muscle weakness
	MIP <60 cm H_2O widely used to identify those at risk of hypoventilation
	Difficult for some patients to perform (eg, bulbar impairment); affected by leaks in those with orofacial muscle weakness
	Reliant on patient effort
	Wide range of normal values
Sniff nasal inspiratory pressure (SNIP)	Normal values >70 cm H_2O (males) and 60 cm H_2O (females)
	Useful when used in conjunction with MIP
	SNIP <30 cm H_2O more sensitive than VC or MIP in identifying patients with amyotrophic lateral sclerosis (ALS) at risk of hypoventilation[9]
	Reliant on patient effort; important learning effect
	Both MIP and SNIP assess global inspiratory muscle function rather than specific diaphragm strength
Clinical assessment of breathing	Dyspnea at rest can occur with severe global respiratory muscle weakness
	Orthopnea and abdominal paradox can occur when diaphragmatic strength is reduced to 25% of normal[50]
	Modified supine Borg score of 3 or greater is a predictor of respiratory muscle weakness in ALS[51]
	Use of accessory muscles at rest[7]

These tests should be considered as complementary investigations in identifying respiratory muscle weakness and likelihood of sleep hypoventilation/daytime hypercapnia to prioritize the use of more complex sleep-breathing monitoring.

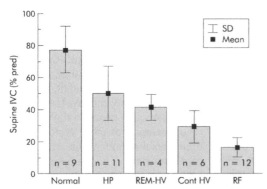

Fig. 1. In patients with neuromuscular disorders, supine inspiratory vital capacity (IVC) is closely associated with the development of various sleep-breathing disturbances. Cont HV, continuous hypoventilation in rapid eye movement (REM) and non-REM sleep; HP, hypopneas in REM sleep; Normal, no sleep-disordered breathing; REM-HV, hypoventilation in REM sleep; RF, diurnal respiratory failure. (*From* Ragette R, Mellies U, Schwake C, et al. Patterns and predictors of sleep disordered breathing in primary myopathies. Thorax 2002;57:726; with permission from the BMJ Publishing Group Ltd.)

40 kg/m^2 are associated with hypercapnia in patients with obesity and obstructive sleep apnea,[10–12] there is no clear threshold value that reliably discriminates individuals with obesity hypoventilation syndrome (OHS) from those with eucapnic obesity. In chronic obstructive pulmonary disease (COPD) and other obstructive lung diseases, daytime hypercapnia is unlikely to occur until the forced expiratory volume in 1 second is less than 30% of predicted, and even then significant variability exists.[13]

ASSESSMENT OF AWAKE GAS EXCHANGE IN IDENTIFYING SLEEP HYPOVENTILATION
Daytime Arterial Blood Gases

Analysis of arterial blood gases (ABGs) is used to determine if $Paco_2$ is elevated and whether this is an acute or chronic situation. With ABGs the pH, $Paco_2$, and Pao_2 are measured values, whereas the bicarbonate (HCO_3^-) is calculated based on the Henderson-Hasselbach equation. The base excess (BE) represents the metabolic (renal) compensation for any acid-base disorder (ie, the number of mmol/L that would have to be added or removed from a given arterial sample to normalize its pH for a given $Paco_2$).

To date, sampling of arterial blood remains the gold standard for assessing daytime hypoventilation. However, repeated nocturnal arterial punctures are neither practical nor an appropriate method of routinely assessing nocturnal

hypoventilation. Of importance is that the procedure itself may alter ventilation because it awakens the patient. Furthermore, a normal morning $Paco_2$ does not exclude significant nocturnal hypoventilation.[14]

Arterialized Capillary Blood Gases

Arterialized capillary blood gas (CBG) sampling has been shown to be a valid substitute for arterial Pco_2 and pH.[15,16] To ensure the sample is arterialized, the area needs to be adequately vasodilated; this is achieved by warming the site with a heater or warm towel, or by applying a topical vasodilatory substance to the skin 10 to 20 minutes before sampling.[17] A meta-analysis found that blood sampled from the earlobe provides a more accurate measure of Pco_2 than fingertip sampling, while sampling from either site closely reflects arterial pH.[16] Of importance, limits of agreement between arterial and capillary samples are wide for Pao_2, with a trend for underestimating arterial values by capillary sampling.[15]

Venous Blood Gases

Some studies have reported acceptable differences between venous and ABGs for assessing Pco_2 and pH in patients with acute respiratory disease, and venous CO_2 is used in some centers to assess efficacy of therapy in patients with hypercapnia.[18] However, results from a meta-analysis found that wide limits of agreement between venous and arterial Pco_2 renders venous Pco_2 an inappropriate substitution for $Paco_2$. In addition, the relationship between venous and arterial Pco_2 was not stable, precluding the use of a conversion factor to predict $Paco_2$ from the venous sample.[19] Consequently, it is currently recommended that a venous Pco_2 sample not be substituted for arterial Pco_2 in identifying hypercapnic respiratory failure.[19,20]

Clinical Implications

Sleep hypoventilation is common in patients with severe COPD and daytime hypercapnia, occurring in 20% to 40% of those who require nocturnal oxygen therapy.[3,21] In both COPD and cystic fibrosis, $Paco_2$ has been found to be a better predictor of nocturnal hypoventilation than simple spirometric indices.[3,22] In patients with OHS, a raised awake $Paco_2$ is mandatory for the diagnosis to be made.

However, there are several technical issues surrounding the use of daytime $Paco_2$ to identify sleep hypoventilation (**Box 4**). Limited skill in performing an arterial puncture, and the potential pain or discomfort arising from an inexpertly performed procedure, are 2 major reasons why clinicians and patients may avoid ABG sampling. Although

---

Box 4
Advantages and precautions of blood gases

Arterial Blood Gases	Arterialized Capillary Blood Gases
Advantages	Advantages
• Considered the gold standard for assessing gas exchange	• Closely reflects
	• Minimal discomfort to subject
• Provides accurate Pao_2 measure	• Minimal procedural or safety concerns
• Derived values can be obtained (base excess, arterial-alveolar difference)	• Requires only a very small sample
Precautions/considerations	Precautions/considerations
• Requires skilled personnel to obtain	• Requires adequate vasodilation
• Can be painful, altering breathing and hence CO_2 and pH values	• No air bubbles
• Bleeding and bruising at the site; potential nerve injury	• Reduced precision for Po_2 compared with Pao_2, but improves under hypoxic conditions
• Difficult access in some individuals (eg, obesity or joint contractures)	• Earlobe more accurate than fingertip for Po_2 and Pco_2. No difference for pH

CBGs cause far less discomfort, some skill in obtaining a sample and analyzing it is still necessary.

In conditions such as neuromuscular and chest wall disorders, awake hypoventilation occurs only after significant sleep hypoventilation is already present. Consequently, waiting until daytime hypoventilation occurs to consider initiating therapy increases the risk of significant morbidity and mortality for the patient.[4,9] Conversely, a normal awake $Paco_2$ cannot exclude sleep hypoventilation.

On the other hand, high bicarbonate values, in the absence of other metabolic abnormalities, reflect chronic hypoventilation, including that occurring during sleep only. Therefore, high bicarbonate despite a normal daytime $Paco_2$ should raise the suspicion of sleep hypoventilation. In patients with ALS, Lyall and colleagues[9] found that nocturnal hypercapnia was invariable when earlobe CBG bicarbonate was raised, even when earlobe CBG Pco_2 and Po_2 were normal. Likewise in patients with OHS, raised bicarbonate either from a CBG or on serum blood is a sensitive predictor of daytime hypercapnia, and has been suggested as a simple screening tool to distinguish patients with OHS from eucapnic obese sleep apneics.[23,24]

Nevertheless, caution is required when interpreting high bicarbonate values, and other common causes responsible for metabolic alkalosis need to be considered:

- Dehydration
- Use of loop diuretics
- Glucocorticoids
- Vomiting and diarrhea

MONITORING OF HYPOVENTILATION DURING SLEEP

Although daytime measures can provide an indication that sleep hypoventilation may be present, more direct monitoring of breathing and gas exchange during sleep is required to confirm that hypoventilation is present and to determine its severity.

Tools available for monitoring are:

- Pulse oximetry
- Polygraphy/polysomnography
- End-tidal carbon dioxide monitoring
- Transcutaneous carbon dioxide monitoring

The sensitivity and usefulness of each of these tools will vary considerably depending on the type of patients being studied and their clinical circumstances (**Fig. 2**).

PULSE OXIMETRY

Pulse oximetry (Spo_2) is a noninvasive method of estimating the percentage of hemoglobin molecules that are bound to oxygen in the arterial blood (Sao_2), and is used to detect the presence of hypoxemia in a wide range of clinical situations including sleep. Hypoventilation and ventilation-perfusion (V/Q) mismatch are the 2 major causes of hypoxemia in respiratory pathology. Both mechanisms decrease Sao_2 and Spo_2, which can be readily detected by pulse oximetry.

This technique has become a popular approach for detecting sleep-disordered breathing and

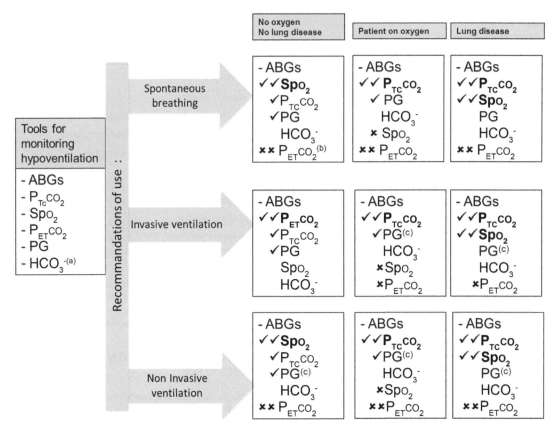

Fig. 2. Flowchart illustrating the most appropriate tools for detecting hypoventilation. The tool chosen varies depending on the clinical situation. In all situations, arterial blood gases (ABGs) provide information about daytime hypoventilation. However, significant nocturnal hypoventilation may be present despite a normal awake ABG measurement. Therefore, supporting measures are necessary to identify and confirm sleep hypoventilation, but the tool chosen needs to be appropriate for the clinical setting, taking into consideration its limitations. ✔✔ plus boldface text, the most appropriate tool(s) for this setting; ✔, acceptable alternatives in this setting; regular text, may be used in this setting; ✗, measurements not useful in this particular setting; ✗✗, tools that should be avoided in this setting. [a] If no diuretics or long-term steroids being used. [b] Except if the patient is tracheostomized with a cuffed tracheostomy. [c] Inbuilt ventilator polygraphic signals can replace the polygraph. ABGs, arterial blood gases; HCO_3^-, bicarbonates; $P_{ET}CO_2$, end-tidal carbon dioxide; PG, polygraphy; $P_{TC}CO_2$, transcutaneous carbon dioxide; SpO_2, pulse oximetry.

hypoxemia because of its low cost, simplicity, and ease of setup. However, there are several technical and practical aspects of pulse oximetry that need to be considered when interpreting oximetry output (**Box 5**). The accuracy of SpO_2 in the 75% to 100% range is around 2% ± 2% when compared with hemoglobin saturation derived from arterial samples.[25] However, at values less than 80% the accuracy can decrease considerably, with a tendency to underread. The SpO_2 values displayed by the device represent an averaging of measurements over a period of time that is user-adjusted, generally in the range of 2 to 16 seconds, with the display value updated every 0.5 to 1 second. The averaging time chosen is an important consideration and can lead to overestimation or

underestimation of desaturation events. Longer averaging times smooth out more transient events, and are useful in reducing motion artifact. However, they will also reduce the detection of more transient changes in oxygenation associated with sleep-disordered breathing.[26] For nocturnal monitoring, an averaging time of 3 seconds is recommended.[27]

Owing to the sigmoidal shape of the oxyhemoglobin dissociation curve, small reductions in SpO_2 can equate to significant increases in $PaCO_2$ associated with hypoventilation, and may be overlooked by the clinician: that is, an SpO_2 of 90% to 92%, which may seem acceptable per se, may be associated with a $PaCO_2$ value of 60 mm Hg (**Fig. 3**). The accuracy and reliability of SpO_2

Box 5
Technical and practical considerations in pulse oximetry monitoring

Technical

- Presence of motion artifact
- Accuracy ±2% for Spo_2 values greater than 90%; decreases markedly for Spo_2 values less than 80%
- Probe site: finger versus earlobe
- Oximeter calibration and accuracy
- Averaging time
- Sample rate used for data playback

Practical

- Measures oxygen saturation, not alveolar ventilation
- Poor sensitivity in patients using oxygen therapy
- Skin and nail conditions (eg, digital clubbing, acrylic or dark nail polishes)
- Low perfusion states
- Poor probe positioning
- Pain or discomfort related to finger probe
- Ambient light interference
- Irregular rhythms
- Absence of specificity for discriminating obstructive from central events
- Prolonged desaturation may reflect hypoventilation or ventilation/perfusion mismatching

Adapted from Pretto JJ, Roebuck T, Beckert L, et al. Clinical use of pulse oximetry: official guidelines from the Thoracic Society of Australia and New Zealand. Respirology 2014;19(1):38–46.

measurements may also be affected by the level of $Paco_2$ such that the agreement between Sao_2 and Spo_2 decreases with increasing $Paco_2$ levels.[28]

Clinical Uses and Interpretation

Daytime oximetry can be easily performed in the home or clinic. Whereas normal values for Spo_2 are lacking and will vary according to factors such as age, altitude, and probe location, expected values for Sao_2 lie within the range of 94% to 97%.[26] In patients with neuromuscular and chest wall disorders, Spo_2 of less than 95% should trigger further investigation of ventilation status. Similarly, Spo_2 of less than 95% in an obese individual can be useful in screening for OHS,[29] but does not predict the presence of daytime hypercapnia or the severity of sleep

hypoventilation and needs to be considered in relation to other clinical and physiologic measures.

Nocturnal oximetry is widely used for screening and diagnosing sleep-disordered breathing in both adults and children. Patients with OHS experience significantly greater degrees of sleep hypoxemia than eucapnic obese sleep apneics, with time spent with Spo_2 less than 90% being a strong predictor of daytime hypercapnia,[11] although no specific threshold separates the 2 groups.

Patterns of desaturation can indicate different types of sleep-breathing events. Cyclical desaturation/resaturation suggests the presence of apneas and hypopneas, and is often used to rule-in obstructive sleep apnea. However, depending on the threshold used, the sensitivity and specificity of pulse oximetry in detecting obstructive sleep apnea can range from 31% to 95% and 41% to 100%, respectively.[30] Furthermore, whether these events are central or obstructive in nature cannot be accurately determined from the oximetry recording alone.[31] Apparent desaturation can arise from movement artifact, poor signal quality, or a poorly placed probe. The oximetry trace needs to be carefully interpreted with these limitations in mind.

Of importance and frequently misunderstood is that pulse oximetry measures oxygen saturation and not alveolar ventilation. Sustained periods of desaturation may reflect alveolar hypoventilation, but equally could represent V/Q mismatch, especially in patients with lung disease or obesity. Oximetry identifies the presence of hypoxemia but not the mechanism, and additional measurements are required to determine whether these changes in oxygenation are associated with hypoventilation. Furthermore, in patients with a brisk arousal response or those who do not attain REM sleep, the potential for sleep hypoventilation may be underestimated by oximetry alone. Finally, the diagnostic usefulness of oximetry alone is severely limited if the patient is receiving supplemental oxygen (**Fig. 4**).[32]

Heart rate variability and variability of pulse-wave amplitude (PWA) can also be derived from the pulse oximeter recording. A high rate of PWA declines (>30% of baseline amplitude, so-called autonomic arousals) may reflect disruption of sleep structure.[33] However, variations in PWA are nonspecific and may be related to sleep-disordered breathing, periodic leg movements, autonomic instability during REM sleep, or severe hypoxemia, and are not specific to nocturnal hypoventilation.

POLYGRAPHY AND POLYSOMNOGRAPHY

Polysomnography (PSG) is often considered the gold standard for identifying the presence of sleep-disordered breathing, with the measurement

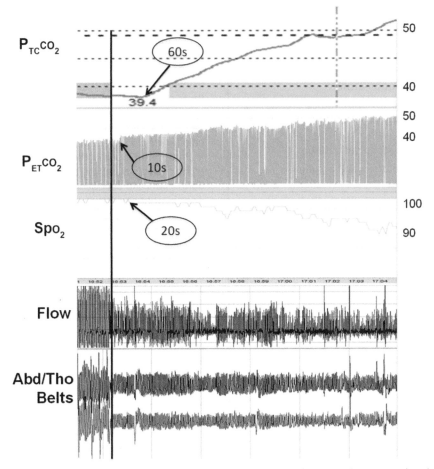

Fig. 3. Monitoring of hypoventilation in a patient with central congenital hypoventilation ventilated through an inflated cuffed tracheostomy. The black vertical bar denotes the beginning of an event, with decreased amplitude of the abdominal and thoracic belts (Abd/Tho Belts) and reduced airflow, resulting in hypoventilation. The circles and arrow illustrate the time differences in response to the event for the various signals. An increase in P_{ETCO_2} is apparent after 10 seconds and Spo_2 decreases after 20 seconds, whereas it is 60 seconds before a change in P_{TCCO_2} occurs. Note that Spo_2 values remain in the 90% to 92% range despite marked hypoventilation ($Paco_2 > 55$ mm Hg).

of various cardiorespiratory and sleep parameters allowing improved characterization of the severity and consequences of sleep-disordered breathing. The evaluation tools discussed previously are frequently seen as a simplified method of screening patients to determine the appropriate time to perform a PSG to document nocturnal hypoventilation and other types of sleep-disordered breathing. However, PSG is not a minor undertaking, especially for patients with high care needs. The procedure often requires a hospital admission or overnight stay in a sleep laboratory, and these environments may not be well suited to caring for individuals with severe physical disability.

Polygraphy (PG) (type III portable monitoring) refers to more abbreviated monitoring channels than PSG, recording at least Spo_2, heart rate, and nasal flow, and most often combining these items with

thoracic and abdominal movements, position detectors, leg movement detectors, and snoring detectors. PG is widely used for the detection of sleep-disordered breathing on an outpatient basis. However, it has several drawbacks:

- Total sleep time cannot be estimated precisely, although the addition of actimetry can be helpful in detecting subtle movements related to wakefulness.
- There is a high interobserver variability regarding quantification of hypopnea and their classification as central or obstructive.[34]
- Flow-limitation and respiratory-related arousals can be markedly underestimated when compared with PSG, underestimating the severity of sleep-disordered breathing in some cases.

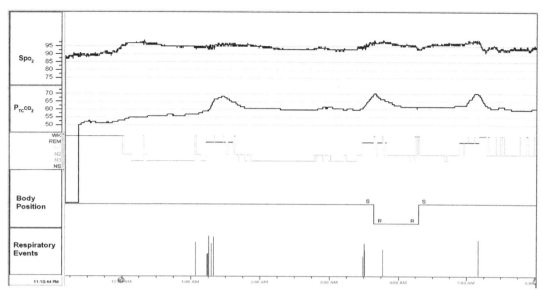

Fig. 4. Overnight summary from an overnight polysomnogram showing oximetry and transcutaneous carbon dioxide ($P_{TC}CO_2$) monitoring in a patient with cystic fibrosis. The patient was receiving supplemental oxygen, so SpO_2 values were well maintained. Baseline $P_{TC}CO_2$ was raised during wakefulness at 50 mm Hg, with an increase of about 5 mm Hg once asleep. However, during periods of REM sleep, further increases of around 10 mm Hg in $P_{TC}CO_2$ occurred. REM hypoventilation may not have been suspected if $P_{TC}CO_2$ monitoring had not been performed. N1, N2, N3, stages of non-REM sleep; NS, no signal; REM, rapid eye movement; WK, wakefulness.

- Sleep stages cannot be determined. Abnormalities are most likely to occur in REM sleep first. Absent or minimal REM may occur in patients with significant diaphragmatic weakness, and without the ability to analyze REM sleep specifically, the degree of sleep hypoventilation may be underestimated.

However, continuous overnight CO_2 recording (most often transcutaneous) is not routinely undertaken in many sleep laboratories. Thus, neither PSG nor PG provide useful additional information for identifying nocturnal hypoventilation without some measure of PCO_2 being undertaken.

CONTINUOUS NOCTURNAL MONITORING OF CARBON DIOXIDE

The limitations of a single or repeated blood sampling to identify sleep hypoventilation can be overcome by continuous nocturnal monitoring of CO_2. However, invasive monitoring by placement of an arterial line for this purpose is neither practical nor desirable. The 2 methods of noninvasive continuous monitoring available are end-tidal CO_2 ($P_{ET}CO_2$) and transcutaneous CO_2 ($P_{TC}CO_2$), both of which have been widely used in the diagnosis of sleep hypoventilation and in gauging response to positive pressure therapy.

End-Tidal Carbon Dioxide Monitoring

The relationship between $PaCO_2$ and $P_{ET}CO_2$ depends on the alveolar dead space (V_{DA}) and the individual's tidal volume (V_T), that is, $P_{ET}CO_2 = PaCO_2 (1 - V_{DA}/V_T)$. In healthy awake individuals, $P_{ET}CO_2$ is largely equivalent to $PaCO_2$ values.[35] However, this is not the case during sleep because of the physiologic decrease in V_T during this state, producing an increase in the $[PaCO_2 - P_{ET}CO_2]$ gradient owing to the higher V_{DA}/V_T ratio. In patients with underlying lung disease and V/Q mismatch, the dissociation between $P_{ET}CO_2$ and alveolar CO_2 widens further. Mouth breathing and the use of supplemental oxygen or positive pressure therapy will also affect the accuracy of $P_{ET}CO_2$ readings.[36] End-tidal CO_2 remains widely used and supported in the evaluation of sleep-disordered breathing in pediatric populations.[37,38] In adults, although increased $P_{ET}CO_2$ is highly suggestive of an increase in $PaCO_2$, biases and limits of agreement between $PaCO_2$ and $P_{ET}CO_2$ are too high to recommend $P_{ET}CO_2$ as a screening technique for nocturnal hypoventilation. Consequently, although $P_{ET}CO_2$ is easily measured using portable devices, it is a poor predictor of $PaCO_2$.

Under volume-cycled noninvasive ventilation (NIV), $P_{ET}CO_2$ is considered unreliable: events such as leaks, upper airway obstruction, or patient-ventilator asynchrony will affect the accuracy of $P_{ET}CO_2$. Furthermore, in pressure support

NIV, the high flows necessary to achieve preset pressure values interfere with the feasibility of $P_{ET}CO_2$ measurements. The exception is invasive ventilation in neuromuscular patients without underlying pulmonary disorders, when a tracheostomy and an inflated cuff are used; in this case $P_{ET}CO_2$ may be reliable.

Transcutaneous Carbon Dioxide Monitoring

Transcutaneous measurement of CO_2 is based on the observation that CO_2 has high tissue solubility and diffuses easily through the skin. Most capnometers use the Severinghaus electrode, which combines a pH-sensitive glass electrode, a silver/silver chloride (Ag/AgCl) reference electrode, and a heater. The electrodes are bathed in an electrolyte solution covered with a gas-permeable membrane. The sensor heats the skin to induce a local hyperemia, which increases the permeability of the skin to gas diffusion and "arterializes" the capillary blood to obtain $P_{TC}CO_2$ readings closer to $Paco_2$ values. The signal produced is the voltage difference between the pH electrode and the Ag/AgCl reference electrode. Transcutaneous CO_2 values displayed by the sensor reflect correction factors used by the system software to compensate for both patient and sensor temperature.

Available data show good agreement between $P_{TC}CO_2$ and $Paco_2$ values,[39] although higher $Paco_2$ values may increase the difference (bias) between $Paco_2$ and $P_{TC}CO_2$ values.[40] Agreement between these 2 measures does not appear to be affected by age-related changes in skin structure or by BMI.[41] However, when using $P_{TC}CO_2$ monitoring to identify sleep hypoventilation, the technical limitations of this technique need to be carefully considered in interpreting the measurements:

- Sensor calibration drift: the change in $P_{TC}CO_2$-$Paco_2$ difference. Compensation of this drift can be achieved by using linear interpolation, with 2 arterial measures of $Paco_2$ at the beginning and at the end of the $P_{TC}CO_2$ recording.[35] Drift can also be estimated using a calibration gas at the beginning and at the end of the recording, and introducing a correction factor. Technological improvements appear to have significantly reduced sensor drift.[42]
- Lag time. A delay of up to 2 minutes between $P_{TC}CO_2$ values best matching $Paco_2$ measures has been identified, which limits its use in detecting very short-lasting changes in $Paco_2$ (see **Fig. 3**).[43] However, in monitoring sleep for hypoventilation, sustained increases in Pco_2 are more important than short transient changes.

Developments in technology mean that recent devices are much more user-friendly, with highly improved software, reduced need for frequent sensor-probe membrane changes, and the capability of connection to portable PG and PSG systems. These devices are providing increasingly reliable and accurate measurements of Pco_2 during sleep.[42] Continuous recordings over 8 to 12 hours are now possible at probe temperatures of 42°C or 43°C, significantly reducing the possibility of inducing thermal injury or local discomfort.[44,45] In many centers and sleep laboratories, $P_{TC}CO_2$ is becoming a more routine procedure for monitoring patients under noninvasive ventilation.[42,46]

Even with these important improvements $P_{TC}CO_2$ devices remain expensive, and fragile. Their use requires expertise, and appropriate maintenance of the sensor and the device. Unexpected errant values occur and are reported in several clinical studies.[43,45] Unexplained drifts also occur. It is therefore important for the clinician to be aware of the limitations of this technique, to have a high degree of suspicion in the presence of unexpected values, and to look for indices suggestive of artifacts.

Clinical Implications

Despite the limitations of the technique, $P_{TC}CO_2$ is considered to be the best available tool for detecting and quantifying nocturnal alveolar hypoventilation. Using $P_{TC}CO_2$ monitoring in patients with restrictive thoracic disorders, Ward and colleagues[4] showed that once nocturnal hypoventilation was present, the risk of daytime respiratory failure developing within 12 months was significant. Transcutaneous CO_2 monitoring is being increasingly utilized for outpatient monitoring in adults and children, thus facilitating the diagnosis of sleep hypoventilation while potentially reducing costs. Several current guidelines advocate the use of $P_{TC}CO_2$ to monitor the adequacy of ventilation during sleep.[2,37,47]

Studies in both adults and children have reported the failure of nocturnal oximetry, even when used in conjunction with daytime blood gases to detect nocturnal hypoventilation in spontaneously breathing patients and those using nocturnal respiratory support. Several transcutaneous CO_2 monitors now have the capability of simultaneously measuring Spo_2 and $P_{TC}CO_2$ with a single sensor. The use of this combined Spo_2/$P_{TC}CO_2$ sensor technology has been shown to improve the detection of sleep hypoventilation in comparison with nocturnal oximetry alone, with nocturnal hypercapnia detected in 30% to 40%

of patients studied in the absence of substantial oxygen desaturation.[14,48,49] Thus a more comprehensive evaluation of nocturnal hypoventilation across a range of clinical settings is now possible. However, the degree to which this will have an impact on management and patient outcomes requires further evaluation.

SUMMARY

Nocturnal hypoventilation is an early manifestation of progressive hypercapnic respiratory failure in a range of disorders affecting the respiratory system. Identifying sleep-breathing abnormalities early can help plan treatment options and avoid unexpected sudden decompensation. Although daytime measures are widely used to identify individuals at high risk of hypoventilating during sleep, they are limited in their ability to detect hypercapnia confined to sleep. However, daytime evaluation can assist in determining the most appropriate time to undertake more complex nocturnal monitoring to achieve a positive finding. Advances in technology, particularly in continuous CO_2 monitoring techniques, are increasing our ability to identify and quantify nocturnal hypoventilation not only in supervised settings but also increasingly in the home.

REFERENCES

1. Becker HF, Piper AJ, Flynn WE, et al. Breathing during sleep in patients with nocturnal desaturation. Am J Respir Crit Care Med 1999;159(1):112–8.
2. Berry RB, Budhiraja R, Gottlieb DJ, et al. Rules for scoring respiratory events in sleep: update of the 2007 AASM Manual for the Scoring of Sleep and Associated Events. Deliberations of the Sleep Apnea Definitions Task Force of the American Academy of Sleep Medicine. J Clin Sleep Med 2012; 8(5):597–619.
3. O'Donoghue FJ, Catcheside PG, Ellis EE, et al. Sleep hypoventilation in hypercapnic chronic obstructive pulmonary disease: prevalence and associated factors. Eur Respir J 2003;21(6): 977–84.
4. Ward S, Chatwin M, Heather S, et al. Randomised controlled trial of non-invasive ventilation (NIV) for nocturnal hypoventilation in neuromuscular and chest wall disease patients with daytime normocapnia. Thorax 2005;60(12):1019–24.
5. Ragette R, Mellies U, Schwake C, et al. Patterns and predictors of sleep disordered breathing in primary myopathies. Thorax 2002;57(8):724–8.
6. Fromageot C, Lofaso F, Annane D, et al. Supine fall in lung volumes in the assessment of diaphragmatic weakness in neuromuscular disorders. Arch Phys Med Rehabil 2001;82(1):123–8.
7. Lechtzin N, Wiener CM, Shade DM, et al. Spirometry in the supine position improves the detection of diaphragmatic weakness in patients with amyotrophic lateral sclerosis. Chest 2002;121(2): 436–42.
8. Poussel M, Kaminsky P, Renaud P, et al. Supine changes in lung function correlate with chronic respiratory failure in myotonic dystrophy patients. Respir Physiol Neurobiol 2014;193(1):43–51.
9. Lyall RA, Donaldson N, Polkey MI, et al. Respiratory muscle strength and ventilatory failure in amyotrophic lateral sclerosis. Brain 2001; 124(Pt 10):2000–13.
10. Akashiba T, Akahoshi T, Kawahara S, et al. Clinical characteristics of obesity-hypoventilation syndrome in Japan: a multi-center study. Intern Med 2006;45(20):1121–5.
11. Kaw R, Hernandez AV, Walker E, et al. Determinants of hypercapnia in obese patients with obstructive sleep apnea: a systematic review and metaanalysis of cohort studies. Chest 2009; 136(3):787–96.
12. Laaban JP, Chailleux E, for the Observatory Group of ANTADIR. Daytime hypercapnia in adult patients with obstructive sleep apnea syndrome in France, before initiating nocturnal nasal continuous positive airway pressure therapy. Chest 2005;127(3):710–5.
13. Bégin P, Grassino A. Inspiratory muscle dysfunction and chronic hypercapnia in chronic obstructive pulmonary disease. Am Rev Respir Dis 1991; 143(5 Pt 1):905–12.
14. Paiva R, Krivec U, Aubertin G, et al. Carbon dioxide monitoring during long-term noninvasive respiratory support in children. Intensive Care Med 2009;35(6):1068–74.
15. Sauty A, Uldry C, Debetaz L, et al. Differences in PO_2 and PCO_2 between arterial and arterialized earlobe samples. Eur Respir J 1996;9(2):186–9.
16. Zavorsky GS, Cao J, Mayo NE, et al. Arterial versus capillary blood gases: a meta-analysis. Respir Physiol Neurobiol 2007;155(3):268–79.
17. Pitkin AD, Roberts CM, Wedzicha JA. Arterialised earlobe blood gas analysis: an underused technique. Thorax 1994;49(4):364–6.
18. Kelly AM, Klim S. Can a change in pH and pCO_2 be used to monitor progress in patients undergoing noninvasive ventilation? A prospective cohort study. Eur J Emerg Med 2014;21(1):69–72.
19. Byrne AL, Bennett M, Chatterji R, et al. Peripheral venous and arterial blood gas analysis in adults: are they comparable? A systematic review and meta-analysis. Respirology 2014;19(2):168–75.
20. Davis MD, Walsh BK, Sittig SE, et al. AARC clinical practice guideline: blood gas analysis and

hemoximetry: 2013. Respir Care 2013;58(10): 1694–703.

21. Tarrega J, Anton A, Guell R, et al. Predicting nocturnal hypoventilation in hypercapnic chronic obstructive pulmonary disease patients undergoing long-term oxygen therapy. Respiration 2011; 82(1):4–9.

22. Milross MA, Piper AJ, Norman M, et al. Predicting sleep-disordered breathing in patients with cystic fibrosis. Chest 2001;120(4):1239–45.

23. Macavei VM, Spurling KJ, Loft J, et al. Diagnostic predictors of obesity-hypoventilation syndrome in patients suspected of having sleep disordered breathing. J Clin Sleep Med 2013; 9(9):879–84.

24. Mokhlesi B, Tulaimat A, Faibussowitsch I, et al. Obesity hypoventilation syndrome: prevalence and predictors in patients with obstructive sleep apnea. Sleep Breath 2007;11(2):117–24.

25. Janssens JP, Borel JC, Pepin JL. Nocturnal monitoring of home non-invasive ventilation: the contribution of simple tools such as pulse oximetry, capnography, built-in ventilator software and autonomic markers of sleep fragmentation. Thorax 2011;66(5):438–45.

26. Pretto JJ, Roebuck T, Beckert L, et al. Clinical use of pulse oximetry: official guidelines from the Thoracic Society of Australia and New Zealand. Respirology 2014;19(1):38–46.

27. Farre R, Montserrat JM, Ballester E, et al. Importance of the pulse oximeter averaging time when measuring oxygen desaturation in sleep apnea. Sleep 1998;21(4):386–90.

28. Munoz X, Torres F, Sampol G, et al. Accuracy and reliability of pulse oximetry at different arterial carbon dioxide pressure levels. Eur Respir J 2008; 32(4):1053–9.

29. Basoglu OK, Tasbakan MS. Comparison of clinical characteristics in patients with obesity hypoventilation syndrome and obese obstructive sleep apnea syndrome: a case-control study. Clin Respir J 2014;8(2):167–74.

30. Netzer N, Eliasson AH, Netzer C, et al. Overnight pulse oximetry for sleep-disordered breathing in adults: a review. Chest 2001;120(2):625–33.

31. Series F, Kimoff RJ, Morrison D, et al. Prospective evaluation of nocturnal oximetry for detection of sleep-related breathing disturbances in patients with chronic heart failure. Chest 2005;127(5):1507–14.

32. Fu ES, Downs JB, Schweiger JW, et al. Supplemental oxygen impairs detection of hypoventilation by pulse oximetry. Chest 2004;126(5):1552–8.

33. Zacharia A, Haba-Rubio J, Simon R, et al. Sleep apnea syndrome: improved detection of respiratory events and cortical arousals using oximetry pulse wave amplitude during polysomnography. Sleep Breath 2008;12(1):33–8.

34. Bridevaux PO, Fitting JW, Fellrath JM, et al. Inter-observer agreement on apnoea hypopnoea index using portable monitoring of respiratory parameters. Swiss Med Wkly 2007;137(43–44): 602–7.

35. Berlowitz DJ, Spong J, O'Donoghue FJ, et al. Transcutaneous measurement of carbon dioxide tension during extended monitoring: evaluation of accuracy and stability, and an algorithm for correcting calibration drift. Respir Care 2011;56(4): 442–8.

36. Sanders MH, Kern NB, Costantino JP, et al. Accuracy of end-tidal and transcutaneous PCO_2 monitoring during sleep. Chest 1994;106(2): 472–83.

37. Hull J, Aniapravan R, Chan E, et al. British Thoracic Society guideline for respiratory management of children with neuromuscular weakness. Thorax 2012;67(Suppl 1):i1–40.

38. Kirk VG, Batuyong ED, Bohn SG. Transcutaneous carbon dioxide monitoring and capnography during pediatric polysomnography. Sleep 2006; 29(12):1601–8.

39. Storre JH, Steurer B, Kabitz HJ, et al. Transcutaneous PCO_2 monitoring during initiation of noninvasive ventilation. Chest 2007;132(6):1810–6.

40. Cuvelier A, Grigoriu B, Molano LC, et al. Limitations of transcutaneous carbon dioxide measurements for assessing long-term mechanical ventilation. Chest 2005;127(5):1744–8.

41. Janssens JP, Laszlo A, Uldry C, et al. Non-invasive (transcutaneous) monitoring of PCO_2 ($TcPCO_2$) in older adults. Gerontology 2005;51(3):174–8.

42. Storre JH, Magnet FS, Dreher M, et al. Transcutaneous monitoring as a replacement for arterial PCO_2 monitoring during nocturnal non-invasive ventilation. Respir Med 2011;105(1):143–50.

43. Janssens JP, Howarth-Frey C, Chevrolet JC, et al. Transcutaneous PCO_2 to monitor noninvasive mechanical ventilation in adults: assessment of a new transcutaneous PCO_2 device. Chest 1998; 113(3):768–73.

44. Janssens JP, Perrin E, Bennani I, et al. Is continuous transcutaneous monitoring of PCO_2 ($TcPCO_2$) over 8 h reliable in adults? Respir Med 2001;95(5): 331–5.

45. Parker SM, Gibson GJ. Evaluation of a transcutaneous carbon dioxide monitor ("TOSCA") in adult patients in routine respiratory practice. Respir Med 2007;101(2):261–4.

46. Berry R, Chediak A, Brown L, et al. Best clinical practices for the sleep center adjustment of noninvasive positive pressure ventilation (NPPV) in stable chronic alveolar hypoventilation syndromes. J Clin Sleep Med 2010;6(5):491–509.

47. Restrepo RD, Hirst KR, Wittnebel L, et al. AARC clinical practice guideline: transcutaneous

monitoring of carbon dioxide and oxygen: 2012. Respir Care 2012;57(11):1955–62.

48. Bauman KA, Kurili A, Schmidt SL, et al. Home-based overnight transcutaneous capnography/pulse oximetry for diagnosing nocturnal hypoventilation associated with neuromuscular disorders. Arch Phys Med Rehabil 2013;94(1):46–52.

49. Nardi J, Prigent H, Adala A, et al. Nocturnal oximetry and transcutaneous carbon dioxide in home-ventilated neuromuscular patients. Respir Care 2012;57(9):1425–30.

50. Mier-Jedrzejowicz A, Brophy C, Moxham J, et al. Assessment of diaphragm weakness. Am Rev Respir Dis 1988;137(4):877–83.

51. Just N, Bautin N, Danel-Brunaud V, et al. The Borg dyspnoea score: a relevant clinical marker of inspiratory muscle weakness in amyotrophic lateral sclerosis. Eur Respir J 2010;35(2):353–60.

Advances in Positive Airway Pressure Treatment Modalities for Hypoventilation Syndromes

Daniel Combs, MD[a,b], Safal Shetty, MD[b],
Sairam Parthasarathy, MD[c],*

KEYWORDS

- Hypoventilation syndrome • Obesity • Sleep • Obstructive sleep apnea
- Continuous positive airway pressure • Positive airway pressure • Artificial respiration • Algorithms

KEY POINTS

- The physiologic rationale for advanced positive airway pressure (PAP) modalities is sound considering the complexity of sleep-disordered breathing in patients with hypoventilation syndromes.
- The therapeutic physiological rationale for the various advanced PAP modalities and the details about the principles of operation and technology implementation need to be well-understood by the prescribing health care provider.
- Sleep-disordered breathing is complex and requires sophisticated devices with algorithms designed to accurately detect and effectively treat respiratory events that include hypoventilation, upper airway obstruction, lower airway obstruction, central apneas, and central hypopneas, and reduce the work of breathing while maintaining breathing comfort.
- There is much opportunity for further refinement of these devices that include the ability of the device to reliably monitor gas exchange, sleep–wakefulness state, and for reducing variability in device efficacy owing to provider-selected device settings.

INTRODUCTION

Positive airway pressure (PAP) therapy for hypoventilation syndromes can significantly improve health-related quality of life (HR-QOL), health care costs, and even mortality.[1–3] Such important, patient-centered and health care–related outcomes are affected by the beneficial effects of PAP therapy on intermediary physiologic endpoints such as improved gas exchange and better sleep quality accomplished during both sleep and wakefulness.[1,4,5] Although different definitions for advanced PAP therapy may exist, for the purposes of this review, advanced PAP modalities refer to modes other than continuous PAP (CPAP) therapy administered by noninvasive mask interface during sleep. They could be broadly categorized into bilevel PAP, automated PAP therapy, volume-targeted pressure assistance (volume assured pressure support), volume control invasive or

Disclosures: See last page of article.
 a Department of Pediatrics, Arizona Respiratory Center, University of Arizona, 1501 North Campbell Avenue, Tucson, AZ, USA; b Division of Pulmonary, Critical Care, Allergy and Sleep Medicine, Department of Medicine, Arizona Respiratory Center, University of Arizona, 1501 North Campbell Avenue, Tucson, AZ, USA; c Division of Pulmonary, Critical Care, Allergy and Sleep Medicine, Department of Medicine, Arizona Respiratory Center, University of Arizona, 1501 North Campbell Avenue, Room 2342D, Tucson, AZ 85724, USA
* Corresponding author.
E-mail address: spartha@arc.arizona.edu

1556-407X/14/$ – see front matter © 2014 Elsevier Inc. All rights reserved.

noninvasive ventilation, or new and emerging devices that administer ventilatory assistance during wakefulness in ambulatory patients. The therapeutic physiological rationale for the various technological options and details about the technology implementation are provided herein. Supporting randomized, clinical trials and other clinical evidence are discussed elsewhere in this issue by Murphy and Hart.

THERAPEUTIC OPTIONS AND PHYSIOLOGIC RATIONALE

The need for advanced PAP modalities should ideally be viewed in the context of the entire gamut of therapeutic options and their respective targets in patients with hypoventilation syndromes (**Fig. 1**). Although conventional CPAP arguably could be effective in most cases of obesity hypoventilation syndrome, there are instances when CPAP may fail to adequately correct sleep-related hypoventilation.[6,7] Specifically, Piper and colleagues[7] performed a head-to-head study comparing CPAP with bilevel PAP therapy and came to the conclusion that both treatments were equally effective in improving daytime hypercapnia in a subgroup of patients with obesity hypoventilation syndrome without severe nocturnal hypoxemia. The seclusion of patients with severe nocturnal hypoxemia identifies the subgroup of patients who need a more advanced form of ventilation. In keeping with such

an observation, Banerjee and colleagues[6] noted that patients with obesity hypoventilation with 4 characteristics that includes severe hypoxemia during sleep—namely, greater levels of morbid obesity, restrictive defect on pulmonary function testing, and greater levels of daytime hypercapnia—are also more likely to fail CPAP therapy. Failure of CPAP therapy may also be attributable to the fact that CPAP therapy may not measure and therefore effectively abrogate other pathophysiologic derangements that underlie the various hypoventilation syndromes (**Fig. 2**). In the case of obesity hypoventilation syndrome, whereas CPAP may have been effective in abrogating the obstructive hypoventilation, the inspiratory assistance required to surmount the chest wall load owing to morbid obesity may have been insufficient (see **Fig. 2**). Such differences in efficacy of various PAP therapy modalities may apply not only to patients with obesity hypoventilation syndrome, but to other causes of hypoventilation syndromes as well (see **Fig. 2**).

Morbid obesity may be associated with expiratory airflow limitation.[8–10] Such expiratory flow limitation can contribute to gas exchange abnormalities that could benefit from the application of positive end-expiratory pressure (PEEP).[10] Such expiratory flow limitation in morbidly obese individuals may be secondary to mechanical compression of the smaller airways. However, different levels of PEEP may be required to provide ventilatory assistance versus adequately treat upper

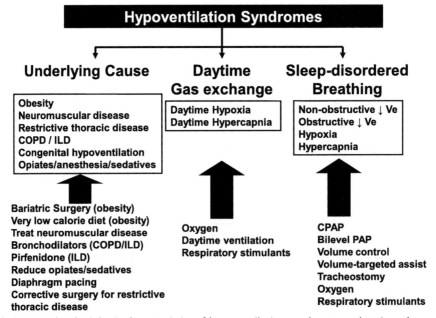

Fig. 1. Underlying pathophysiologic characteristics of hypoventilation syndromes and various therapeutic interventions that could be used to provide targeted treatment. Positive airway pressure therapy is one of many available treatment modalities.

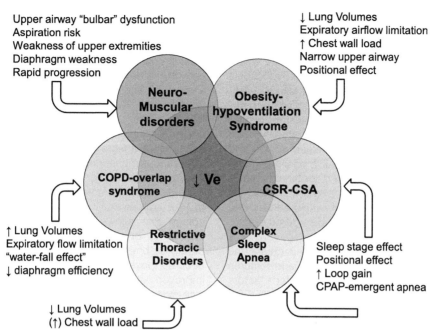

Upper airway "bulbar" dysfunction
Aspiration risk
Weakness of upper extremities
Diaphragm weakness
Rapid progression

↓ Lung Volumes
Expiratory airflow limitation
↑ Chest wall load
Narrow upper airway
Positional effect

Neuro-Muscular disorders

Obesity-hypoventilation Syndrome

COPD-overlap syndrome

↓ Ve

CSR-CSA

↑ Lung Volumes
Expiratory flow limitation
"water-fall effect"
↓ diaphragm efficiency

Restrictive Thoracic Disorders

Complex Sleep Apnea

Sleep stage effect
Positional effect
↑ Loop gain
CPAP-emergent apnea

↓ Lung Volumes
(↑) Chest wall load

Fig. 2. Overlapping pathophysiologic traits that may manifest in patients with hypoventilation syndromes of various causes.

airway obstruction during inspiration. However, excessive administration of PEEP may cause hyperinflation and a consequent increase in the inspiratory threshold load. To make matters more complex, such pressure requirements may differ with body position and sleep stage. Advanced PAP modalities may potentially be able to measure and target such physiologic variables; however, the additional benefit gained needs to translate into clinically significant outcomes.

A similar situation can be said to exist in sleep-related hypoventilation secondary to chronic obstructive pulmonary disease (COPD) in whom significant expiratory flow limitation occurs.[11] In patients with COPD, however, there is greater end-expiratory lung volume or hyperinflation, which, in turn, exerts a certain level of increased traction on the upper airway that could conceivably protect against inspiratory flow limitation and obstruction.[12] Such a physiologic "traction" effect on the upper airway of the increased lung volume (hyperinflation) in patients with COPD may be a potential mechanism for the lack of an association between mild COPD and obstructive sleep apnea in a community-based population.[13] It follows that application of moderate levels of PEEP that does not exceed the level of intrinsic PEEP (PEEP$_i$; "waterfall effect") would be more relevant in this population than the level of PAP needed to treat upper airway obstruction. However, current technology in advanced PAP

modalities cannot measure PEEP$_i$ or titrate pressure levels in an automated manner. Conceivably, such advanced PAP modalities that are capable of measuring and treating PEEP$_i$ would constitute an improvement over current technology, but whether such advanced PAP modalities can effect improvements in relevant patient outcomes remain to be seen. For example, in patients with COPD, nocturnal noninvasive ventilation in addition to long-term oxygen therapy seemed to reduce mortality compared with those treated with long-term oxygen therapy alone, but such an intervention was accompanied by reduced HR-QOL.[14] The mechanisms for such reduced HR-QOL (manifesting as confusion and reduced vigor) was variably attributed to survivor effect and complexity of device therapy, but additional factors such as worsening hyperinflation owing to excessive application of PEEP may be additional and unmeasured contributors. Noninvasive ventilation does not improve lung function, gas exchange, or sleep efficiency in patients with COPD.[15] A knowledge gap exists in this area of study, in that despite multiple clinical trials of nocturnal noninvasive ventilation, whether physiologically titrated PEEP and pressure assist aimed at alleviating PEEP$_i$ and inspiratory work of breathing can effect improvements in clinical outcomes remains unclear.

Central apneas may complicate the management of sleep-disordered breathing in patients with obesity hypoventilation syndrome, neuromuscular disease, or concomitant heart failure (see **Fig. 2**).[16–19] Central apneas in the setting of hypoventilation syndromes could occur in the setting of hypercapnia (owing to respiratory muscle weakness or restrictive thoracic disease) or hypocapnia (in the setting of concomitant heart failure). Additionally, patients with severe obstructive sleep apnea may suffer from unstable ventilatory control (high loop gain) and manifest central apneas during PAP therapy (termed complex sleep apnea) and therefore require advanced PAP modality to more effectively treat their sleep-disordered breathing.[16,20,21] Specifically, advanced modes such as servo ventilation or bilevel PAP with a backup rate can help to abrogate the sleep-disordered breathing in such instances.[22]

Other disease-related factors that create the need for advanced PAP modalities and features responsive to specific disease-related factors include bulbar involvement by neuromuscular diseases, diaphragm weakness, weakness of upper extremities, and rate of disease progression (see **Fig. 2**). Bulbar involvement and accompanying aspiration risk owing to dysphagia requires the need for invasive ventilation through a tracheostomy and attendant features to advanced PAP modalities, such as the ability to switch between modes of ventilation (pressure- or volume-assisted modes), active or passive exhalation ports, and sip and puff features for triggering ventilators. Disease progression in neuromuscular conditions such as amyotrophic lateral sclerosis could predicate the need for "volume-assured" advanced modality of ventilation that would guarantee adequate ventilator assistance despite worsening neuromuscular weakness over the 1- to 2-month period between provider visits. In such instances, volume-assured modality adjusts the level of pressure assist to ensure that minute ventilation is above a threshold determined as a function of ideal body weight and ensuring a minimum level of adequate ventilation.[17,23]

The Achilles heel of advanced PAP modalities are the presence of air leak (usually from noninvasive mask or mouthpiece interface) and failure to sense the trigger that switches the ventilator from exhalation to inhalation mode. Advanced PAP modalities have tackled such limitation by tracking basal flow (leak) rates, tracking flow contours, and other sophisticated algorithms aimed at assessing the state of the air column connecting the device and the patient. However, knowledge of the nuances of how a device is set is important to enable such advanced features of leak detection and compensation.[24] Flow contours allow devices to "anticipate" when the next inspiratory breath is going to occur and allow triggering of a device-delivered breath in a timely manner to enable adequate and comfortable ventilatory assistance.[25]

Although the technology of advanced PAP modalities continues to evolve significantly with efficacy of the device in sharp focus, there has been a renewed and well-justified push for improving adherence to PAP therapy that includes advanced PAP modalities. A major limitation of any PAP technology is adherence to such therapy, which in turn deleteriously affects the effectiveness of such therapy. Various monitoring connectivity through wireless, modem-based, or SD card–based technology have allowed for remote monitoring and facilitation of PAP adherence.[26] Additionally, tracking technology that allows for reminders and remote monitoring of mask fit, leak levels, and even breath-by-breath visualization of breathing have become possible.[27,28] PAP adherence can be improved with the use of a web-based telemedicine system at the initiation of treatment.[26] With such a physiologic and psychological rationale in mind, we now consider each of the advanced PAP technologies and assess the technology.

BILEVEL PAP TECHNOLOGY

Bilevel PAP therapy varies the airway pressure with a greater inspiratory pressure level and lower expiratory pressure level with algorithms that cycle the device from inspiratory-to-expiratory mode.[29] The decreased pressure during exhalation decreases the amount of pressure against which the patient exhales and consequently reduces respiratory discomfort during the expiratory cycle (**Fig. 3**). Moreover, during the inspiratory cycle, the greater level of pressure assist increases tidal volume and therefore the minute ventilation in patients suffering from hypoventilation syndromes (see **Fig. 3**). The difference between inspiratory PAP (IPAP) and expiratory PAP (EPAP) could be considered the pressure support level. The implementation of bilevel PAP in hypoventilation requires careful titration during polysomnography to treat persistent hypoventilation that manifests as reduced oxygen saturation ($\leq$88% by pulse oximetry) in the absence of evidence of obstruction. Generally, in adults with neuromuscular disorders, the IPAP and EPAP levels are initiated from arbitrary levels of IPAP of 8 cm H_2O and EPAP of 4 cm H_2O and titrated upwards based on symptomatic improvement in symptoms of hypoventilation such as early morning headache and patient comfort. Others prefer that such titration be performed under the auspices of polysomnography, confirmed by polysomnography, or by utilizing other advanced PAP modalities such as volume-assured pressure assist methods.[30] In

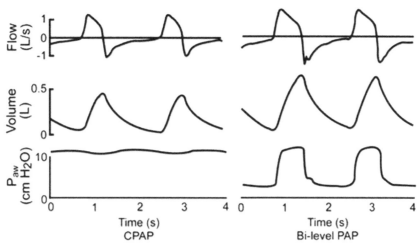

Fig. 3. Representative tracings of flow, tidal volume, and airway pressure (P_{aw}) during administration of continuous positive airway pressure (CPAP) and bilevel PAP. *Left,* Small undulations in the CPAP level generated by the patient's inspiratory and expiratory effort, and the consequent displacement of inspiratory and expiratory tidal volume. Such inflections are usually negligible in a responsive CPAP device. In this instance, the CPAP is set at 14 cm H_2O. *Right,* Large decrements in the pressure during exhalation (expiratory positive airway pressure [EPAP], which is set at 4 cm H_2O), whereas during inspiration the inspiratory positive airway pressure (IPAP) is set at 14 cm H_2O, which would conceivably provide the same level of airway splinting as a CPAP of 14 cm H_2O. Note the larger tidal volumes and flow patterns consequent to the pressure assist provided by the bilevel PAP device that would benefit a patient suffering from hypoventilation. In this instance, a pressure support or assist level of 10 cm H_2O (IPAP minus EPAP) is being administered, with consequently greater tidal volume and inspiratory flow. (*From* Antonescu-Turcu A, Parthasarathy S. CPAP and bi-level PAP therapy: new and established roles. Respir Care 2010;55(9):1217; with permission.)

general, the maximum pressure setting for bilevel PAP is not to exceed 30 cm H_2O in adults (20 cm H_2O in children), and the minimum difference between IPAP and EPAP level should not be less than 4 cm H_2O.[31] The goals of such titration include improving oxygen saturation through increments in tidal volume and minute ventilation while providing comfort, relieving nocturnal dyspnea, improving daytime gas exchange, providing respiratory muscle rest, and prolonging life.[1,30,32] The cycling of the device from the inspiratory phase (IPAP) to the expiratory phase (EPAP) and vice versa may be triggered by the spontaneously breathing patient (spontaneous mode) or by a set respiratory rate programmed into the device (timed mode). The device can be set to cycle from the inspiratory to the expiratory mode based on pressure inflections, flow contour, set timing for inspiratory time, or a combination of such measures. In the spontaneous timed or timed mode, a backup respiratory rate of 10 breaths per minute could be initiated and titrated upward by one to two increments and generally do not exceed 16 breaths per minute. The backup respiratory rate could be initiated when a patient with hypoventilation syndrome manifests central apneas or inappropriately low respiratory rate and consequent low minute ventilation.[30]

Dyssynchronous cycling between the patient and the device can be uncomfortable and in the presence of COPD could lead to hyperinflation and further dyssynchrony.[33,34] In the past, the triggering sensitivities for cycling of the device between inspiration and expiration could be adjusted by the therapist or physician, but in most modern bilevel PAP devices the technology has been automated with an emphasis on remaining resilient to air leaks. Similarly, the rate of pressurization ("rise time") from EPAP to IPAP level can be adjusted to make the pressure increase briskly or slowly, but beyond individual patient comfort, the clinical implications of such adjustments is less clear.

AUTOMATION

Self-adjusting, automatic, or autoadjusting PAP devices are considered an advanced PAP modality; although they could be utilized in hypoventilation syndromes, there are few data regarding the use of such a device in this particular condition. However, it is worth considering the technological approach of the automation involved in managing hypoventilation syndromes that includes respiratory events such as hypoventilation, obstructive events (apneas and hypopneas), central apneas, and central hypopneas.

The purposes of such automation may be to serve as an alternative to in-laboratory manual titration to determine adequate pressure setting[31]; to achieve lower mean pressures levels that may conceivably promote adherence[35]; or for affecting therapy on a long-term basis while being responsive to various aspects of sleep-disordered breathing events (hypoventilation, obstruction, and central) that occur and that include changes in weight, sleep state, body position, or even alcohol ingestion.

The principles of automation have evolved, and continue to evolve, over multiple generations and comprises enhancements to sensing events of sleep-disordered breathing (sensors), automated computing and analysis of the sensed signals (analysis), and hierarchical set of algorithms that will determine the action taken by the device in response to the conditions exposed (effectors). The sensors include measurement of changes in pressure and flow that can detect snoring (as pressure oscillations) to signify obstructive events and flattening of inspiratory flow curves (indicating inspiratory flow limitation of the upper airway). Devices can even send pulses of air or oscillations to detect the state of the upper airway (open or closed) based on the presence or absence of reflected (echo) pressure waves to differentiate central from obstructive apneas. They can identify Cheyne–Stokes respiration (by detecting breath-by-breath variation in peak flow), identify hypoventilation (by measuring tidal volume or minute ventilation using calibrated flow sensors), and compensate for air leaks (using sophisticated flow-based algorithms).[36]

The effector arm of the auto PAP device has undergone changes as well. Newer generation devices can not only increase the CPAP level, but can also increase the IPAP alone to ameliorate obstructive events (auto bilevel PAP), correct hypoventilation (averaged volume-assured pressure support, or intelligent volume-assured pressure support), or combat central apneas in patients with complex sleep apnea or CPAP-emergent central apneas (servo ventilation).[17,37–39] The servo ventilators may also introduce a backup rate to prevent central apneas, and even though they are not called auto PAP devices, they function using similar principles and can be judged as the latest generation of auto PAP devices.[38,39]

An important aspect of such technology is that different manufacturers of such devices may incorporate different algorithms that lead to significant differences in performance. Bench studies have consistently shown varied performance when comparing devices made by different manufacturers.[40–44] We have shown,

for instance, that the range of pressure response of 4 automated PAP devices was as large as 10 cm H_2O.[40] Moreover, bench studies have shown that some devices are more resilient to the effects of air leak than others.[40] Despite such bench studies, the clinical implication of such differential performance of various manufacturers is less clear. It should be noted that most of the randomized, controlled trials that involved the utilization of automatic CPAP devices excluded patients with hypoventilation syndromes such as obesity hypoventilation syndrome, coexistent heart failure, neuromuscular weakness, and COPD.[45,46]

VOLUME-ASSURED PRESSURE ASSISTANCE

Advanced PAP modalities that targets minute ventilation and tidal volume are ideal for patients with hypoventilation syndromes.[17,37] These devices are unlike auto bilevel PAP device, which target obstructive events like the auto PAP, and the servo ventilator that targets central apneas and Cheyne–Stokes respiration. Volume-assured pressure support technology has been used in critically ill patients receiving mechanical ventilation before it made inroads into managing patients with sleep-disordered breathing and hypoventilation syndromes.[47] In patients with acute respiratory failure, volume-assured pressure support ventilation was able to ensure a minimum preset target tidal volume and reduced patient workload while improving synchrony between the patient and the ventilator.[47] Although such technology was geared to assess tidal volume breath by breath, the devices that address hypoventilation in patients with hypoventilation syndromes assesses the tidal volume (or minute ventilation) over a variable (1–5 minutes) time window. Specifically, the principles of operation of volume-assured pressure support or assist is shown in **Fig. 4**. Essentially, when the patient's tidal volume (or minute ventilation) decreases below a certain threshold it is detected by the device that correspondingly responds by increasing the IPAP or pressure support and restores the tidal volume (or minute ventilation; measured over a certain time window) to approximate that of the selected target volume. Previous versions of these devices required an EPAP level setting, but more recent versions have combined the automated PAP therapy technology for optimal EPAP setting determination. Therefore, such devices have a minimum and maximum EPAP range that needs to be prescribed. The pressure assistance delivered during inspiratory phase, which is above the operating EPAP level, is aimed at ensuring a certain tidal

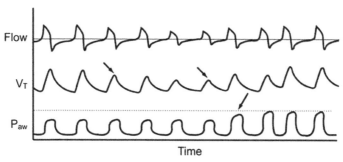

Fig. 4. Principles of operation of volume-assured pressure support or assist. Flow, tidal volume (V_T), and airway pressure (P_{aw}) tracings are shown. Note that in this instance the V_T and flow decrease progressively between the 2 *shorter arrows*. The device detects such a V_T drop and responds by increasing the inspiratory positive airway pressure (IPAP; *longer arrow*) and restores the V_T to near the target. The new, yet higher, IPAP is better shown by the difference between the *dashed line* and the preexisting IPAP before the increment. Conversely, the IPAP could decrease if the measured V_T were to exceed the target V_T prescribed by the provider. (*From* Antonescu-Turcu A, Parthasarathy S. CPAP and bi-level PAP therapy: new and established roles. Respir Care 2010;55(9):1225; with permission.)

volume calculated as a function of ideal body weight (usually 8 mL/kg ideal body weight or at 110% of patient's tidal volume).[17] The operating IPAP (or pressure assist) level is then allowed to fluctuate between a minimum and maximum pressure support level to ensure the target tidal volume.

The selection of target tidal volume is left to the provider with variable targets of 8 to 10 mL/kg ideal body weight or as a function of patient's own ambient tidal volume. Notably, the choice of tidal volume may be influenced by the sleep–wakefulness state of the patient.[17,48] In patients with chronic respiratory insufficiency (obesity hypoventilation and neuromuscular disease) receiving averaged volume-assured pressure support, patients preferred (measured as dyspnea score) 110% of ambient tidal volume during wakefulness, but the patients slept better (when measured as sleep efficiency) when receiving tidal volume based on ideal body weight.[48] Such data suggest that the choice of device setting is to a certain extent arbitrary and, conceivably, devices that can measure the sleep–wakefulness state and adjust their algorithms may be superior to the current conventional devices that operate in a similar fashion regardless of the sleep or wakefulness state of the patient. Additional settings may include spontaneous or timed respiratory rate settings, and some newer technology has automated the respiratory rate selection based on the patient's minute ventilation and proportion of breaths that are triggered versus spontaneous over a period of time.

Laboratory-based, short-term efficacy studies using volume-assured pressure support devices have failed to demonstrate advantages over conventional bilevel PAP settings with regard to improvements in sleep quality.[17,37,49] Some of the lack of demonstrable difference between such an advanced PAP modality and bilevel PAP may be owing to the carefully adjusted "optimized" bilevel PAP setting in research study conditions. Studies that assess the performance of such devices in less expert hands (in the "real world") may identify differences that were not discerned in such controlled experiments. Additionally, the advantage of such advanced PAP modalities in adjusting for changes in clinical situations needs to be further explored. Such clinical situations may include rapid weight loss in morbidly obese individuals after bariatric surgery or patients with amyotrophic lateral sclerosis who are experiencing rapidly progressive respiratory muscle weakness. Nevertheless, even current data seem to suggest that such assurance of tidal volume has advantages with regard to lower transcutaneous P_{CO_2} readings[37] and greater minute ventilation,[17] and that they afford resilience against changes attributable to changes in body position and sleep state. More research of these devices, however, needs to be performed to better understand the role of these devices.

SERVO VENTILATION

Servo ventilation devices can identify and treat central apneas and periodic breathing. Servo ventilation can treat Cheyne–Stokes respiration, central sleep apnea, and emergent central apneas in patients with hypoventilation syndromes. The principle of operation of such technology is a servo-controlled pressure support adjustment (effector) that is inversely related to the changes in peak flow levels over a moving time window (sensor; **Fig. 5**). The device calculates an average peak flow level over a period of time; subsequently, if the instantaneous peak flows are lower than such an average peak flow rate that was derived from the previous moving time window, the device recognizes this as the decrescendo pattern that precedes a central apnea, and responds by increasing the pressure support level. Conversely, when the peak flow rate is significantly higher than the previously calculated average peak flow levels, the device assumes that the patient is manifesting a hyperpneic phase, and correspondingly reduces the level of pressure assist. Therefore, the servo system dampens the inherent oscillatory behavior of the patient's breathing pattern and smoothes respiration (see **Fig. 5**).

The instantaneous IPAP level is determined by the device algorithm within a set range of minimum and maximum pressure support levels. Previously, the terminology for servo ventilation was based on minimum and maximum IPAP (see **Fig. 5**). However, considering that the EPAP level can change in later generation of the devices, the corresponding PS levels are better descriptors of the setting because PS levels are a function of the EPAP levels. Essentially, the instantaneous IPAP level minus the instantaneous EPAP is the instantaneous pressure support level. Generally, the maximum pressure levels are not to exceed 30 cm H_2O in these advanced PAP devices. The backup rate can either be set to adjust automatically or be set at a manually determined rate, which is usually determined during a sleep study. Servo ventilation can successfully treat central apneas, central hypopneas, and Cheyne–Stokes respiration.[38,39,50–56] Investigators have variably used manual backup rates set at 15 breaths per minute[39,51] or employed an automatic backup rate.[38,50] They have used EPAP levels of 5 cm H_2O in patients with Cheyne–Stokes respiration and central sleep apnea[39,51] or titrated the EPAP

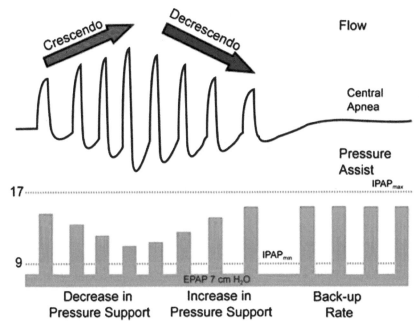

Fig. 5. Principles of operation of servo ventilation. The air flow tracing depicts a classical crescendo (*orange arrow*) and decrescendo (*red arrow*) pattern of Cheyne–Stokes respiration, followed by an ensuing central apnea. The servo-controlled automatic adjustment of the inspiratory positive airway pressure (IPAP) level is inversely related to the changes in peak flow over a moving time window. Specifically, during the crescendo pattern of peak flow rates (*orange arrow*) the pressure assist (or IPAP) level decreases to dampen the rise in inspiratory peak flow rate (or tidal volume). Conversely, during the decrescendo pattern of peak flow rates (*red arrow*) the pressure assist (or IPAP) level increases to dampen the fall in inspiratory peak flow rate (or tidal volume). Therefore, the servo system dampens the inherent oscillatory behavior of the patient's breathing pattern and smoothes respiration. During a central apnea, however, the device backup rate kicks in and ventilates the patient (*right side* of the figure). The maximum and minimum IPAP (IPAP$_{max}$ and IPAP$_{min}$) are set at 17 and 9 cm H_2O, respectively (*dashed blue lines*). The expiratory positive airway pressure (EPAP) is set at 7 cm H_2O. During any given breath, the pressure assist or pressure support is equal to the IPAP minus the EPAP. (*From* Antonescu-Turcu A, Parthasarathy S. CPAP and bilevel PAP therapy: new and established roles. Respir Care 2010;55(9):1224; with permission.)

level to treat obstructive apneas in patients with emergent central apneas.[38,50] Although small studies have demonstrated improvement in physiologic measures, such as sleepiness and urinary levels of catecholamines in patients with Cheyne–Stokes respiration and central sleep apnea,[51] larger studies on tangible patient outcomes such as hospitalization or all-cause mortality are awaited.

SUMMARY

The physiologic rationale for advanced PAP modalities is sound considering the complexity of sleep-disordered breathing in patients with hypoventilation syndromes. Various advanced PAP devices are available to assist breathing during sleep and wakefulness in patients with hypoventilation syndromes. Although such devices are increasingly used in clinical practice, the supporting clinical evidence warranting the use of such devices needs further study. Currently, there is an evolving body of literature that supports the beneficial effect of advanced PAP modalities on HR-QOL, physiologic endpoints, and even mortality. However, more comparative effectiveness research of such advanced PAP modality devices against conventional CPAP therapy in "real-world" situations and without the requirement of titration polysomnography need to be conducted. Moreover, there is much opportunity for further refining these devices, including the ability of the device to reliably monitor gas exchange, sleep–wakefulness state, and reducing variability in device efficacy owing to provider-selected device settings.

DISCLOSURES

Drs D. Combs and S. Shetty do not have any disclosures. Dr S. Parthasarathy reports current grants awarded to University of Arizona from (a) NIH/NHLBI (Grant No. HL095748), (b) Patient-Centered Outcomes Research Institute (PCORI; IHS-1306-02505), (c) Younes Sleep Technologies, Ltd, and (d) Johrei Institute (non-profit foundation); personal fees from American Academy of Sleep Medicine for lectures ($600 in 2013); non-financial support from National Center for Sleep Disorders Research of the NIH/NHLBI for travel; personal fees from UpToDate Inc ($600 in 2013); personal fees from Philips-Respironics, Inc ($750 in 2013), previous grant from Philips-Respironics, Inc awarded to Dr S. Parthasarathy's institution (for AVAPS study in 2007–2008 and AVAPS-AE in 2011–2013).

REFERENCES

1. Carrillo A, Ferrer M, Gonzalez-Diaz G, et al. Noninvasive ventilation in acute hypercapnic respiratory failure caused by obesity hypoventilation syndrome and chronic obstructive pulmonary disease. Am J Respir Crit Care Med 2012;186(12):1279–85.
2. Vrijsen B, Testelmans D, Belge C, et al. Non-invasive ventilation in amyotrophic lateral sclerosis. Amyotroph Lateral Scler Frontotemporal Degener 2013;14(2):85–95.
3. Geiseler J, Karg O, Borger S, et al. Invasive home mechanical ventilation, mainly focused on neuromuscular disorders. GMS Health Technol Assess 2010;6:Doc08.
4. Kelly JL, Jaye J, Pickersgill RE, et al. Randomized trial of 'intelligent' autotitrating ventilation versus standard pressure support non-invasive ventilation: impact on adherence and physiological outcomes. Respirology 2014;19(4):596–603.
5. Held M, Walthelm J, Baron S, et al. Functional impact of pulmonary hypertension due to hypoventilation and changes under noninvasive ventilation. Eur Respir J 2014;43(1):156–65.
6. Banerjee D, Yee BJ, Piper AJ, et al. Obesity hypoventilation syndrome: hypoxemia during continuous positive airway pressure. Chest 2007;131(6):1678–84.
7. Piper AJ, Wang D, Yee BJ, et al. Randomised trial of CPAP vs bilevel support in the treatment of obesity hypoventilation syndrome without severe nocturnal desaturation. Thorax 2008;63(5):395–401.
8. Ferretti A, Giampiccolo P, Cavalli A, et al. Expiratory flow limitation and orthopnea in massively obese subjects. Chest 2001;119(5):1401–8.
9. Rubinstein I, Zamel N, DuBarry L, et al. Airflow limitation in morbidly obese, nonsmoking men. Ann Intern Med 1990;112(11):828–32.
10. Koutsoukou A, Koulouris N, Bekos B, et al. Expiratory flow limitation in morbidly obese postoperative mechanically ventilated patients. Acta Anaesthesiol Scand 2004;48(9):1080–8.
11. O'Donoghue FJ, Catcheside PG, Ellis EE, et al. Sleep hypoventilation in hypercapnic chronic obstructive pulmonary disease: prevalence and associated factors. Eur Respir J 2003;21(6):977–84.
12. Van de Graaff WB. Thoracic traction on the trachea: mechanisms and magnitude. J Appl Physiol (1985) 1991;70(3):1328–36.
13. Sanders MH, Newman AB, Haggerty CL, et al. Sleep and sleep-disordered breathing in adults with predominantly mild obstructive airway disease. Am J Respir Crit Care Med 2003;167(1):7–14.
14. McEvoy RD, Pierce RJ, Hillman D, et al. Nocturnal non-invasive nasal ventilation in stable hypercapnic COPD: a randomised controlled trial. Thorax 2009;64(7):561–6.

15. Wijkstra PJ, Lacasse Y, Guyatt GH, et al. A meta-analysis of nocturnal noninvasive positive pressure ventilation in patients with stable COPD. Chest 2003;124(1):337–43.

16. Younes M, Ostrowski M, Thompson W, et al. Chemical control stability in patients with obstructive sleep apnea. Am J Respir Crit Care Med 2001; 163(5):1181–90.

17. Ambrogio C, Lowman X, Kuo M, et al. Sleep and non-invasive ventilation in patients with chronic respiratory insufficiency. Intensive Care Med 2009; 35(2):306–13.

18. Kiyan E, Okumus G, Cuhadaroglu C, et al. Sleep apnea in adult myotonic dystrophy patients who have no excessive daytime sleepiness. Sleep Breath 2010;14(1):19–24.

19. Aboussouan LS, Lewis RA, Shy ME. Disorders of pulmonary function, sleep, and the upper airway in Charcot-Marie-Tooth disease. Lung 2007; 185(1):1–7.

20. Parthasarathy S. Complex sleep apnea. In: Basner RC, editor. UpToDate. Waltham (MA): UpToDate; 2013.

21. Antonescu-Turcu A, Parthasarathy S. CPAP and bilevel PAP therapy: new and established roles. Respir Care 2010;55(9):1216–29.

22. Javaheri S, Goetting MG, Khayat R, et al. The performance of two automatic servo-ventilation devices in the treatment of central sleep apnea. Sleep 2011;34(12):1693–8.

23. Vagiakis E, Koutsourelakis I, Perraki E, et al. Average volume-assured pressure support in a 16-year-old girl with congenital central hypoventilation syndrome. J Clin Sleep Med 2010;6(6): 609–12.

24. Carlucci A, Schreiber A, Mattei A, et al. The configuration of bi-level ventilator circuits may affect compensation for non-intentional leaks during volume-targeted ventilation. Intensive Care Med 2013;39(1):59–65.

25. Parthasarathy S. Effects of sleep on patient-ventilator interaction. Respir Care Clin N Am 2005;11(2):295–305.

26. Fox N, Hirsch-Allen AJ, Goodfellow E, et al. The impact of a telemedicine monitoring system on positive airway pressure adherence in patients with obstructive sleep apnea: a randomized controlled trial. Sleep 2012;35(4):477–81.

27. Valentin A, Subramanian S, Quan SF, et al. Air leak is associated with poor adherence to autoPAP therapy. Sleep 2011;34(6):801–6.

28. Schwab RJ, Badr SM, Epstein LJ, et al. An official American Thoracic Society statement: continuous positive airway pressure adherence tracking systems. The optimal monitoring strategies and outcome measures in adults. Am J Respir Crit Care Med 2013;188(5):613–20.

29. Sanders MH, Kern N. Obstructive sleep apnea treated by independently adjusted inspiratory and expiratory positive airway pressures via nasal mask. Physiologic and clinical implications. Chest 1990;98(2):317–24.

30. Berry RB, Chediak A, Brown LK, et al. Best clinical practices for the sleep center adjustment of noninvasive positive pressure ventilation (NPPV) in stable chronic alveolar hypoventilation syndromes. J Clin Sleep Med 2010;6(5):491–509.

31. Kushida CA, Chediak A, Berry RB, et al. Clinical guidelines for the manual titration of positive airway pressure in patients with obstructive sleep apnea. J Clin Sleep Med 2008;4(2):157–71.

32. Aboussouan LS, Khan SU, Meeker DP, et al. Effect of noninvasive positive-pressure ventilation on survival in amyotrophic lateral sclerosis. Ann Intern Med 1997;127(6):450–3.

33. Parthasarathy S, Jubran A, Tobin MJ. Cycling of inspiratory and expiratory muscle groups with the ventilator in airflow limitation. Am J Respir Crit Care Med 1998;158(5 Pt 1):1471–8.

34. Younes M, Kun J, Webster K, et al. Response of ventilator-dependent patients to delayed opening of exhalation valve. Am J Respir Crit Care Med 2002;166(1):21–30.

35. Smith I, Lasserson TJ. Pressure modification for improving usage of continuous positive airway pressure machines in adults with obstructive sleep apnoea. Cochrane Database Syst Rev 2009;(4):CD003531.

36. Ficker JH, Clarenbach CF, Neukirchner C, et al. Auto-CPAP therapy based on the forced oscillation technique. Biomed Tech (Berl) 2003;48(3):68–72.

37. Storre JH, Seuthe B, Fiechter R, et al. Average volume-assured pressure support in obesity hypoventilation: a randomized crossover trial. Chest 2006;130(3):815–21.

38. Morgenthaler TI, Gay PC, Gordon N, et al. Adaptive servoventilation versus noninvasive positive pressure ventilation for central, mixed, and complex sleep apnea syndromes. Sleep 2007;30(4): 468–75.

39. Teschler H, Dohring J, Wang YM, et al. Adaptive pressure support servo-ventilation: a novel treatment for Cheyne-Stokes respiration in heart failure. Am J Respir Crit Care Med 2001;164(4):614–9.

40. Coller D, Stanley D, Parthasarathy S. Effect of air leak on the performance of auto-PAP devices: a bench study. Sleep Breath 2005;9(4):167–75.

41. Lofaso F, Desmarais G, Leroux K, et al. Bench evaluation of flow limitation detection by automated continuous positive airway pressure devices. Chest 2006;130(2):343–9.

42. Farre R, Montserrat JM, Rigau J, et al. Response of automatic continuous positive airway pressure devices to different sleep breathing patterns: a bench

study. Am J Respir Crit Care Med 2002;166(4): 469–73.

43. Hirose M, Honda J, Sato E, et al. Bench study of auto-CPAP devices using a collapsible upper airway model with upstream resistance. Respir Physiol Neurobiol 2008;162(1):48–54.

44. Rigau J, Montserrat JM, Wohrle H, et al. Bench model to simulate upper airway obstruction for analyzing automatic continuous positive airway pressure devices. Chest 2006;130(2):350–61.

45. Parthasarathy S. CON: thoughtful steps informed by more comparative effectiveness research is needed in home testing. J Clin Sleep Med 2013; 9(1):9–12.

46. Morgenthaler TI, Aurora RN, Brown T, et al. Practice parameters for the use of autotitrating continuous positive airway pressure devices for titrating pressures and treating adult patients with obstructive sleep apnea syndrome: an update for 2007. An American Academy of Sleep Medicine report. Sleep 2008;31(1):141–7.

47. Amato MB, Barbas CS, Bonassa J, et al. Volume-assured pressure support ventilation (VAPSV). A new approach for reducing muscle workload during acute respiratory failure. Chest 1992;102(4): 1225–34.

48. Williams K, Hinojosa-Kurtzberg M, Parthasarathy S. Control of breathing during mechanical ventilation: who is the boss? Respir Care 2011;56(2):127–36.

49. Murphy PB, Davidson C, Hind MD, et al. Volume targeted versus pressure support non-invasive ventilation in patients with super obesity and chronic respiratory failure: a randomised controlled trial. Thorax 2012;67(8):727–34.

50. Arzt M, Wensel R, Montalvan S, et al. Effects of dynamic bilevel positive airway pressure support on central sleep apnea in men with heart failure. Chest 2008;134(1):61–6.

51. Pepperell JC, Maskell NA, Jones DR, et al. A randomized controlled trial of adaptive ventilation for Cheyne-Stokes breathing in heart failure. Am J Respir Crit Care Med 2003;168(9):1109–14.

52. Randerath WJ, Galetke W, Kenter M, et al. Combined adaptive servo-ventilation and automatic positive airway pressure (anticyclic modulated ventilation) in co-existing obstructive and central sleep apnea syndrome and periodic breathing. Sleep Med 2009;10(8):898–903.

53. Garber AM, Tunis SR. Does comparative-effectiveness research threaten personalized medicine? N Engl J Med 2009;360(19):1925–7.

54. Garber AM. Modernizing device regulation. N Engl J Med 2010;362(13):1161–3.

55. Miller RG, Jackson CE, Kasarskis EJ, et al. Practice parameter update: the care of the patient with amyotrophic lateral sclerosis: drug, nutritional, and respiratory therapies (an evidence-based review): report of the Quality Standards Subcommittee of the American Academy of Neurology. Neurology 2009;73(15):1218–26.

56. Parthasarathy S, Habib M, Quan SF. How are automatic positive airway pressure and related devices prescribed by sleep physicians? A web-based survey. J Clin Sleep Med 2005;1(1):27–34.

Scoring Abnormal Respiratory Events on Polysomnography During Noninvasive Ventilation

Jean-Louis Pepin, MD, PhD[a],*, Jean-Christian Borel, PhD[b],
Olivier Contal, PhD[c], Jésus Gonzalez-Bermejo, MD, PhD[d],
Claudio Rabec, MD[e], Renaud Tamisier, MD, PhD[a],
Dan Adler, MD[f], Jean-Paul Janssens, MD[f]

KEYWORDS

- Noninvasive ventilation • Settings • Polysomnography • Titration

KEY POINTS

- Monitoring of nocturnal NIV is required to determine if NIV is correctly adapted to detect residual or de novo respiratory events and patient-ventilator asynchrony.
- Understanding and classifying the mechanisms involved in respiratory events under NIV is crucial for adapting appropriate NIV settings or interfaces.
- Periodic polysomnography is recommended by experts in the follow-up of home-ventilated patients.
- Future studies are needed to establish whether recognition and correction of these abnormalities during sleep positively impact long-term efficacy of NIV, compliance, or quality of life.

INTRODUCTION

Noninvasive ventilation (NIV) is widely accepted as a long-term treatment of chronic hypercapnic respiratory failure. NIV is predominantly applied at night, when profound changes in ventilatory patterns, respiratory drive, and respiratory and upper airway muscle recruitment occur. These physiologic conditions promote sleep hypoventilation and upper airway obstruction particularly in patients with chronic respiratory failure. NIV per se may also induce de novo undesirable respiratory events.[1,2] Positive pressure ventilation–induced hyperventilation has been shown to promote active periodic breathing and glottic closures. NIV is also inevitably associated with unintentional leaks, which have been shown to alter not only efficacy of ventilation, but also quality of sleep.

There are simple tools, such as oximetry, transcutaneous Pco_2, and device software, available to assess NIV efficacy during sleep.[2] However, increasing awareness of nocturnal respiratory events occurring under NIV has led to a wider use of respiratory polygraphy and polysomnography (PSG) to improve adjustment of long-term

Conflict of Interest Statement: None of the authors has a conflict of interest regarding this article.
[a] INSERM U 1042, Sleep Laboratory, Grenoble University Hospital, CHU de Grenoble, Grenoble 38043, France;
[b] Research and Development Department, AGIR à dom, Meylan 38240, France; [c] Department of Physiotherapy, HESAV School of Health Sciences, University of Applied Sciences Western Switzerland, Lausanne 1011, Switzerland; [d] Service de Pneumologie et Réanimation Respiratoire, Hôpital de la Pitié-Salpêtrière, Assistance Publique-Hôpitaux de Paris, Paris 75013, France; [e] Service de Pneumologie et Réanimation Respiratoire, Centre Hospitalier et Universitaire de Dijon, Dijon 21033, France; [f] Division of Pulmonary Diseases, Geneva University Hospitals, Geneva 1211, Switzerland
* Corresponding author. Laboratoire EFCR, CHU de Grenoble, CS 10 217, 38043 Grenoble Cedex 9, France.
E-mail address: JPepin@chu-grenoble.fr

sleep.theclinics.com

NIV settings.[3] Whether systematic PSG is necessary for titrating NIV, as suggested by the American Academy of Sleep Medicine,[3] remains a subject of debate, but the first step is to improve knowledge about a correct classification of abnormal respiratory events under NIV. Appropriate analysis of polygraphic or polysomnographic recordings must take into account the type of ventilator used (volume- or pressure-cycled), ventilator settings (ventilatory mode, triggers), and type of interface (nasal or full face mask).

During NIV, there is a continuous interaction between the ventilator, generating an intermittent positive pressure, and the patient's neural respiratory drive. Therefore, events can result from the patient, the ventilator, or poor patient-ventilator coordination. This article summarizes how to score abnormal respiratory events on PSG during NIV. The most frequent problems detected are unintentional leaks (ie, not related to exhalation valve of interface), central or obstructive events (either residual or induced by NIV), persistent rapid eye movement (REM) hypoventilation, and patient-ventilator asynchrony. In this article we limit our description to pressure support ventilators with intentional leaks, which are by far the most widely used in chronic respiratory failure.

POLYSOMNOGRAPHIC FEATURES OF ABNORMAL RESPIRATORY EVENTS UNDER NIV
Unintentional Leaks

Detrimental effects of unintentional leaks
Leaks are by far the most common event occurring during NIV.[4] It has been demonstrated that major leaks cause microarousals and disrupt patients' sleep and conversely, that correction of mouth leaks is associated with improved sleep structure.[5] Leaks increase the probability of poor or nondetection of inspiratory efforts and may lead to unrewarded inspiratory efforts, or to other forms of patient-ventilator asynchrony with or without prolonged episodes of desaturation and hypoventilation.[1] Although home bilevel positive airway pressure (PAP) ventilators have a high capacity of leak compensation, increased flow related to leak compensation can also be a source of discomfort. In presence of leaks, we recently demonstrated that a higher percentage of cycles triggered by the ventilator occur and that there is a marked increase in respiratory effort proportional to the amount of the leaks.[6]

Recent ventilators designed for home care have built-in software that provides potentially useful information for the clinician in terms of monitoring NIV. Clinicians need to know if values of tidal volume (V_T), leaks, or apnea-hypopnea index recorded by built-in software are reliable and can be used. There is large variability in the reliability of the results particularly for V_T and this is specially the case with major leaks.[7] This means that V_T can be overestimated when associated with important leaks and this can lead clinicians to improperly adjust the ventilator settings.

Polysomnographic features of unintentional leaks occurring under NIV
The importance of the leak and the ability of the ventilator to compensate for leaks determines whether the pressure signal amplitude remains stable or decreases. A fall in positive pressure (inspiratory and expiratory) indicates major unintentional leaks (Fig. 1). With pressure-controlled ventilators, an increase in ventilator flow signal during insufflation with a simultaneous decrease in thoracic and abdominal belt signal amplitude is suggestive of unintentional leaks (see Fig. 1). Ventilator flow increases to compensate for drop in pressure, but leaks result in decreased effective V_T delivered to the patient. If present on baseline tracing (pneumotachograph between mask and expiratory valve), an amputation of the expiratory part of the flow curve indicates the loss of expiratory flow in the circuit and thus leaks (see Fig. 1).

Additionally, leaks may promote the nondetection of the patient's inspiratory efforts by the ventilator. This may result in patient-ventilator asynchrony with a switch to back-up respiratory frequency in assist-controlled mode or to autotriggering of the ventilator (Fig. 2).

Central Events Under NIV: Partial or Total Upper Airway Obstruction with Reduction of Ventilatory Drive

Physiologic and mechanistic background
Ventilatory control is physiologically altered during sleep, with a decreased responsiveness to chemical, mechanical, and cortical inputs.[1] The $Paco_2$ apneic threshold is unmasked, at 1.5 to 5.8 mm Hg below eupneic $Paco_2$.[8] If NIV settings lead to hyperventilation, bursts of central apnea or hypopnea can occur, particularly during transitions between sleep onset and wakefulness. Furthermore, NIV has the potential to induce periodic breathing during sleep (Fig. 3).[9] In a PSG study, 40% of obese patients using NIV showed a high index of periodic breathing, mostly occurring in light stages of sleep and associated with severe nocturnal hypoxemia.[10] The susceptibility to induction of periodic breathing varies considerably among subjects; its occurrence under NIV is thus difficult to predict and needs to be specifically monitored. It is possible that not only hyperventilation, but

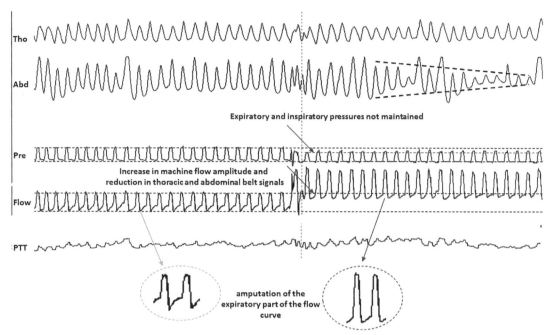

Fig. 1. Nonintentional leaks with pressure-controlled ventilator (3-minute epoch). Abd, abdominal movements; Flow, flow signal measured using a pneumotachograph; Pre, pressure; PTT, pulse transit time; Tho, thoracic movements.

also NIV-induced decreases in $Paco_2$ in subjects who nevertheless remain hypercapnic may generate central apneas or hypopneas.

Adduction of the vocal cords resulting in progressive closure of the glottis has also been described in response to ventilator-induced hyperventilation.[11] Glottic closure was shown to be proportional to total ventilation and inversely proportional to end-tidal CO_2. These events are characterized by a simultaneous reduction or abolition of inspiratory effort (ie, reduction or abolition of thoracoabdominal movements), most probably reflecting a decrease in ventilatory command (**Fig. 4**).

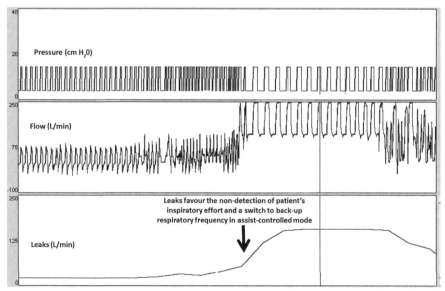

Fig. 2. Leaks favor the nondetection of patient's inspiratory efforts by the ventilator and a switch to back-up respiratory frequency in assist-controlled mode.

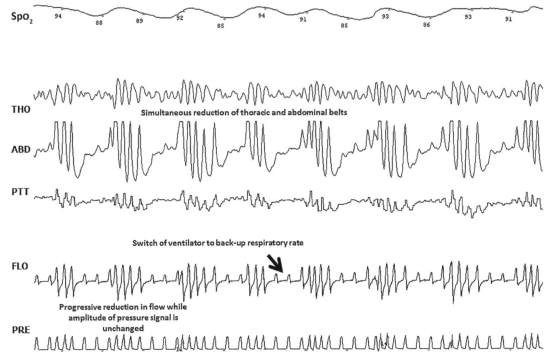

Fig. 3. Excess ventilatory support producing periodic breathing (3-minute epoch). Abd, abdominal movements; Flow, flow signal measured using a pneumotachograph; Pre, pressure; PTT, pulse transit time; Spo₂, oxygen saturation as measured by pulse oximetry; Tho, thoracic movements.

The main polysomnographic patterns suggestive of central events under NIV (ie, airway closure with reduced ventilatory drive) are depicted in **Figs. 3–5**:

1. Progressive and smooth reduction in flow amplitude while amplitude of pressure signal is unchanged (see **Fig. 3**).
2. Simultaneous reduction or disappearance of thoracic and abdominal belt signals (see **Fig. 3**).

3. Switch of ventilator to back-up respiratory rate (BURR; assist-control mode and ST mode) (see **Fig. 3**).

Home bilevel ventilators provide three different modes: (1) an "S" (spontaneous) mode in which each pressurization by the ventilator is triggered and cycled by the patient; (2) an "S/T" (spontaneous/timed) mode in which, if the patient fails to initiate a pressurization within a time frame based

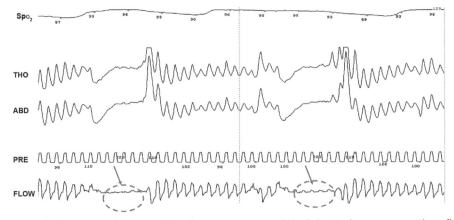

Fig. 4. Excess ventilatory support causes reflex glottic narrowing. Abd, abdominal movements; Flow, flow signal measured using a pneumotachograph; Pre, pressure; PTT, pulse transit time; Spo₂, oxygen saturation as measured by pulse oximetry; Tho, thoracic movements.

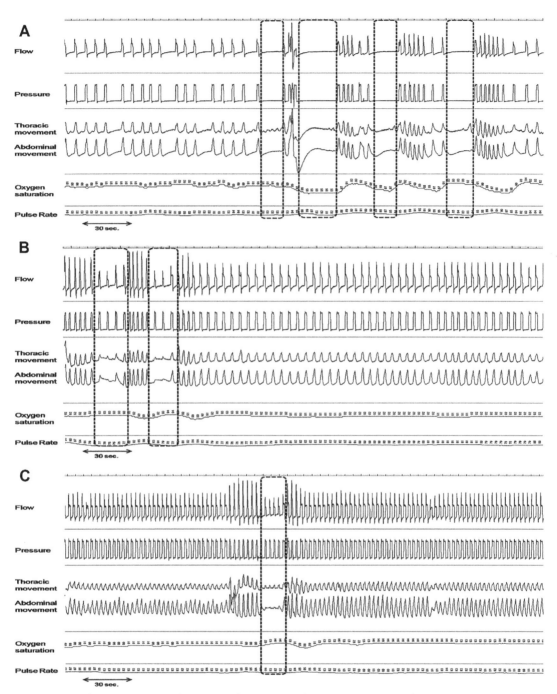

Fig. 5. Impact of spontaneous mode on central events. In a homogenous group of patients treated with long-term noninvasive positive pressure ventilation for obesity hypoventilation, the spontaneous (S) mode (*A*) was associated with the occurrence of a highly significant increase in respiratory events, mainly of central and mixed origin, when compared with both spontaneous/timed (S/T) modes at low (*B*) or high back-up respiratory rate (*C*).

on a BURR, the device delivers a machine-triggered cycle for a defined inspiratory time (ie, between TI_{MIN} and TI_{MAX}); and (3) a "T" (timed) mode in which the NIV device delivers pressurizations at a preset respiratory rate, during a preset

inspiratory time, without taking into account the patients' inspiratory efforts. Recent guidelines published by the American Academy of Sleep Medicine for the adjustment of NIV in chronic alveolar hypoventilation syndromes recommend the

S mode as default setting, unless patients have a significant number of central apneas, a low spontaneous respiratory rate, or are unable to trigger the ventilator.[3] We performed the first study to analyze the impact on treatment efficacy of changes in BURR performed in a random order (three consecutive PSGs) in a group of patients on chronic noninvasive positive pressure ventilation (NPPV) treatment, all suffering from obesity hypoventilation syndrome (OHS) and treated with the same bilevel NPPV device.[7] No other ventilator setting was modified. Results showed that changing BURR from an S/T mode with a high or low BURR to an S mode was associated with the occurrence of a highly significant increase in respiratory events, mainly central and mixed events (see **Fig. 5**).[7] One possible hypothesis is that a first central event in S mode generates successive arousals causing further increases in ventilation, and driving the Pa_{CO_2} below the apneic threshold, thus triggering a vicious cycle of central events. Indeed, although respiratory drive and ventilator response to CO_2 are blunted in subjects with OHS, these parameters improve under NPPV, thus re-establishing the normal reactivity of respiratory centers to changes in Pa_{CO_2}. Other non–chemoreceptor dependent mechanisms may be relevant. In isocapnic conditions, increasing V_T or respiratory rate per se could reduce respiratory motor output or induce central apnea. These data strongly question the systematic use of an S mode during initiation of bilevel NPPV in this particular OHS population.

Polysomnographic Features of Obstructive Events: Partial or Total Upper Airway Obstruction Without Reduction of Ventilatory Drive Under NIV

These events are comparable with what occurs in obstructive sleep apnea. Upper airway patency decreases at the end of expiration. During inspiration, a further reduction in upper airway patency can lead to a complete collapse. Inspiratory efforts increase, reflecting persistent respiratory drive against the obstacle. These efforts continue until a microarousal occurs, reestablishing upper airway muscular tone and patency and thus ending the event.

With a pressure-controlled ventilator, a sudden reduction in flow amplitude during insufflation while inspiratory positive pressure is maintained suggests upper airway obstruction or instability (**Fig. 6**). A phase opposition or a phase angle between thoracic and abdominal belt signals suggests partial or total closure of the upper airways with persistence or increase of respiratory drive

and efforts (see **Fig. 6**). A phase opposition with a negative inflexion of the thoracic belt signal on inspiration associated with a positive inflexion of the abdominal belt signal suggests fighting against upper airway obstruction. A progressive increase of abdominal and thoracic belt signals, with an increase in respiratory rate of the patient caused by increasing efforts to open the airways, also suggests upper airway obstruction. However, the sensitivity and specificity of abdomen and thoracic movement signals is limited particularly in obese patients and additional tools for identifying respiratory efforts are desirable (see below). As mentioned previously, upper airway obstruction is associated with poor detection of patient's inspiratory efforts; thus a switch to BURR in assist-controlled mode can be observed (see **Fig. 6**).

POLYSOMNOGRAPHIC FEATURES OF MIXED EVENTS: PARTIAL OR TOTAL CLOSURE OF THE UPPER AIRWAYS AND REDUCED VENTILATORY DRIVE FOLLOWED BY PASSIVE CLOSURE OF THE UPPER AIRWAYS AND RESUMPTION OF RESPIRATORY DRIVE

A synchronous reduction in flow, thoracic and abdominal movements, and respiratory rate with resumption of thoracic and abdominal movements before restoration of normal flow suggests initial obstruction of the upper airway with reduced ventilatory drive, followed by persistent obstruction of upper airways despite resumption of ventilatory drive (**Fig. 7**).

DIFFERENTIATING BETWEEN CENTRAL AND OBSTRUCTIVE EVENTS ON PSG TRACINGS UNDER NIV IS A MAJOR CHALLENGE

Differentiating between central and obstructive events on polygraphy or PSG tracings under NIV is even more complex than in spontaneous breathing and requires appropriate measurements of respiratory effort. Esophageal pressure is the gold standard for quantifying variations in intrathoracic pressure resulting from respiratory efforts (**Fig. 8**). However, measuring esophageal pressure is invasive, frequently unaccepted or poorly tolerated by the patients, interferes with sleep quality, and generates leaks around the mask under NIV. Pulse transit time (PTT) has been proposed as an alternate tool for quantifying respiratory effort by detecting changes in blood pressure oscillations associated with pleural pressure swings. PTT refers to the time it takes for a pulse wave to travel between two arterial sites. The speed at which this arterial pressure wave travels is inversely

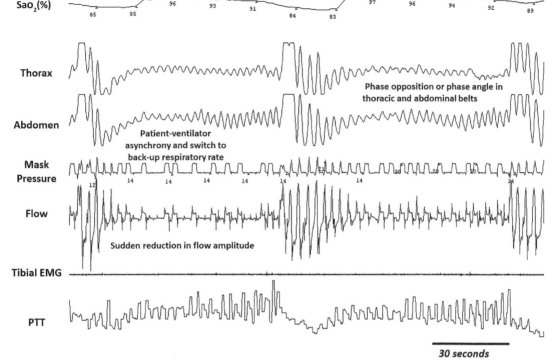

Fig. 6. Recurrent obstructive events occurring on bilevel ventilation support. Note total loss of synchronism (patient/ventilator) during obstruction and increases in pulse transit time (PTT) variations between inspiration and expiration. Sao₂, arterial oxygen saturation.

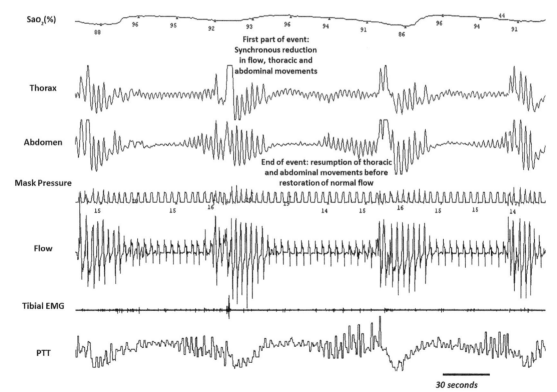

Fig. 7. Recurrent mixed events (central then obstructive) occurring on bilevel ventilation support. Note total loss of synchronism (patient/ventilator) and artifacts during obstructive phase. EMG, electromyogram; Sao₂, arterial oxygen saturation.

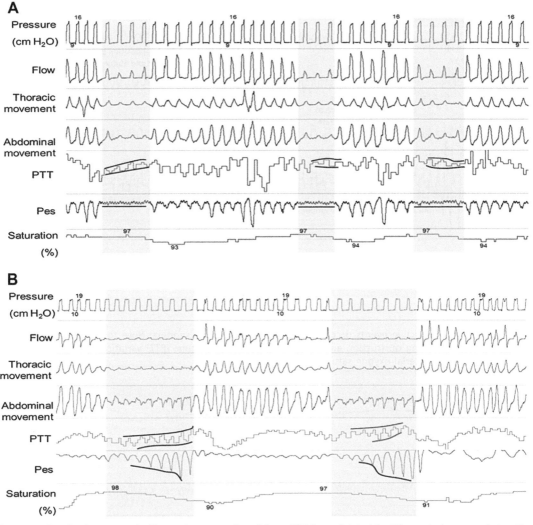

Fig. 8. During 3-minute epoch, illustrative examples of how PTT is useful to identify central versus obstructive events using PTT (see esophageal pressure as the reference signal [Pes]). (*A*) Central respiratory event: for both Pes and PTT signals, respiratory oscillations are markedly reduced or disappear. (*B*) Obstructive respiratory event: swings of Pes become increasingly negative during an obstructive event, with a simultaneous increase in oscillations of PTT between inspiration and expiration (*dark lines*). (*From* Contal O, Carnevale C, Borel JC, et al. Pulse transit time as a measure of respiratory effort under noninvasive ventilation. Eur Respir J 2013;41:348; with permission.)

proportional to blood pressure. The variation of PTT between inspiration and expiration thus reflects the intensity of corresponding changes in intrathoracic pressure. Our group has previously demonstrated that PTT can be used during PSG to analyze respiratory effort and, moreover, that it is specific when defining certain respiratory events occurring during spontaneous breathing (hypopneas, upper airway resistance episodes, and central events).[12–14] We have also shown that despite the changes in intrathoracic pressure and hemodynamics induced by positive pressure ventilation, PTT accurately reflects the unloading

of respiratory muscles induced by NIV and the increase in respiratory effort accompanying leaks during NIV.[6] Analysis of PTT during sleep studies allows an appropriate classification of respiratory events occurring under NIV as being either central or obstructive in nature (ie, partial or complete upper airway obstruction with or without reduction of ventilatory drive). These results support the use of PTT as a surrogate marker of inspiratory muscle effort under NIV (see **Fig. 8**). Other examples of the usefulness of PTT to document respiratory effort under NIV are displayed in **Figs. 3**, **6** and **7**. **Fig. 9** illustrates an obstructive event followed by an arousal and marked hyperventilation, then a consecutive central event on bilevel PAP ventilation. PTT is very helpful for characterizing these two types of events.

POLYSOMNOGRAPHIC FEATURES OF PERSISTENT HYPOVENTILATION UNDER NIV

A major goal of NIV is prevention of worsening of hypoventilation during sleep. It is common for patients in chronic respiratory failure to have the most severe degree of hypoventilation during REM sleep. Therefore, it is important to document that NIV settings selected for chronic treatment are effective during this period.[3] Recently, new rules for defining nocturnal hypoventilation have been established by the American Academy of Sleep Medicine.[15] For adults, sleep hypoventilation is scored when the arterial P_{CO_2} (or surrogate) is greater than 55 mm Hg for greater than or equal to 10 minutes or there is an increase in the arterial P_{CO_2} (or surrogate) greater than or equal to 10 mm Hg (in comparison with an awake supine value) to a value exceeding 50 mm Hg for greater than or equal to 10 minutes. These rules have been

proposed for PSG in spontaneous breathing and no specific recommendations were provided for PSG under NIV. Persistent hypoventilation during REM sleep under NIV (**Fig. 10**) may warrant either increasing level of pressure support or implementing a volume-targeted mode, which has been proposed to decrease transcutaneous P_{CO_2} more efficiently during sleep (**Fig. 11**).[16] It has been proposed that pressure support may be increased if the oxygen saturation as measured by pulse oximetry remains below 90% for 5 minutes or more and V_T is low (<6–8 mL/kg).[3] The rationale behind this recommendation is that an increase in pressure support may increase V_T and reduce or eliminate residual hypoventilation thereby improving oxygenation. Volume-targeted NIV has the potential advantage of automatically varying the pressure support to deliver a targeted V_T. For example, if respiratory muscle strength declined and the V_T decreased, the device would deliver higher pressure support to return the delivered V_T to the targeted level (see **Fig. 11**). New modes and features, such as target V_T, might give the impression of improved alveolar ventilation control but whether this is a great progress or just

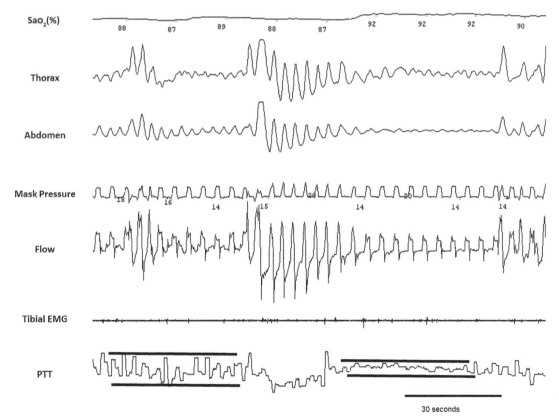

Fig. 9. Illustration of an obstructive event followed by an arousal and marked hyperventilation, then a consecutive central event on bilevel pressure support ventilation. See PTT signal nicely allowing separating the central and obstructive nature of the events. EMG, electromyogram; Sao_2, arterial oxygen saturation.

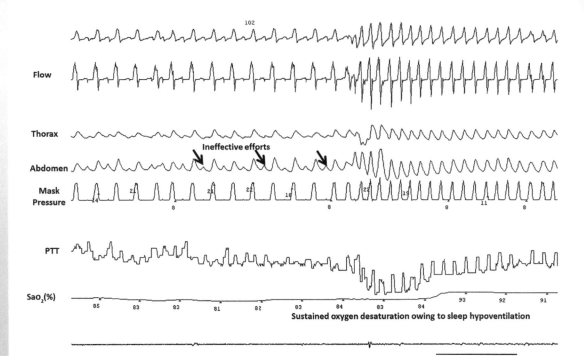

Fig. 10. Sleep hypoventilation under NIV. Illustration of sleep hypoventilation under bilevel pressure support. Note the sustained desaturation with loss of patient/ventilator synchrony ended by an arousal allowing returning to patient/ventilator synchrony and effective NIV. This patient with severe chronic obstructive pulmonary disease, did not produce a high enough inspiratory effort during sleep to trigger the ventilator when compared with the wake period. Sao$_2$, arterial oxygen saturation.

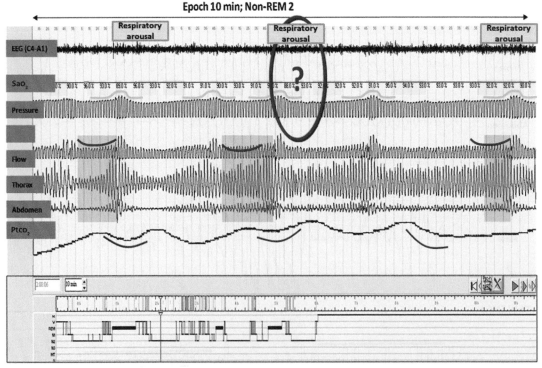

Fig. 11. Volume-ensured ventilation is a hybrid mode of ventilation that ensures a defined preset tidal volume during pressure support ventilation. Volume targeted NIV has the potential advantage of automatically varying the pressure support to deliver a targeted tidal volume. For example, if tidal volume decreases, the device would deliver higher pressure support to return the delivered tidal volume to the targeted level. Note the associated variations in Ptcco$_2$. This figure highlights a possible risk of sleep fragmentation during volume-ensured ventilation, especially when a sudden increase of inspiratory pressure occurs. EEG, electroencephalogram; Ptcco$_2$, transcutaneous Pco$_2$; Sao$_2$, arterial oxygen saturation.

a gadget remains an open question.[17] Large-scale validation studies are lacking and there are still debated issues regarding the risk of impairment in sleep quality and occurrence of microarousals related to constant variations in pressure (see **Fig. 11**).[18,19] It is probably more a careful NIV titration rather than the mode of ventilation that seems to matter the most to attain appropriate alveolar ventilation in different sleep stages.[20]

POLYSOMNOGRAPHIC FEATURES OF PATIENT-VENTILATOR ASYNCHRONY

Profound modifications in the recruitment of respiratory muscles may occur during the various stages of sleep potentially leading to inappropriate triggering. Patient-ventilator dyssynchrony may lead to suboptimal ventilation and sleep fragmentation (**Fig. 12**). In a study involving a cohort of OHS patients evaluated by PSG, 55% of the patients exhibited desynchronization occurring mostly in slow-wave sleep and REM sleep and associated with arousals.[10] Autotriggering was more sporadic and usually limited to one or two breaths.[10] Similarly, Fanfulla and colleagues,[21] studying 48 patients enrolled in a long-term

home NIV program, found a mean of 48 ± 37 ineffective efforts per hour during sleep compared with none during wakefulness. Adler and colleagues[22] suggested that in patients with chronic obstructive pulmonary disease too much pressure support is associated with more asynchrony. Reducing pressure support from an average of 13.6 ± 1.8 to 10.3 ± 1.7 cm H_2O decreased significantly patient ventilator-asynchrony, without any repercussion on arterial blood gases and sleep structure assessed by PSG. The latter study was neither randomized nor controlled, but impact on symptoms and patient-ventilator synchrony were remarkable. Patient-ventilator dyssynchrony is frequently associated with a switch to back-up respiratory frequency in assist-controlled mode (see **Figs. 6** and **10**).

SUMMARY, PERSPECTIVES, AND RESEARCH AGENDA

Monitoring of nocturnal NIV is required to determine if NIV is correctly adapted to detect residual or de novo respiratory events and patient-ventilator asynchrony. Indeed, Rabec and colleagues[4] showed in a cohort of 169 patients that

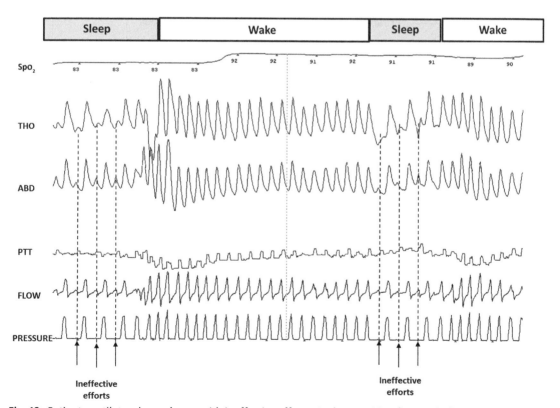

Fig. 12. Patient-ventilator dyssynchrony with ineffective efforts. At the transition from wakefulness to sleep, ineffective efforts occur being a cause of suboptimal ventilation (see oxygen desaturation) and sleep fragmentation. Spo_2, oxygen saturation as measured by pulse oximetry.

66% of their patients had abnormalities during nocturnal NIV; leaks and desaturation dips were the most frequent findings. Various tools can be used for monitoring NIV. Although the gold standard PSG is more systematically used in the United States, in Europe clinicians use simpler tools before implementing a full sleep study. Janssens and colleagues[2] proposed an algorithm for monitoring NIV, recommending PSG only when simple monitoring tools fail to help physicians identify correct NIV settings (**Fig. 13**).

Understanding and classifying the mechanisms involved in respiratory events under NIV is crucial for adapting appropriate NIV settings or interfaces. Thus, documenting residual obstructive events in an obese patient leads to an increase in positive expiratory pressure. Persistent hypoventilation during REM sleep may warrant either increasing level of pressure support or implementing a volume-targeted mode. Periodic breathing and glottic closure, which are frequently associated with hypocapnia and hyperventilation, might be diminished by

reducing pressure support with or without increasing BURR. Finally, patient-ventilator asynchrony may require adjusting inspiratory and expiratory triggers and reducing nonintentional leaks when present. Leaks increase the probability of most abnormal respiratory events under NIV, thus reducing the efficacy of ventilatory support. It must be kept in mind that relationships between these events and quality of sleep are extremely complex. For example, volume targeting may improve ventilation across the different sleep stages while concurrently impairing sleep quality. Moreover, increasing ventilation to correct residual REM sleep hypoventilation can favor the emergence of periodic breathing particularly in non-REM sleep.

For all these reasons, periodic PSG is recommended by experts in the follow-up of home-ventilated patients. However, in sleep medicine, scoring and interpreting PSG under NIV is probably one of the most difficult tasks. Resulting flow and pressure signals are influenced not only by the patients' ventilation but also by the technical

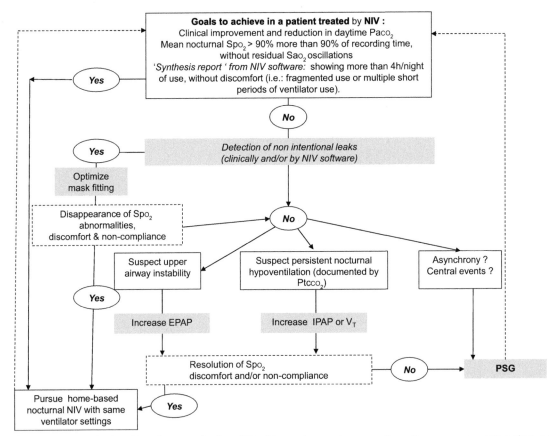

Fig. 13. Proposed algorithm for monitoring NIV. Ptcco$_2$, transcutaneous Pco$_2$; Spo$_2$, oxygen saturation as measured by pulse oximetry. EPAP, expiratory positive airway pressure; IPAP, inspiratory positive airway pressure; Vt, tidal volume. (*From* Janssens JP, Borel JC, Pepin JL. Nocturnal monitoring of home non-invasive ventilation: the contribution of simple tools such as pulse oximetry, capnography, built-in ventilator software and autonomic markers of sleep fragmentation. Thorax 2011;66:442; with permission.)

specifications of the device and the ventilatory mode. Specific recommendations regarding the channels that need to be recorded and consensus criteria for scoring are highly desirable. A European multicentre group (SomnoNIV) has proposed minimal requirements for analysis and a standardized scoring under NIV.[1] Further studies are now needed to evaluate this standardized scoring in different centers and to establish the prevalence of residual events according to patient diagnosis. This might be an exciting task for a joint European and US panel of experts. Finally, future studies are needed to establish whether recognition and correction of these abnormalities during sleep positively impact long-term efficacy of NIV, compliance, or quality of life.

ACKNOWLEDGMENT

Research for this article was provided by the SomnoNIV group.

REFERENCES

1. Gonzalez-Bermejo J, Perrin C, Janssens JP, et al. Proposal for a systematic analysis of polygraphy or polysomnography for identifying and scoring abnormal events occurring during non-invasive ventilation. Thorax 2012;67:546–52.
2. Janssens JP, Borel JC, Pepin JL. Nocturnal monitoring of home non-invasive ventilation: the contribution of simple tools such as pulse oximetry, capnography, built-in ventilator software and autonomic markers of sleep fragmentation. Thorax 2011;66:438–45.
3. Berry RB, Chediak A, Brown LK, et al. Best clinical practices for the sleep center adjustment of noninvasive positive pressure ventilation (NPPV) in stable chronic alveolar hypoventilation syndromes. J Clin Sleep Med 2010;6:491–509.
4. Rabec C, Georges M, Kabeya NK, et al. Evaluating NIV using a monitoring system coupled to a ventilator: a bench to bedside study. Eur Respir J 2009; 34(4):902–13.
5. Teschler H, Stampa J, Ragette R, et al. Effect of mouth leak on effectiveness of nasal bilevel ventilatory assistance and sleep architecture. Eur Respir J 1999;14:1251–7.
6. Contal O, Carnevale C, Borel JC, et al. Pulse transit time as a measure of respiratory effort under noninvasive ventilation. Eur Respir J 2013;41:346–53.
7. Contal O, Adler D, Borel JC, et al. Impact of different backup respiratory rates on the efficacy of noninvasive positive pressure ventilation in obesity hypoventilation syndrome: a randomized trial. Chest 2013; 143:37–46.
8. Douglas NJ, White DP, Pickett CK, et al. Respiration during sleep in normal man. Thorax 1982;37:840–4.
9. Jounieaux V, Aubert G, Dury M, et al. Effects of nasal positive-pressure hyperventilation on the glottis in normal sleeping subjects. J Appl Phys 1995;79:186–93.
10. Guo YF, Sforza E, Janssens JP. Respiratory patterns during sleep in obesity-hypoventilation patients treated with nocturnal pressure support: a preliminary report. Chest 2007;131:1090–9.
11. Parreira VF, Jounieaux V, Aubert G, et al. Nasal two-level positive-pressure ventilation in normal subjects. Effects of the glottis and ventilation. Am J Respir Crit Care Med 1996;153:1616–23.
12. Argod J, Pepin JL, Levy P. Differentiating obstructive and central sleep respiratory events through pulse transit time. Am J Respir Crit Care Med 1998;158:1778–83.
13. Argod J, Pepin JL, Smith RP, et al. Comparison of esophageal pressure with pulse transit time as a measure of respiratory effort for scoring obstructive nonapneic respiratory events. Am J Respir Crit Care Med 2000;162:87–93.
14. Smith RP, Argod J, Pepin JL, et al. Pulse transit time: an appraisal of potential clinical applications. Thorax 1999;54:452–7.
15. Berry RB, Budhiraja R, Gottlieb DJ, et al. Rules for scoring respiratory events in sleep: update of the 2007 AASM Manual for the Scoring of Sleep and Associated Events. Deliberations of the Sleep Apnea Definitions Task Force of the American Academy of Sleep Medicine. J Clin Sleep Med 2012;8:597–619.
16. Storre JH, Steurer B, Kabitz HJ, et al. Transcutaneous PCO2 monitoring during initiation of noninvasive ventilation. Chest 2007;132:1810–6.
17. Windisch W, Storre JH. Target volume settings for home mechanical ventilation: great progress or just a gadget? Thorax 2012;67:663–5.
18. Carlucci A, Fanfulla F, Mancini M, et al. Volume assured pressure support ventilation–induced arousals. Sleep Med 2012;13:767–8.
19. Janssens JP, Metzger M, Sforza E. Impact of volume targeting on efficacy of bi-level non-invasive ventilation and sleep in obesity-hypoventilation. Respir Med 2009;103:165–72.
20. Murphy PB, Davidson C, Hind MD, et al. Volume targeted versus pressure support non-invasive ventilation in patients with super obesity and chronic respiratory failure: a randomised controlled trial. Thorax 2012;67:727–34.
21. Fanfulla F, Taurino AE, Lupo ND, et al. Effect of sleep on patient/ventilator asynchrony in patients undergoing chronic non-invasive mechanical ventilation. Respir Med 2007;101:1702–7.
22. Adler D, Bridevaux PO, Contal O, et al. Pulse wave amplitude reduction: a surrogate marker of micro-arousals associated with respiratory events occurring under non-invasive ventilation? Respir Med 2013;107(12):2053–60.

Obesity Hypoventilation Syndrome
Epidemiology and Diagnosis

 CrossMark

Jay S. Balachandran, MD[a],*,
Juan Fernando Masa, MD, PhD[b,c], Babak Mokhlesi, MD, MSc[a]

KEYWORDS

- Sleep-disordered breathing • Obesity hypoventilation syndrome • Sleep hypoventilation
- Obstructive sleep apnea • Obesity • Morbid obesity

KEY POINTS

- Obesity hypoventilation syndrome (OHS) is defined as daytime alveolar hypoventilation (awake, sea-level, arterial Pco_2>45 mm Hg) among patients with body mass index $\geq$30 kg/m^2 in the absence of other causes of hypoventilation.
- Ninety percent of OHS patients have concomitant obstructive sleep apnea (OSA).
- Incorporating elevated serum bicarbonate levels and/or low finger pulse oximetry may augment OHS screening among obese OSA patients.
- The overall prevalence of OHS is estimated to be approximately 0.6% of the general adult population.
- OHS prevalence increases as the degree of obesity increases.

INTRODUCTION

The drumbeats have been sounding for some time now—the obesity epidemic has become a pandemic. By 2015, nearly 1 of 3 adults in the world are expected to be overweight (body mass index [BMI] $\geq$25 kg/m^2) and almost 1 in 10 adults will be obese (BMI $\geq$30 kg/m^2).[1] The health consequences of this "Obesity Era" are becoming more and more apparent. Among the myriad comorbidities associated with obesity is obesity hypoventilation syndrome (OHS), defined as the presence of diurnal alveolar hypoventilation (awake arterial Pco_2>45 mm Hg) among obese patients in the absence of other possible causes of hypoventilation.

Patients with OHS have higher rates of hospitalization and health care utilization, greater cardiorespiratory comorbidities, and higher mortality than obese-matched patients with obstructive sleep apnea (OSA) without hypoventilation.[2,3] In light of these consequences, it seems imperative for clinicians to recognize and treat this condition appropriately, yet OHS remains frequently overlooked.[4,5]

The aim of this article is to therefore increase clinician awareness of OHS by reviewing diagnostic criteria and current data on disease prevalence.

DEFINITION

Initial reports of OHS by Auchincloss and colleagues[6] and Bickelmann and colleagues[7] described patients with obesity, hypersomnolence, secondary erythrocytosis, pulmonary hypertension, and cor pulmonale. Nocturnal observation

Conflict of Interest: None of the authors have a conflict of interest to disclose.
[a] Sleep Disorders Center, Section of Pulmonary and Critical Care, Department of Medicine, University of Chicago, 5841 South Maryland Avenue, Chicago, IL 60637, USA; [b] Pulmonary Division, San Pedro de Alcantara Hospital, Avda. Pablo Naranjo s/n, Caceres 10003, Spain; [c] CIBERES National Research Network, Avd. Montforte de Lemos 5, Pabellon 11, Madrid 28029, Spain
* Corresponding author.
E-mail address: jsbalach@uchicago.edu

of these patients led to the first description of OSA[8] and it was soon noted that a consistent proportion of OSA patients also exhibited daytime hypoventilation.[9,10] During this period of investigation, considerable variation existed with respect to the definition of hypoventilation and OSA, and to establish standardized descriptions of sleep-breathing disorders, a task force of the American Academy of Sleep Medicine established a definition of OHS as the presence of daytime alveolar hypoventilation (awake, sea-level, arterial $P_{CO_2} > 45$ mm Hg) among patients with BMI ≥ 30 kg/m^2 in the absence of other causes of hypoventilation.[11] This definition also incorporated the observation that, although most patients with OHS had concurrent OSA, approximately 10% had no evidence of nocturnal OSA; these patients developed sleep-related hypoventilation, particularly during REM sleep.[12,13] This point is relevant because, although the definition suggests a diurnal pathologic abnormality, overnight polysomnography is required to determine the pattern of nocturnal hypoventilation (obstructive or nonobstructive) and to individualize therapy based on an adequate titration study.

DIAGNOSIS

Importantly, OHS is a diagnosis of exclusion, and suspected patients should be evaluated for other possible causes of hypoventilation, such as underlying obstructive respiratory disease, mechanical respiratory limitations (eg, kyphoscoliosis), neuropathic and myopathic conditions, and central causes (eg, cerebrovascular disease, severe hypothyroidism) (**Box 1**).[14,15] Furthermore, suspected patients should be screened for factors that can exacerbate hypoventilation, such as the use of sedative-hypnotics, opiates, or alcohol.[13]

OHS is frequently first diagnosed either when an afflicted patient reaches a high state of acuity, in the form of acute-on-chronic hypoventilatory failure, or alternatively, when ambulatory care is escalated to evaluation by pulmonary or sleep specialists.[2,4,16] Unfortunately, a delay in diagnosis is common; the diagnosis typically occurs during the fifth and sixth decades of life,[5] and during that delay, OHS patients use more health care resources than comparably obese normocapneic patients.[3]

Patients with OHS tend to be morbidly obese (BMI ≥ 35 kg/m^2), have severe OSA (≥ 30 obstructive respiratory events per hour of sleep), and are typically hypersomnolent. Compared with patients with OSA, patients with OHS are more likely to report dyspnea and manifest cor pulmonale. **Table 1** paints the typical portrait of an OHS patient, based on the clinical features[16–19] of a large combined cohort of OHS patients reported in the literature.[5]

Box 1
Diagnostic features of OHS

Obesity

- BMI ≥ 30 kg/m^2

Chronic hypoventilation

- Awake daytime hypercapnia (sea-level arterial $P_{CO_2} \geq 45$ mm Hg, $P_{O_2} < 70$ mm Hg)
- Possible role of serum venous bicarbonate or calculated capillary blood gas bicarbonate greater than 27 mEq/L*

Sleep-disordered breathing[†]

- Obstructive sleep apnea (apnea-hypopnea index [AHI] ≥ 5 event/h)
- Nonobstructive sleep hypoventilation (AHI <5 events/h, P_{CO_2} increases by ≥ 7 mm Hg during sleep or oxygen saturation $\leq 88\%$ for at least 5 min without obstructive respiratory events)

Exclusion of other causes of hypoventilation

- Severe obstructive respiratory disease
- Severe interstitial lung disease
- Severe chest-wall disorders (eg, kyphoscoliosis)
- Severe hypothyroidism
- Neuromuscular disease
- Congenital hypoventilation syndromes

  * Serum bicarbonate level assessment is not part of the definition but advocates suggest using this for screening.
  [†] OSA is present in 90% of cases, with the remaining cases featuring nonobstructive sleep hypoventilation.

Several investigators have suggested incorporating serum bicarbonate (HCO_3^-) levels into the definition of OHS, particularly given that using a single measurement of arterial P_{CO_2} for OHS diagnosis is susceptible to several confounding factors, including the impact of periprocedural patient anxiety leading to hyperventilation.[17] Mokhlesi and colleagues[18] first demonstrated that a venous serum bicarbonate threshold of 27 mEq/L, suggestive of chronic respiratory acidemia from hypoventilation, could be used for OHS diagnosis. Their data demonstrated that among obese patients with OSA, a serum bicarbonate level less than 27 mEq/L had a 97% negative predictive value for excluding a diagnosis of OHS. Macavei and colleagues[19] assessed earlobe capillary blood gas samples from patients referred to a sleep center and determined that bicarbonate values calculated from the Henderson-Hasselbach formula have similar predictive value. A calculated serum bicarbonate level of ≥ 27 mEq/L had a

Table 1
Clinical features of patients with OHS

Clinical Features	Mean (Range)
Age (y)	52 (42–61)
Male (%)	60 (49–90)
BMI (kg/m^2)	44 (35–56)
Neck circumference (cm)	46.5 (45–47)
pH	7.38 (7.34–7.40)
Arterial P_{CO_2} (mm Hg)	53 (47–61)
Arterial P_{O_2} (mm Hg)	56 (46–74)
Serum bicarbonate (mEq/L)	32 (31–33)
Hemoglobin (g/dL)	15 (ND)
Apnea-hypopnea index (events/h)	66 (20–100)
Oxygen nadir during sleep (%)	65 (59–76)
Percentage time S_pO_2 <90%	50 (46–56)
FVC (% predicted)	68 (57–102)
FEV$_1$ (% predicted)	64 (53–92)
FEV$_1$/FVC	0.77 (0.74–0.88)
Medical Research Council dyspnea class 3 or 4 (%)	69 (ND)
Epworth sleepiness scale score (out of 24)	14 (12–16)

Features are based on aggregated sample of 757 patients from 15 studies.

Abbreviations: FEV$_1$, forced expiratory volume in first second; FVC, forced vital capacity; ND, no data to calculate a range.

Data from Mokhlesi B. Obesity hypoventilation syndrome: a state-of-the-art review. Respir Care 2010;55(10):1347–65.

sensitivity of 85% and a specificity of 89% for the diagnosis of OHS among their patient sample.

In addition to blood gas sampling and venous bicarbonate assessments, daytime finger pulse oximetry may be a valuable tool for clinicians in screening for possible OHS. Hypoxemia during wakefulness is not a typical feature of patients with either OSA or obesity. Therefore, abnormal pulse oximetry during wakefulness should prompt an evaluation for OHS among obese OSA patients.[13]

RISK FACTORS

Obesity, and in particular, morbid obesity, is a predominant risk factor for OHS.[20] However, although all OHS patients are obese, not all patients with obesity, or even morbid obesity, develop OHS. It is worth noting that there are significant differences between obese patients who develop OHS compared with similarly obese patients without OHS, as summarized in **Table 2**.[20]

Table 2
Physiologic differences between morbidly obese patients and those with OHS

	Normocapnic Morbid Obesity	Obesity Hypoventilation Syndrome
Waist:hip ratio	↑	↑↑
FEV$_1$/FVC	Normal	Normal/↓
Total lung capacity	Normal	Slight ↓
Functional residual capacity	↓	↓
Vital capacity	Normal/↓	↓↓
Expiratory reserve volume	↓	↓↓
Work of breathing	↑	↑↑
Hypercapnic/ hypoxic ventilatory drive	Normal	↓
Inspiratory muscle strength	Normal	↓

Abbreviations: FEV$_1$, forced expiratory volume in first second; FVC, forced vital capacity.

In the same light, the severity of concurrent OSA also appears to be a significant risk factor for OHS,[20] but not all patients with even extremely severe OSA have OHS. In fact, even among patients with an apnea-hypopnea index ≥100/h and serum bicarbonate ≥27 mEq/L, 24% do *not* meet criteria for OHS,[18] suggesting nonobstructive pathophysiologic factors for OHS even among these very severe OSA patients.

Male gender does *not* appear to confer a significant risk for OHS, in contrast to uncomplicated OSA.[21] Similarly, no race-specific or ethnic-specific risk has been demonstrated thus far, although it has been speculated[5] that African Americans might have a higher risk for OHS simply because of the higher prevalence of morbid obesity in this race compared with others.[22,23]

PREVALENCE

More than 20 studies regarding the prevalence of OHS have been published since the syndrome was first described. Prevalence estimates for OHS vary significantly across studies, owing partly to differences in sample characteristics, disease definitions, and assessment procedures.

Because most OHS patients have coexisting OSA, most prevalence studies have focused on patients referred to sleep centers for evaluation of sleep-disordered breathing, and a reasonable prevalence estimate among OSA patients has emerged. At least 20 studies have examined this prevalence. Of these, only approximately 10 studies either included coprevalence data for obstructive pulmonary disease[9,18,19,24–26] or excluded these patients entirely[4,27–29] and allow for an assessment of the prevalence of OHS without these patients (**Table 3**). From these 10 studies, the aggregate prevalence of OHS among OSA patients referred to a sleep disorder center is 17% (range 4%–50%). The considerable range in prevalence reflects varying patient populations across studies. For example, the mean BMI of patients in the 2 studies with the lowest prevalence[25,28] was 34 kg/m^2 and was considerably lower than the mean BMI of 59 kg/m^2 from the study with the highest prevalence.[29]

The total prevalence of OHS in the general population is unknown but can be estimated using OSA prevalence data, as illustrated by Mokhlesi.[5] If approximately 6% of the general US population has severe obesity (BMI $\geq$40 kg/m^2),[22] and if it is conservatively estimated that half of patients with

this degree of obesity will have OSA (although some studies actually suggest a prevalence of OSA >70% in patients with this degree of obesity who are referred for bariatric surgery)[30–32] and that approximately 20% of these OSA patients will have OHS, then the estimated prevalence of OHS can be estimated as roughly 0.6% (approximately 1 in 160 adults in the US population; **Fig. 1**). This estimate does not take into account the ~10% of OHS patients who do not have significant OSA, but this figure may also overestimate the frequency of OHS in countries where the prevalence of severe obesity is lower.

Several studies have shed light on the increasing prevalence of OHS as the degree of obesity worsens (**Fig. 2**). Among patients with OSA, the prevalence of OHS at a BMI of 30 to 35 kg/m^2 is 8% to 11% among non-Asian populations and increases to 18% to 31% at a BMI $\geq$40 kg/m^2.[5,18,19,28] At the extreme, Banerjee and colleagues[29] evaluated patients referred for overnight polysomnography with a BMI $\geq$50 kg/m^2 and found an OHS prevalence of 50% in this cohort.

East Asian populations are known to develop OSA at a lower BMI compared with other populations because of cephalometric differences.[33]

Table 3
OHS prevalence and characteristics among patients with OSA[a]

Author, Country	Year	Patients (No.)	Male (%)	Age (y)	BMI (kg/m^2)	AHI (Events/hr)	OHS (No.)	OHS (%)
Leech,[b,c] US[9]	1987	111	68	47	0.71[d]	58	41	37
Resta,[b,c] Italy[24]	2000	219	64	50	40	45	38	17
Verin,[b,c] France[25]	2001	218	92	55	34	51	21	10
Akashiba,[b] Japan[27]	2002	143	100	48	30	55	55	38
Nowbar,[b,e] US[4]	2004	150	53	53	43	N/R	47	31
Laaban & Chailleux,[b] France[28]	2005	1141	83	56	34	55	126	11
Mokhlesi,[b,c] US[18]	2007	522	56	48	44	59	124	24
Kawata,[b,c] Japan[26]	2007	1227	89	50	29	42	168	14
Banerjee,[b,f] Australia[29]	2007	74	54	43	59	62	23	31
Macavei,[b,c] UK[19]	2013	344	64	52	39	25	71	21
Aggregate		4149					714	17

Data are mean or median values provided in each article. Aggregate prevalence calculated by dividing total patients diagnosed with OHS by total patients studied.

Abbreviations: AHI, apnea-hypopnea index; BMI, body mass index; N/R, not reported; OHS, Obesity hypoventilation syndrome; UK, United Kingdom; US, United States.

  [a] OSA defined variably as between AHI $\geq$5 up to AHI $\geq$15.
  [b] Gender, Age, BMI, and AHI values are given as the mean of all patients (ie, OSA and OHS patients) and were calculated from the data provided by the authors in the article.
  [c] Did not exclude patients with obstructive deficits on spirometry in data presented here.
  [d] BMI not reported; value given as weight/ height ratio reported in kg/cm.
  [e] Study population comprised of patients hospitalized in medical non-ICU setting with BMI $\geq$35 kg/m^2.
  [f] Enrolled consecutive patients with BMI $\geq$50 and OSA (defined as AHI $\geq$5).

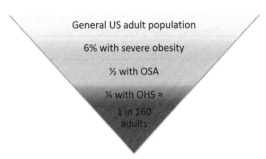

Fig. 1. Estimated prevalence of OHS in the US adult population. The overall prevalence of OHS can be estimated using severe obesity (BMI >40 kg/m^2) and OSA prevalence data. This estimate is likely conservative, because it does not take into account the roughly 10% of OHS patients who do not have OSA. OHS may be more prevalent in the United States because of the higher prevalence of severe obesity than other countries.

Therefore, in these populations, OHS may be more prevalent at a lower BMI range than in non-Asian populations. Indeed, the average BMI of 291 OHS patients from 4 studies involving Japanese subjects was 32 kg/m^2,[26,27,34,35] compared with an average BMI of 44 kg/m^2 from 757 OHS patients from 10 studies involving mostly non-Asian subjects.[5]

Because patients undergoing bariatric surgery are generally more obese, the prevalence of OHS might be expected to be higher among these patients and, indeed, 2 studies support this notion. Sugerman and colleagues[36] found that 65% of their bariatric surgery OSA patients had OHS.

Domínguez-Cherit and colleagues[37] found that 18 of 37 (49%) patients undergoing bariatric surgery in their cohort had either hypercapnia or hypercapnia + hypoxemia; the mean BMI in their study was 50 kg/m^2. In contrast, however, Lecube and colleagues[38] evaluated asymptomatic women referred to a bariatric clinic. Of 66 of these subjects diagnosed with OSA based on limited polygraphy, their study found that only 7 (11%) had OHS; the lower prevalence in the study could be attributed to recruitment of only asymptomatic subjects as well as OSA diagnosis based on limited polygraphy.

Hospitalized patients are also known to have a higher prevalence of OHS and may suffer excess morbidity and mortality because of a lack of appropriate OHS therapy. Of 277 patients with a BMI ≥35 kg/m^2 admitted to an inpatient medical service, Nowbar and colleagues[4] found that 31% met criteria for OHS. Reinforcing the association with obesity, when a subgroup of patients with BMI greater than 50 kg/m^2 was examined, OHS was found in 48%. Of particular concern, (though likely representative of many hospitals), effective therapy for hypoventilation was only instituted in 13% of these patients. This lack of recognition may have important consequences: compared with patients with simple obesity, OHS patients in this study were more likely to require intensive care and invasive mechanical ventilation, and strikingly, these patients had nearly twice the mortality 1.5 years after hospital discharge. Marik and Desai[39] found that 8% of *all admissions* to a general ICU met criteria for OHS. All OHS patients

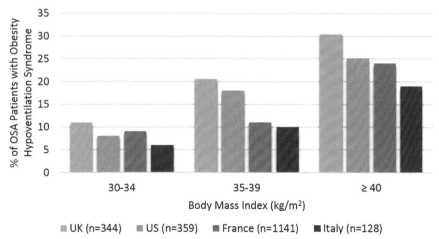

Fig. 2. Prevalence of OHS in patients with OSA, sorted by BMI. In the UK study, the mean BMI was nearly 40 kg/m^2 and 38% of subjects had a BMI greater than 40 kg/m^2.[19] Similarly, in the US study, the mean BMI was 43 kg/m^2 and 60% of subjects had a BMI greater than 40 kg/m^2.[18] In contrast, the mean BMI in the French study was 34 kg/m^2 and only 15% of subjects had a BMI greater than 40 kg/m^2.[28] Italian data were provided by Onofrio Resta, personal communication.[5]

had been admitted with acute on chronic hypercarbic respiratory failure, and of these patients, *nearly 75% were misdiagnosed and treated for obstructive lung disease* despite having no evidence of obstruction on pulmonary function testing.

ASSOCIATED MORBIDITY

As already noted, most OHS patients are morbidly obese and have severe OSA.[18] Although obesity[40] and severe OSA[41] are associated with decreases in quality of life, OHS may contribute to further quality-of-life decrements.[42] Furthermore, quality-of-life ratings among OHS patients appear to be lower than those with hypoventilatory respiratory disorders, such as obstructive lung disease.[43]

The medical morbidity associated with a diagnosis of OHS can be quite varied as illustrated by Jennum and colleagues,[44] who evaluated 755 patients with a diagnosis of OHS from a Danish national patient registry and found that, in the 3 years before OHS diagnosis, these patients were more likely than age-matched and gender-matched controls to be diagnosed with many conditions, including cellulitis, carpal tunnel syndrome, diabetes, congestive heart failure, obstructive lung disease, and arthritis of the knee. It remains unclear if these conditions would be more prevalent than in an obese-matched cohort with uncomplicated OSA.

Cardiovascular morbidity is of particular concern in OHS. Kessler and colleagues[2] found a pulmonary hypertension prevalence of 58% among a cohort of 34 OHS patients compared with just 9% among a sample of similar OSA patients. Similarly, Berg and colleagues[3] evaluated 20 OHS patients from a Canadian health registry and compared them with obese matched controls. OHS patients in their study were 9 times more likely to have a diagnosis of cor pulmonale and 9 times more likely to have a diagnosis of congestive heart failure.

SUMMARY

OHS prevalence is expected to increase, following global trends in obesity, and because significant morbidity is associated with this disease, timely diagnosis and appropriate therapy are imperative. The traditional criteria for OHS diagnosis include the presence of daytime alveolar hypoventilation (awake, sea-level, arterial P_{CO_2} >45 mm Hg) among patients with BMI $\geq$30 kg/m^2 in the absence of other causes of hypoventilation, and incorporating finger pulse oximetry and serum bicarbonate screening will likely aid in improving diagnosis. The major risk factors for OHS include obesity and OSA; therefore, a high index of suspicion is needed in these patients, particularly in the inpatient setting and before bariatric surgery.

REFERENCES

1. World Health Organization. Preventing chronic diseases: a vital investment. Geneva: World Health Organization; 2005.
2. Kessler R, Chaouat A, Schinkewitch P, et al. The obesity-hypoventilation syndrome revisited: a prospective study of 34 consecutive cases. Chest 2001;120(2):369–76.
3. Berg G, Delaive K, Manfreda J, et al. The use of health-care resources in obesity-hypoventilation syndrome. Chest 2001;120(2):377–83.
4. Nowbar S, Burkart KM, Gonzales R, et al. Obesity-associated hypoventilation in hospitalized patients: prevalence, effects, and outcome. Am J Med 2004;116(1):1–7.
5. Mokhlesi B. Obesity hypoventilation syndrome: a state-of-the-art review. Respir Care 2010;55(10):1347–65.
6. Auchincloss JH Jr, Cook E, Renzetti AD. Clinical and physiological aspects of a case of obesity, polycythemia and alveolar hypoventilation. J Clin Invest 1955;34(10):1537.
7. Bickelmann AG, Burwell CS, Robin ED, et al. Extreme obesity associated with alveolar hypoventilation; a Pickwickian syndrome. Am J Med 1956;21(5):811–8.
8. Gastaut H, Tassinari CA, Duron B. Polygraphic study of diurnal and nocturnal (hypnic and respiratory) episodal manifestations of Pickwick syndrome. Rev Neurol (Paris) 1965;112(6):568–79 [in French].
9. Leech JA, Onal E, Baer P, et al. Determinants of hypercapnia in occlusive sleep apnea syndrome. Chest 1987;92(5):807–13.
10. Javaheri S, Colangelo G, Lacey W, et al. Chronic hypercapnia in obstructive sleep apnea-hypopnea syndrome. Sleep 1994;17(5):416–23.
11. Sleep-related breathing disorders in adults: recommendations for syndrome definition and measurement techniques in clinical research. The Report of an American Academy of Sleep Medicine Task Force. Sleep 1999;22(5):667–89.
12. Kessler R, Chaouat A, Weitzenblum E, et al. Pulmonary hypertension in the obstructive sleep apnoea syndrome: prevalence, causes and therapeutic consequences. Eur Respir J 1996;9(4):787–94.
13. Olson AL, Zwillich C. The obesity hypoventilation syndrome. Am J Med 2005;118(9):948–56.
14. Glauser FL, Fairman RP, Bechard D. The causes and evaluation of chronic hypercapnea. Chest 1987;91(5):755–9.
15. Chebbo A, Tfaili A, Jones SF. Hypoventilation syndromes. Med Clin North Am 2011;95(6):1189–202.

16. Quint JK, Ward L, Davison AG. Previously undiagnosed obesity hypoventilation syndrome. Thorax 2007;62(5):462–3.

17. Hart N, Mandal S, Manuel A, et al. Obesity hypoventilation syndrome: does the current definition need revisiting? Thorax 2014;69(1):83–4.

18. Mokhlesi B, Tulaimat A, Faibussowitsch I, et al. Obesity hypoventilation syndrome: prevalence and predictors in patients with obstructive sleep apnea. Sleep Breath 2006;11(2):117–24.

19. Macavei VM, Spurling KJ, Loft J, et al. Diagnostic predictors of obesity-hypoventilation syndrome in patients suspected of having sleep disordered breathing. J Clin Sleep Med 2013;9(9):879–84.

20. Piper AJ, Grunstein RR. Obesity hypoventilation syndrome: mechanisms and management. Am J Respir Crit Care Med 2011;183(3):292–8.

21. Kaw R, Hernandez AV, Walker E, et al. Determinants of hypercapnia in obese patients with obstructive sleep apnea: a systematic review and metaanalysis of cohort studies. Chest 2009;136(3):787–96.

22. Flegal KM, Carroll MD, Kit BK, et al. Prevalence of obesity and trends in the distribution of body mass index among US adults, 1999-2010. JAMA 2012; 307(5):491.

23. Freedman DS, Khan LK, Serdula MK, et al. Trends and correlates of class 3 obesity in the United States from 1990 through 2000. JAMA 2002;288(14):1758–61.

24. Resta O, Foschino Barbaro MP, Bonfitto P, et al. Hypercapnia in obstructive sleep apnoea syndrome. Neth J Med 2000;56(6):215–22.

25. Verin E, Tardif C, Pasquis P. Prevalence of daytime hypercapnia or hypoxia in patients with OSAS and normal lung function. Respir Med 2001;95(8):693–6.

26. Kawata N, Tatsumi K, Terada J, et al. Daytime hypercapnia in obstructive sleep apnea syndrome. Chest 2007;132(6):1832–8.

27. Akashiba T, Kawahara S, Kosaka N, et al. Determinants of chronic hypercapnia in Japanese men with obstructive sleep apnea syndrome. Chest 2002;121(2):415–21.

28. Laaban JP, Chailleux E. Daytime hypercapnia in adult patients with obstructive sleep apnea syndrome in France, before initiating nocturnal nasal continuous positive airway pressure therapy. Chest 2005;127(3):710–5.

29. Banerjee D, Yee BJ, Piper AJ, et al. Obesity hypoventilation syndrome: hypoxemia during continuous positive airway pressure. Chest 2007;131(6):1678–84.

30. Lee W, Nagubadi S, Kryger MH, et al. Epidemiology of obstructive sleep apnea: a population-based perspective. Expert Rev Respir Med 2008;2(3):349–64.

31. Sareli AE, Cantor CR, Williams NN, et al. Obstructive sleep apnea in patients undergoing bariatric surgery—a tertiary center experience. Obes Surg 2009;21(3):316–27.

32. Lopez PP, Stefan B, Schulman CI, et al. Prevalence of sleep apnea in morbidly obese patients who presented for weight loss surgery evaluation: more evidence for routine screening for obstructive sleep apnea before weight loss surgery. Am Surg 2008; 74(9):834–8.

33. Yu X, Fujimoto K, Urushibata K, et al. Cephalometric analysis in obese and nonobese patients with obstructive sleep apnea syndrome. Chest 2003; 124(1):212–8.

34. Chin K, Hirai M, Kuriyama T, et al. Changes in the arterial PCO2 during a single night's sleep in patients with obstructive sleep apnea. Intern Med 1997;36(7):454–60.

35. Akashiba T, Akahoshi T, Kawahara S, et al. Clinical characteristics of obesity-hypoventilation syndrome in Japan: a multi-center study. Intern Med 2006; 45(20):1121–5.

36. Sugerman HJ, Fairman RP, Baron PL, et al. Gastric surgery for respiratory insufficiency of obesity. Chest 1986;90(1):81–6.

37. Domínguez-Cherit G, Gonzalez R, Borunda D, et al. Anesthesia for morbidly obese patients. World J Surg 1998;22(9):969–73.

38. Lecube A, Sampol G, Lloberes P, et al. Asymptomatic sleep-disordered breathing in premenopausal women awaiting bariatric surgery. Obes Surg 2009;20(4):454–61.

39. Marik PE, Desai H. Characteristics of patients with the "malignant obesity hypoventilation syndrome" admitted to an ICU. J Intensive Care Med 2012; 28(2):124–30.

40. Flegal KM, Graubard BI, Williamson DF, et al. Excess deaths associated with underweight, overweight, and obesity. JAMA 2005;293(15):1861–7.

41. Young T, Finn L, Peppard PE, et al. Sleep disordered breathing and mortality: eighteen-year follow-up of the Wisconsin sleep cohort. Sleep 2008;31(8):1071–8.

42. Hida W. Quality of life in obesity hypoventilation syndrome. Sleep Breath 2003;7(1):1–2.

43. Budweiser S, Hitzl AP, Jörres RA, et al. Health-related quality of life and long-term prognosis in chronic hypercapnic respiratory failure: a prospective survival analysis. Respir Res 2007;8:92.

44. Jennum P, Ibsen R, Kjellberg J. Morbidity prior to a diagnosis of sleep-disordered breathing: a controlled national study. J Clin Sleep Med 2013;9(2): 103–8.

Outcomes for Obese Patients with Chronic Respiratory Failure
Results from Observational and Randomized Controlled Trials

Patrick B. Murphy, MRCP, PhD[a,b,*],
Nicholas Hart, FRCP, PhD[a,b,c]

KEYWORDS

- Continuous positive airway pressure • Noninvasive ventilation • Chronic respiratory failure • Obesity
- Outcomes

KEY POINTS

- Observational cohort data support the clinical effectiveness of positive airway pressure (PAP) therapy in improving clinical outcome in obese patients with chronic respiratory failure.
- There are limited data to recommend a single PAP strategy, and a considered approach to the phenotype of sleep-disordered breathing must be applied.
- Phenotyping of sleep-disordered breathing resulting in obesity-related chronic respiratory failure is essential for interpreting the current published data and clinical decision making on which PAP strategy to employ.
- Reversal of chronic respiratory failure should be the long-term aim of PAP therapy.
- 4 hours per night use of PAP therapy should be targeted for treatment of obese patients with chronic respiratory failure.
- Physical activity should be augmented following initiation of PAP therapy to improve long-term obesity-related morbidity.

INTRODUCTION

Obesity hypoventilation syndrome (OHS) was originally reported by Auchincloss and colleagues[1] in 1955, with the term Pickwickian syndrome coined the following year.[2] Although the use of mechanical ventilatory support to manage the acute decompensated episodes was described some years later,[3] the first report of the use of positive airway pressure (PAP) to improve sleep-disordered breathing and reverse the associated daytime chronic respiratory failure as a clinical outcome was not reported until several decades later.[4] Despite the increasing global prevalence of this condition across Europe, North America, and Australasia, there are still few randomized controlled trials to support and direct clinical decision making. Currently, clinicians are required to

[a] Lane Fox Clinical Respiratory Physiology Research Centre, Guy's & St Thomas' NHS Foundation Trust, Westminster Bridge Road, London SE1 7EH, UK; [b] Division of Asthma, Allergy and Lung Biology, King's College London, Strand, London WC2R 2LS, UK; [c] Lane Fox Respiratory Unit, Guy's & St Thomas' NHS Foundation Trust, Westminster Bridge Road, London SE1 7EH, UK
* Corresponding author. Lane Fox Respiratory Unit, St Thomas' Hospital, Westminster Bridge Road, London SE1 7EH, UK.
E-mail address: patrick.b.murphy@kcl.ac.uk

Sleep Med Clin 9 (2014) 349–356
http://dx.doi.org/10.1016/j.jsmc.2014.05.003
1556-407X/14/$ – see front matter © 2014 Elsevier Inc. All rights reserved.

develop their own clinical practice primarily based on limited physiologic and clinical data. This article will emphasize the important outcome parameter that the clinician needs to consider.

TARGET POPULATIONS AND THE PHENOTYPE OF PATIENTS WITH SLEEP-DISORDERED BREATHING

In the current definition of OHS, chronic respiratory failure as a consequence of sleep-disordered breathing is an essential component.[5] Although this is predominantly manifested as obstructive sleep apnea (OSA), lone hypoventilation can be the cause in around 10% of cases,[6] highlighting the complexities with physiologic phenotyping of sleep-disordered breathing in clinical practice. There is a requirement, when considering patient-centered, clinician-centered, and health care utilization outcomes, of reflecting on 3 patterns of sleep-disordered breathing that cause obesity-related chronic respiratory failure from severe OSA to a combination of OSA and OHS overlap and lone OHS. This will allow a comprehensive evaluation of the outcome data from the clinical trials, because although a trial may be reported as negative, the clinician must judge whether this is a failure of the treatment, a failure of delivery of the treatment, or that the target population was poorly defined or indeed inappropriate to test the trial hypothesis.

PHYSIOLOGIC AND CLINICAL AND OUTCOMES
Sleep Quality, Gas Exchange, Pulmonary Function, Drive to Breathe, and Mortality

Correction of sleep-disordered breathing associated with obesity-related chronic respiratory failure has been demonstrated in small non-randomized studies with both continuous PAP (CPAP) and noninvasive ventilation (NIV). These have both been shown to abolish apneic events, consolidate sleep architecture with improvements in slow wave and rapid eye movement (REM) sleep, and improve oxygenation.[7,8] CPAP and NIV have also been shown in these studies to reduce the arousal index and to improve subjective sleep quality.[9] However, there have been no sham-controlled trials and only a single randomized controlled trial that investigated the effect of NIV on sleep quality.[10] Borel and colleagues compared life style advice to treatment with NIV in 35 patients with mild OHS over a 4-week period. The authors demonstrated improvements in the apnea–hypopnea index (AHI), nadir oxygen saturation, mean oxygen saturation, stage 1–2

sleep, REM sleep, and respiratory arousals in the patients randomized to receive NIV (**Fig. 1**). Interestingly, there was no difference in total sleep time (TST) between the groups, but there was an increase in nonrespiratory arousals in the NIV group compared with those patients who received lifestyle counseling alone. This was explained by mask leak-related arousals, and although the difference in nonrespiratory arousals reached statistical significance, the magnitude of difference was small and was greatly outweighed by the clinical improvements in other sleep parameters.

Several studies have compared the efficacy of NIV or CPAP, but only 1 randomized controlled trial has directly compared the 2 modes in terms of the effect on sleep quality, suggesting some subtle benefits in favor of NIV over CPAP.[11] The study, however, was not designed or powered to test for these effects, so other data must be examined to evaluate the potential advantages of each form of PAP in the different manifestations of sleep-disordered breathing in OHS. Banerjee and colleagues[7] used a case-controlled approach to compare the efficacy of CPAP in patients who predominantly had OSA compared to those with OSA plus OHS. Patients were matched for severity of OSA, degree of obesity, and lung volumes based on spirometry. Not unexpectedly, the combined OSA plus OHS group had lower resting daytime and nocturnal oxyhemoglobin saturation by pulse oximetry (SpO_2) levels, and a higher arousal index on diagnostic polysomnography. Despite a similar level of control of upper airway obstruction between the groups in a single-night in-hospital monitored study (AHI OSA group 3.7 ± 0.9/h vs OSA plus OHS group 3.7 ± 1.2/h; P = ns), the OSA plus OHS group had more pronounced nocturnal hypoxemia (Nadir SpO_2 OSA group 87 ± 1% vs OSA plus OHS group 75 ± 4%, P = .015; %TST SpO_2<90% OSA group 1% [0%–5%] vs OSA plus OHS group 18% [1%–54%], P = .015). The increased nocturnal hypoxemia in this group did not translate into a difference in sleep efficiency between the groups (sleep efficiency OSA group 75 ± 3% vs OSA plus OHS group 79 ± 3%; P = ns).

Data suggest that the best predictor of CPAP failure in patients with accompanying OHS is persistent nocturnal hypoxemia despite adequate relief of upper airway obstruction.[12,13] The degree of nocturnal hypoxemia is associated with the ventilatory response to carbon dioxide as evidenced by the assessment hypercapnic ventilatory response (HCVR) before treatment.[8] Indeed, this simple daytime test could be used to clinically stratify patients to optimize treatment with CPAP

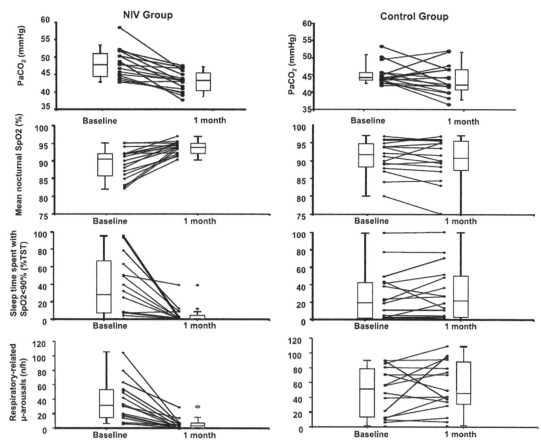

Fig. 1. Difference in gas exchange and sleep quality between NIV group and control group who received lifestyle advice only. $P<.05$, $P<.001$. (*From* Borel JC, Tamisier R, Gonzalez-Bermejo J, et al. Noninvasive ventilation in mild obesity hypoventilation syndrome: a randomized controlled trial. Chest 2011;141(3):698; with permission.)

or NIV when used in combination with home nocturnal monitoring. This approach could be used to validate the increasing prevalence of outpatient setup for such patients in Europe, albeit this would require prospective evaluation.

To support the approach of in-depth patient characterization to optimize the treatment delivered, there is evidence to show that sleep-disordered breathing is better controlled by strategies that guarantee delivery of nocturnal ventilation with either the use of a higher mandatory backup rate on the ventilator[14] or the use of pressure volume hybrid modes.[15] However, with the latter, there was initial concern that the variation in pressure delivery throughout the night would itself cause sleep disruption.[16] The early data investigating the relationship between guaranteed targeted volume pressure support ventilation and sleep quality employed target tidal volumes based on actual rather ideal body weight. This, therefore, resulted in target volumes and pressure support delivery well above the physiologic requirement, resulting in a not unexpected adverse effect on

sleep quality. Subsequent studies have, employing a more physiologic approach to ventilator setup, subsequently failed to show a difference in sleep quality.[17,18]

Daytime Gas Exchange

There is consistent demonstration of a sustained effect on daytime gas exchange from the use of nocturnal NIV with improvements in the partial pressure of oxygen (P_aO_2), partial pressure of carbon dioxide (P_aCO_2), and arterial bicarbonate concentration.[19–21] The improvements demonstrated from observational data have been confirmed from randomized controlled trial data showing that patients treated with NIV demonstrated a mean reduction of 0.7 kPa or 5.3 mm Hg (95% confidence interval [CI] 0.4–0.9 kPa; $P = .015$) in P_aCO_2, compared with patients receiving lifestyle advice, over the 1 month,[10] observational data have demonstrated greater improvements, with a change in P_aCO_2 on the order of 1.5 kPa or 11.4 mm Hg over the first 6 months of therapy.

Importantly, however, there is little further reduction with longer-term follow-up.[19,22] Of major importance, when evaluating success of the treatment in clinical practice, the baseline P_aCO_2 holds no relationship with long-term outcomes, whereas a reduction of greater than 23% in P_aCO_2 is associated with an improved prognosis.[23] Adherence to PAP therapy is essential to achieve these clinical outcomes. In obese patients with chronic respiratory failure secondary to OSA, OHS, or a combination of both, the current data available support a minimum adherence level of treatment of 4 hours per night to reduce P_aCO_2.[20,24] As expected, there is a dose response, with greater adherence associated with enhanced effects. One study showed NIV use of 4 hours per night NIV was associated with a 0.5 kPa or 3.8 mm Hg reduction in P_aCO_2 at 3 months.[18] In addition to the beneficial effects of long-term use of NIV to stabilize gas exchange, in selected patients, stability is maintained even with short periods of NIV withdrawal.[24] This has implications in the clinical setting, and clinicians can confidently reassure patients that in the event of machine failure in the home, the requirement to replace the device is important, but replacement need not necessarily be immediate. Of importance in the long-term management and follow-up of patients are the data showing the importance of reduction in daytime P_aCO_2 as an important measure of clinical efficacy. Not only does the reduction in daytime P_aCO_2 correlate with all of the other clinically significant outcomes such as health-related quality of life, but it also reflects improved prognosis.[18,23]

Pulmonary Function

It has been established that patients with obesity have an associated restrictive ventilatory defect, but it must also be acknowledged that there are other important adverse effects on pulmonary mechanics. In obesity, as the functional residual capacity (FRC) approaches residual volume (RV), there will be a subsequent increase mechanical work of breathing resulting in breathlessness.[25,26] The level of ventilatory restriction is potentially important to identify obese patients with sleep-disordered breathing and chronic respiratory failure. A recent study has shown that the simple measurements of forced vital capacity (FVC) and SpO_2 can predict chronic respiratory failure in obese patients with sleep-disordered breathing. Specifically, an FVC less than 3.5 L and a daytime clinic SpO_2 less than 95% in men and an FVC less than 2.3 L and an SpO_2 less than 93% in women predict a daytime P_aCO_2 above 6 kPa or 45 mm Hg.[27] In part, these changes are reversible, with

long-term treatment with NIV associated with improvements in the restrictive spirometric defect and static lung volumes, such as total lung capacity (TLC), FRC, and RV.[19,22]

Drive to Breathe

Although there are data suggesting the pivotal role of reduced respiratory drive in the pathophysiology of chronic respiratory failure in obese patients, there are conflicting data on the effect of NIV on measures of respiratory drive. Previous data have shown low levels of respiratory drive, as measured by pressure generation over the first 100 milliseconds ($P_{0.1}$) and HCVR, at initiation of treatment, with drive reaching levels comparable with eucapnic OSA following 1 month of therapy.[28] Furthermore, a small study in a subpopulation of patients with OHS but without OSA at diagnosis demonstrated an improvement in $P_{0.1}$ following NIV.[29] However, other studies have not shown a change in measures of respiratory drive, such $P_{0.1}$ and HCVR, following 3-month NIV withdrawal in patients who had been shown to have clinical stability following at least 1 year of NIV.[24] Other long-term observational data have also failed to demonstrate improvements in measures of respiratory drive following prolonged use of domiciliary NIV,[22] and further work is required to both clearly categorize the patients and also employ the advanced modes of measuring neural respiratory drive now available.[30]

Mortality

Both historic and contemporary data show that acute decompensated chronic respiratory failure in hospitalized OHS patients has a significant associated mortality.[31,32] Interestingly, less than half the mortality is reported to be related to hypoventilation, with a larger proportion of the deaths related to pulmonary emboli or other organ failure.[33] Following successful treatment of an acute decompensated episode of OHS, it has been demonstrated that there are concerning high levels of mortality, in excess of 50%, in those patients who declined NIV compared with less than 5% for those who accommodated NIV.[21] Furthermore, patients failing to receive NIV treatment at discharge following an acute presentation with an incidental admission finding of an elevated P_aCO_2 above 6 kPa or 45 mm Hg have an 18-month posthospital discharge mortality rate of 23%.[34] The long-term cohort studies of patients with OHS treated with NIV have reported low levels of mortality compared with these untreated cohorts (**Fig. 2**).[19,35]

Perhaps unsurprisingly, parameters such as more severe hypoxemia and markers of systemic

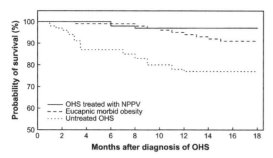

Fig. 2. Composite Kaplan-Meier plot of mortality in eucapnic obesity, untreated OHS and treated OHS. Survival curves for patients with untreated OHS (n = 47; mean age 55 ± 14 years; mean body mass index [BMI] 45 ± 9 kg/m²; mean P_aCO_2, 52 ± 7 mm Hg) and eucapnic, morbidly obese patients (n = 103; mean age 53 ± 13 years; mean BMI 42 ± 8 kg/m²) as reported by Nowbar and colleagues,[34] compared to patients with OHS treated with noninvasive positive pressure ventilation (NPPV) therapy (n = 126; mean age 55.6 ± 10.6 years; mean BMI 44.6 ± 7.8 kg/m²; mean P_aCO_2 55.5 ± 7.7 mm Hg; mean adherence with NPPV, 6.5 ± 2.3 h/d). Data for patients with OHS treated with NPPV were provided by Budweiser and colleagues.[23] (*From* Mokhlesi B, Kryger MH, Grunstein RR. Assessment and management of patients with obesity hypoventilation syndrome. Proc Am Thorac Soc 2008;5(2):221; with permission.)

inflammation (elevated c-reactive protein [CRP] and leukocytosis) are associated with a higher mortality in OHS.[23] Factors that would be expected to be improved by ameliorating sleep-disordered breathing and reversing respiratory failure such as polycythemia and $Paco_2$ are associated with improved prognosis, supporting the consensus that domiciliary PAP with either CPAP or NIV alters the natural history of OHS and reduces mortality.[23] Given the overwhelming observational and nonrandomized data for improved morbidity and mortality in OHS with PAP, long-term randomized controlled trials concerning efficacy are likely to be judged as unethical.

PATIENT-CENTERED OUTCOMES
Daytime Symptoms

There is currently only a single randomized controlled trial comparing CPAP and NIV in obese patients with chronic respiratory failure.[11] Entry criteria into this trial included a satisfactory single-night response to CPAP therapy in terms of maintaining oxygen saturations, which is important to highlight so that a comprehensive critique of the results can be undertaken. Thirty-six patients were randomized to CPAP or spontaneous-mode NIV for 3 months. Both groups had similar

anthropometric and physiologic phenotype in terms of severity of sleep-disordered breathing and impairment of gas exchange at baseline, although there was a nonsignificant gender imbalance between groups (CPAP 14M:4F vs NIV group 9M:9F; P = .09). Both groups showed similar improvements in weight reduction and daytime gas exchange over the trial period. There was no difference in daytime somnolence, as measured by the Epworth Sleepiness Score (ESS), between the groups (ESS CPAP group −6 ± 8 vs NIV group −9 ± 5; P = .21), but there was greater improvement in subjective sleep quality, as measured by the Pittsburgh Sleep Quality Index (PSQI), in the NIV group (PSQI CPAP group −2 ± 4 vs NIV group −6 ± 4; P = .013). The trial demonstrated the clinical efficacy of CPAP, compared with NIV, in the medium-term treatment of obese patients with chronic respiratory failure who have an adequate single-night response to CPAP, although these data lack generalizability. It is necessary to highlight that these data need to be fully interpreted so that the clinician does not consider CPAP as a useful treatment for all obese patients with chronic respiratory failure, as the patients in this trial had predominantly OSA without significant uncorrected hypoventilation. Those patients with OSA plus OHS or lone OHS phenotype were effectively excluded after failing the first-night CPAP assessment.

Data from nonrandomized trials have shown improvement in subjective sleepiness when using both CPAP and NIV in the appropriate selected target populations. However, data from the only randomized study, comparing NIV and lifestyle advice, failed to demonstrate an improvement in daytime somnolence in the NIV group.[10] This lack of response can be explained, in part, by the strong influence of the lifestyle advice as a placebo effect and also the relatively mild phenotype of patients who were recruited into the trial. One study has investigated the effects of NIV on objective markers of vigilance.[8] Specifically, Chouri-Pontarollo and colleagues[8] investigated the effect of NIV on subjective and objective somnolence in a group of 15 patients with OHS following 5 days of treatment. The study used the Oxford Sleep Resistance (OSLER) test as a measure of vigilance and also assessed HCVR, using the technique originally described by Read.[36] Interestingly, only the patients with a low HCVR had impairment of daytime vigilance at enrollment, and these patients had a subsequent significant improvement in vigilance following 5 days of treatment with NIV. Again, HCVR could be considered in future studies to stratify those patients most likely to benefit from the treatment.

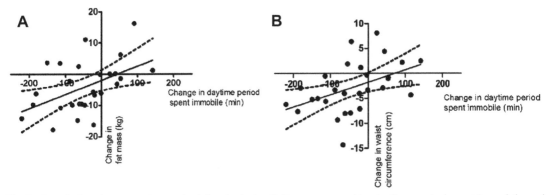

Fig. 3. Correlations between change in daily physical activity as measured by daytime period spent immobile and (*A*) change in fat mass (r = 0.48, P = .01) and (*B*) change in waist circumference (r = 0.46, P = .01).

Health-Related Quality of Life

Several generic and disease-specific health-related quality of life measures have been used to assess the disease burden in obese patients with chronic respiratory failure. Generic measures such as the 36-Item Short Form Health Survey (SF-36) have been used to demonstrate greater impairment in quality of life in patients with OHS compared with eucapnic obese OSA patients, eucapnic nonobese OSA patients, and age-matched controls.[37] Furthermore, treatment of such patients with CPAP led to significant improvements in the SF-36.[37] Similar levels of improvement in the SF-36 are observed in patients with OHS treated with either CPAP or NIV.[11] The severe respiratory insufficiency questionnaire (SRI) has been validated in patients with chronic respiratory failure in a number of languages.[38–40] The SRI has shown the quality of life to be impaired in patients with OHS, albeit less so than in patients with chronic respiratory failure associated with chronic obstructive pulmonary disease (COPD),[41] with improvements following treatment with NIV, either in standard or volume target modes.[15,18] Interestingly, unlike in chronic respiratory failure associated with COPD, the quality of life is a predictor of mortality.[41]

Physical Activity

Physical activity has a causal relationship with obesity (**Fig. 3**). Furthermore, physical activity has a relationship with sleep quality and severity of OSA, as evidenced by a trial that demonstrated that participation in an exercise program resulted in improvements in both objective sleep quality and severity of OSA when compared with a control group.[42] Of clinical relevance, NIV treatment for obesity-related chronic respiratory failure improved objective and subjective markers of physical activity, which are correlated with the magnitude of weight loss.[11,18] Interestingly, this association between physical activity and weight reduction has not been observed in eucapnic OSA patients treated with CPAP therapy, and indeed such patients neither lose weight nor increase their level of physical activity in response to CPAP treatment.[43] The role of obesity in the pathogenesis of chronic respiratory failure and the other adverse changes, such as insulin insensitivity and poor glucose control, is indicated by data that have shown weight loss in these patients is associated with improvements in metabolic outcomes and sleep-disordered breathing.[44,45] In 1 clinical trial, the magnitude of change in physical activity following 3 months of NIV treatment correlated with a change in total bodyweight, and of critical importance, the change in physical activity correlated with a change in fat mass, as measured by bioelectrical impedance, confirming that the change in body mass is not a consequence of simply managing fluid overload and cor pulmonale associated with chronic respiratory failure in obese patients.[18]

Augmenting physical activity provides a range of clinical benefits to these obese patients with chronic respiratory failure, but interestingly, the baseline exercise capacity at the time of initiation of NIV does not appear to relate to long-term prognosis.[46] Future work focusing on exercise therapy in addition to NIV treatment is required.

SUMMARY

This article highlighted the physiological-centered, clinician-centered, and patient-centered outcomes that clinicians must consider in the management of patients with chronic respiratory failure as a consequence of obesity. Indeed, one must be cognizant of the 3 different phenotypes of sleep-disordered breathing, including predominantly obstructive sleep apnea, lone obesity hypoventilation, and a combination of obstructive sleep apnea and obesity hypoventilation syndrome, as these will potentially warrant different treatment strategies. In the future, it is essential that clinical trials that will combine both patient-centered outcomes and health care utilization outcomes as the primary endpoints are initiated. In addition to understanding the physiologic effect of treatment, trials need to be designed that incorporate physical activity, weight reduction, and cost-effectiveness which in itself integrates health-related quality of life and cost.

REFERENCES

1. Auchincloss JH Jr, Cook E, Renzetti AD. Clinical and physiological aspects of a case of obesity, polycythemia and alveolar hypoventilation. J Clin Invest 1955;34(10):1537–45.
2. Burwell CS, Robin ED, Whaley RD, et al. Extreme obesity associated with alveolar hypoventilation; a Pickwickian syndrome. Am J Med 1956;21(5):811–8.
3. Abrahamsen AM, Nitter-Hauge S. Extreme obesity with respiratory failure, necessitating artificial ventilation. Acta Med Scand 1966;180(1):113–6.
4. Sullivan CE, Berthon-Jones M, Issa FG. Remission of severe obesity-hypoventilation syndrome after short-term treatment during sleep with nasal continuous positive airway pressure. Am Rev Respir Dis 1983;128(1):177–81.
5. Sleep-related breathing disorders in adults: recommendations for syndrome definition and measurement techniques in clinical research. The report of an American Academy of Sleep Medicine Task Force. Sleep 1999;22(5):667–89.
6. Kessler R, Chaouat A, Schinkewitch P, et al. The obesity-hypoventilation syndrome revisited: a prospective study of 34 consecutive cases. Chest 2001;120(2):369–76.
7. Banerjee D, Yee BJ, Piper AJ, et al. Obesity hypoventilation syndrome: hypoxemia during continuous positive airway pressure. Chest 2007;131(6):1678–84.
8. Chouri-Pontarollo N, Borel JC, Tamisier R, et al. Impaired objective daytime vigilance in obesity-hypoventilation syndrome: impact of noninvasive ventilation. Chest 2007;131(1):148–55.
9. Piper AJ, Sullivan CE. Effects of short-term NIPPV in the treatment of patients with severe obstructive sleep apnea and hypercapnia. Chest 1994;105(2):434–40.
10. Borel JC, Tamisier R, Gonzalez-Bermejo J, et al. Noninvasive ventilation in mild obesity hypoventilation syndrome: a randomized controlled trial. Chest 2011;141(3):692–702.
11. Piper AJ, Wang D, Yee BJ, et al. Randomised trial of CPAP vs bilevel support in the treatment of obesity hypoventilation syndrome without severe nocturnal desaturation. Thorax 2008;63(5):395–401.
12. Schafer H, Ewig S, Hasper E, et al. Failure of CPAP therapy in obstructive sleep apnoea syndrome: predictive factors and treatment with bilevel-positive airway pressure. Respir Med 1998;92(2):208–15.
13. Salord N, Mayos M, Miralda RM, et al. Continuous positive airway pressure in clinically stable patients with mild-to-moderate obesity-hypoventilation syndrome and obstructive sleep apnea. Respirology 2013;18(7):1135–42.
14. Contal O, Adler D, Borel JC, et al. Impact of different backup respiratory rates on the efficacy of noninvasive positive pressure ventilation in obesity hypoventilation syndrome: a randomized trial. Chest 2013;143(1):37–46.
15. Storre JH, Seuthe B, Fiechter R, et al. Average volume-assured pressure support in obesity hypoventilation: a randomized crossover trial. Chest 2006;130(3):815–21.
16. Janssens JP, Metzger M, Sforza E. Impact of volume targeting on efficacy of bi-level non-invasive ventilation and sleep in obesity-hypoventilation. Respir Med 2009;103(2):165–72.
17. Ambrogio C, Lowman X, Kuo M, et al. Sleep and non-invasive ventilation in patients with chronic respiratory insufficiency. Intensive Care Med 2009;35(2):306–13.
18. Murphy PB, Davidson C, Hind MD, et al. Volume targeted versus pressure support non-invasive ventilation in patients with super obesity and chronic respiratory failure: a randomised controlled trial. Thorax 2012;67(8):727–34.
19. Priou P, Hamel JF, Person C, et al. Long-term outcome of noninvasive positive pressure ventilation for obesity hypoventilation syndrome. Chest 2010;138(1):84–90.
20. Mokhlesi B, Tulaimat A, Evans AT, et al. Impact of adherence with positive airway pressure therapy on hypercapnia in obstructive sleep apnea. J Clin Sleep Med 2006;2(1):57–62.
21. Perez de Llano LA, Golpe R, Ortiz Piquer M, et al. Short-term and long-term effects of nasal intermittent positive pressure ventilation in patients with obesity-hypoventilation syndrome. Chest 2005;128(2):587–94.
22. Heinemann F, Budweiser S, Dobroschke J, et al. Non-invasive positive pressure ventilation improves lung volumes in the obesity hypoventilation syndrome. Respir Med 2007;101(6):1229–35.
23. Budweiser S, Riedl SG, Jorres RA, et al. Mortality and prognostic factors in patients with obesity-hypoventilation syndrome undergoing noninvasive ventilation. J Intern Med 2007;261(4):375–83.

24. De Miguel Diez J, De Lucas Ramos P, Perez Parra JJ, et al. Analysis of withdrawal from noninvasive mechanical ventilation in patients with obesity-hypoventilation syndrome. Medium term results. Arch Bronconeumol 2003;39(7):292–7.

25. Jones RL, Nzekwu MM. The effects of body mass index on lung volumes. Chest 2006;130(3):827–33.

26. Ofir D, Laveneziana P, Webb KA, et al. Ventilatory and perceptual responses to cycle exercise in obese women. J Appl Physiol (1985) 2007;102(6): 2217–26.

27. Mandal S, Suh ES, Boleat E, et al. A cohort study to identify simple clinical tests for chronic respiratory failure in obese patients with sleep disordered breathing. BMJ Open Resp Res 2014;1:e000022. http://dx.doi.org/10.1136/bmjresp-2014-000022.

28. Lin CC. Effect of nasal CPAP on ventilatory drive in normocapnic and hypercapnic patients with obstructive sleep apnoea syndrome. Eur Respir J 1994;7(11):2005–10.

29. Redolfi S, Corda L, La Piana G, et al. Long-term non-invasive ventilation increases chemosensitivity and leptin in obesity-hypoventilation syndrome. Respir Med 2007;101(6):1191–5.

30. Murphy PB, Kumar A, Reilly C, et al. Neural respiratory drive as a physiological biomarker to monitor change during acute exacerbations of COPD. Thorax 2011;66(7):602–8.

31. MacGregor MI, Block AJ, Ball WC Jr. Topics in clinical medicine: serious complications and sudden death in the Pickwickian syndrome. Johns Hopkins Med J 1970;126(5):279–95.

32. Marik PE, Desai H. Characteristics of patients with the "malignant obesity hypoventilation syndrome" admitted to an ICU. J Intensive Care Med 2013; 28(2):124–30.

33. Miller A, Granada M. In-hospital mortality in the Pickwickian syndrome. Am J Med Genet 1974;56: 144–50.

34. Nowbar S, Burkart KM, Gonzales R, et al. Obesity-associated hypoventilation in hospitalized patients: prevalence, effects, and outcome. Am J Med Genet 2004;116:1–7.

35. Budweiser S, Murbeth RE, Jorres RA, et al. Predictors of long-term survival in patients with restrictive thoracic disorders and chronic respiratory failure undergoing non-invasive home ventilation. Respirology 2007;12(4):551–9.

36. Read DJ. A clinical method for assessing the ventilatory response to carbon dioxide. Australas Ann Med 1967;16(1):20–32.

37. Hida W, Okabe S, Tatsumi K, et al. Nasal continuous positive airway pressure improves quality of life in obesity hypoventilation syndrome. Sleep Breath 2003;7(1):3–12.

38. Windisch W, Freidel K, Schucher B, et al. The severe respiratory insufficiency (SRI) questionnaire: a specific measure of health-related quality of life in patients receiving home mechanical ventilation. J Clin Epidemiol 2003;56(8):752–9.

39. Ghosh D, Rzehak P, Elliott MW, et al. Validation of the English severe respiratory insufficiency questionnaire. Eur Respir J 2012;40(2):408–15.

40. Lopez-Campos JL, Failde I, Masa JF, et al. Transculturally adapted Spanish SRI questionnaire for home mechanically ventilated patients was viable, valid, and reliable. J Clin Epidemiol 2008;61(10):1061–6.

41. Budweiser S, Hitzl AP, Jorres RA, et al. Health-related quality of life and long-term prognosis in chronic hypercapnic respiratory failure: a prospective survival analysis. Respir Res 2007;8:92.

42. Kline CE, Crowley EP, Ewing GB, et al. The effect of exercise training on obstructive sleep apnea and sleep quality: a randomized controlled trial. Sleep 2011;34(12):1631–40.

43. West SD, Kohler M, Nicoll DJ, et al. The effect of continuous positive airway pressure treatment on physical activity in patients with obstructive sleep apnoea: a randomised controlled trial. Sleep Med 2009;10(9):1056–8.

44. Anderson JW, Kendall CW, Jenkins DJ. Importance of weight management in type 2 diabetes: review with meta-analysis of clinical studies. J Am Coll Nutr 2003;22(5):331–9.

45. Sugerman HJ, Fairman RP, Sood RK, et al. Long-term effects of gastric surgery for treating respiratory insufficiency of obesity. Am J Clin Nutr 1992; 55(Suppl 2):597S–601S.

46. Budweiser S, Heidtkamp F, Jorres RA, et al. Predictive significance of the six-minute walk distance for long-term survival in chronic hypercapnic respiratory failure. Respiration 2008;75(4):418–26.

Non-PAP Treatment Modalities in Obesity-Hypoventilation Syndrome

Role of Exercise, Nonsurgical and Surgical Weight Reduction, Tracheostomy, Respiratory Stimulants, and Oxygen

CrossMark

Jean-Paul Janssens, MD[a],*, Jean-Christian Borel, PhD[b],
Jean-Louis Pepin, MD, PhD[c]

KEYWORDS

- Obesity-hypoventilation syndrome • Exercise • Bariatric surgery • Weight reduction
- Tracheostomy • Respiratory stimulants • Oxygen

KEY POINTS

- Although NIV is an efficient symptomatic treatment of OHS, a multidisciplinary management of OHS is important to maximize the impact of treatment as much as possible on the cause of OHS (ie, obesity).
- Rehabilitation programs offer the possibility of adapted exercise programs, increasing exercise capacity and decreasing dyspnea.
- Medical and supportive management of weight loss often has limited results, but bariatric surgery can induce significant weight loss in selected individuals, contributing to an improvement in AHI and hypoventilation.
- A few drugs have been shown to have a modest effect on respiratory drive in OHS, but their impact is marginal and no medication is presently recommended for the treatment of OHS.
- Long-term oxygen therapy must not be considered as an alternative to positive pressure therapy (CPAP or NIV), and may have deleterious effects.
- Oxygen supplementation may be indicated after optimal titration of NIV.

INTRODUCTION

Obesity hypoventilation syndrome (OHS) is preferably treated by noninvasive positive pressure ventilation (NIV). NIV improves obstructive sleep apnea hypopnea syndrome (OSAHS), which is frequently associated with OHS, and associated symptoms, and improves symptoms of hypercapnia, quality of sleep, daytime arterial blood gases (ABG), and probably survival. NIV does not, however, treat the underlying cause of OHS (ie, obesity). Furthermore, NIV may be poorly tolerated in a subset of patients, may fail because of poor adherence, and more importantly may not reduce

Conflict of Interest Statement: The authors have no conflict of interest regarding this article.
[a] Division of Pulmonary Diseases, Hôpital Cantonal, Geneva University Hospitals, 4-6 Rue Gabrielle-Perret-Gentil, Geneva 14 1211, Switzerland; [b] Research and Development Department, AGIR à dom, 15, chemin du Vieux Chêne, Meylan 38240, France; [c] Laboratoire EFCR, INSERM Unit N° 1042, Grenoble University Hospital, CHU de Grenoble, CS 10 217, 38043 Grenoble, Cedex 9, France
* Corresponding author.
E-mail address: jean-paul.janssens@hcuge.ch

Sleep Med Clin 9 (2014) 357–364
http://dx.doi.org/10.1016/j.jsmc.2014.05.013
1556-407X/14/$ – see front matter © 2014 Elsevier Inc. All rights reserved.

significantly the comorbidities associated with obesity.[1] Therefore exploring alternative (or complementary) options to NIV is important. Among these options, the contribution of exercise, surgical or nonsurgical weight reduction, tracheostomy, respiratory stimulants, and oxygen are discussed in this article (**Box 1**).

ROLE OF EXERCISE AND REHABILITATION PROGRAMS IN THE MANAGEMENT OF OHS

Although patients with OHS have a relatively preserved functional capacity (ie, performance during a 6-minute walk test) compared with patients with other causes of chronic respiratory failure treated with long-term NIV, their exercise tolerance is lower than that of obese eucapnic patients with OSAHS.[2,3] Little is known about daytime activity of patients with OHS. Murphy and colleagues[4] assessed daytime activity during the week following initiation of NIV in patients with OHS. Daytime activity improved significantly after 3 months of nocturnal NIV, but in a significant percentage of patients, NIV was initiated in acute conditions and the improvement in activity can also be interpreted as a return to baseline level of performance. The authors of the Murphy study hypothesized that there was a relationship between enhanced nocturnal ventilation and improvement in daytime symptoms, which in turn had a direct relationship with the observed increase in daytime physical activity. Conversely, in the only randomized

controlled trial available, West and colleagues,[5] found no increase in activity after 3 months of treatment with nocturnal continuous positive airway pressure (CPAP) in patients with OSAHS, despite improvements in daytime sleepiness. The hypothesis of a relationship between improved daytime symptoms and an increase in daytime physical activity is, however, supported by two earlier studies: in patients with hypercapnic chronic obstructive pulmonary disease (COPD), nocturnal NIV combined with pulmonary rehabilitation enhanced the benefits of pulmonary rehabilitation, reduced fatigue, and increased daily activity compared with rehabilitation alone.[6,7] Improvement in the perception of dyspnea and fatigue may be a key factor for improving daily activity: fatigue and dyspnea could be, for instance, a determinant of the reduction in time spent outdoors.[8]

Patients with OHS often have a very limited social activity; they also lack motivation regarding rehabilitation programs.[9,10] As mentioned, fatigue could contribute to this lack of motivation. Thus, although rehabilitation programs are likely to benefit patients with OHS, optimal modalities and timing for starting such programs must be determined to reinforce motivation, adherence, and long-term benefits. The onset of nocturnal NIV could be the appropriate time to start a rehabilitation program because nocturnal NIV itself may increase exercise tolerance.[11] Regarding modalities of exercise training, few data are available.[12,13] Exercise training in patients with OHS often requires expensive devices adapted to the increased weight load. Beyond these practical aspects, specific strategies may improve exercise training in OHS. For example, despite correction of diurnal $Paco_2$ after 3 months of nocturnal NIV, patients with OHS may continue to hypoventilate during exercise.[12] In this situation, NIV during exercise training may increase performance and efficacy of training.[14] Also, combining respiratory muscle training with a low-calorie diet and a physical activity program has been shown to induce a greater improvement in dyspnea and exercise capacity than physical activity and diet alone.[15] Finally, home-based neuromuscular electrical stimulation previously used in severely disabled patients with COPD might be of interest to allow morbidly obese patients to return to at least a minimal level of physical activity.

In summary, (1) rehabilitation programs are likely to benefit patients with OHS but this must be confirmed by well-designed randomized controlled trials; (2) the onset of nocturnal NIV could be the appropriate time to start a rehabilitation program; and (3) programs have to be

---

Box 1
Treatments for obesity-hypoventilation other than noninvasive positive pressure ventilation

- Rehabilitation programs are recommended for increasing exercise tolerance and daily activity

- The onset of nocturnal NIV could be the appropriate time to start a rehabilitation program

- Contrasting with medical and supportive management of weight loss, bariatric surgery induces more effective weight loss, improves sleep apnea indices and hypoventilation in subjects with OHS and OSAHS

- Respiratory stimulant drugs have a marginal impact in OHS and cannot be recommended

- Long-term oxygen therapy must not be considered as an alternative to positive pressure therapy but may be indicated after optimal titration of NIV for "resistant hypoxemia," although its long-term benefit has yet to be established through randomized trials.

adapted to improve motivation, adherence, and long-term benefits.

ROLE OF NONSURGICAL AND SURGICAL WEIGHT REDUCTION

Although weight loss is the obvious etiologic treatment of OHS, there are remarkably few studies addressing this issue in a strictly defined population of patients with OHS. Of course, inducing a significant weight loss is a major challenge for clinicians and patients. Inducing significant benefits on apnea-hypopnea index (AHI) and nocturnal or diurnal hypoventilation requires a substantial weight loss that is seldom obtained through medical and supportive treatment alone. This is well illustrated by the two following studies. In a prospective randomized controlled trial, Dobbin and colleagues[16] compared the results of medical treatment alone versus laparoscopic adjustable gastric banding (GB); endpoints were weight loss, health-related quality of life (HRQL), and sleep apnea indices. Patients with documented OHS and/or requiring NIV were excluded from this study. Sixty patients with a body mass index (BMI) between 35 and 55 kg/m^2 were included. Weight loss stabilized at 5.1 kg (95% confidence interval [CI], 0.8–9.3) for subjects under medical treatment versus 27.8 kg (95% CI, 20.9–34.7) for the surgical group. Decrease in AHI was substantially more important in the surgical group (25.5 events per hour; 95% CI, 14.2–36.7) than in the control group (14 events per hour; 95% CI, 3.3–24.6); HRQL also improved more significantly in the GB group. Another large observational multicentric nonrandomized study, performed in Sweden,[17] followed 4047 obese subjects, comparing the outcome of 2010 subjects who underwent bariatric surgery with that of 2037 receiving conventional therapy. Average follow-up was 10.9 years. Maximal weight loss was recorded after 1 to 2 years: −32 ± 8% versus baseline for Roux-en-Y gastric bypass (RYGBP), −25 ± 9% for vertical banded gastroplasty (VBG), and −20 ± 10% for GB. After 10 years, weight loss was −25 ± 11% for RYGBP, −16 ± 11% for VBG, and −14 ± 14% for GB. Subjects receiving conventional treatment maintained their weight within ±2% of baseline. There were 129 deaths in the conventional treatment group versus 101 in the surgery group. Most frequent causes of death were myocardial infarction and cancer. Globally, 23.8% of the "surgery" group versus 22.4% of the "conventional treatment" group had OSAHS. However, the study does not describe outcome of OSAHS or treatment of subjects with OSAHS. Furthermore, ABG and prevalence of OHS are not mentioned.

SURGICAL WEIGHT REDUCTION

There is a general consensus that obese subjects with a BMI greater than 40 kg/m^2 in whom dietary changes, medical therapy, and physical activity have failed or subjects with a BMI greater than 35 kg/m^2 and weight-related comorbidities (metabolic and/or respiratory comorbidities, atherosclerosis, hypertension, high low-density lipoprotein cholesterol, type II diabetes, hypoventilation, and/or OSAHS) are candidates for bariatric surgery. Contraindications for surgery vary from country to country, and include age (<18 or >60 years of age, although debated), unstabilized psychiatric disorders, compulsive nutritional disorders, alcohol abuse, and active smoking. Surgical procedures include VBG, adjustable GB, and RYGBP, and the "malabsorbative procedures" of biliopancreatic diversion and biliopancreatic diversion with duodenal switch. RYGBP is by far the most popular procedure in the United States and considered as the gold standard bariatric procedure with the best results in terms of long-term weight loss.[17] The mortality and morbidity associated with the procedure is low in expert centers: in a large Swedish study including 3412 patients who underwent an RYGBP, 30-day death rate was 0.3% and 4.3% of patients reported one major adverse outcome.[18]

A few studies describe the impact of bariatric surgery on OSAHS and OHS. In 1992, Sugerman and colleagues[19] analyzed the outcome of 126 patients with morbid obesity and respiratory failure (pickwickian syndrome). Sixteen (12.6%) had OHS without evidence of OSAHS, 65 (51.6%) had OSAHS, and 45 (35.7%) had OHS with OSAHS; all underwent bariatric surgery (several different procedures). BMI decreased from 56 ± 12 kg/m^2 (baseline) to 37 ± 8 kg/m^2 (after 1 year) and 38 ± 9 kg/m^2 (last visit). In 40 patients with presurgery and postsurgery polysomnograms, AHI decreased from 64 ± 39 events per hour (baseline) to 33 ± 27 events per hour (after 1 year) and 32 ± 32 events per hour (last visit). For patients for whom ABG was available, Paco$_2$ was as follows: at baseline, 53 ± 9 mm Hg; after 1 year, 44 ± 8 mm Hg; and at last visit, 47 ± 12 mm Hg. Of those with OHS, 38 were followed 5.8 ± 2.4 years after surgery; 29 (76%) became asymptomatic. The only treatment provided for OHS was CPAP: there is no mention of NIV either before or after surgery.

A descriptive, uncontrolled study by Boone and coworkers[20] included 35 obese patients with OSAS with or without OHS undergoing VBG. Use of CPAP decreased after VBG from 68% to 22%

of subjects studied. For patients with OSAS, AHI was 45 ± 11 events per hour at baseline and 12 ± 6 events per hour after surgery. Average $Paco_2$ decreased from 55 ± 4 to 41 ± 3 mm Hg after VBG.

Marti-Valeri and colleagues[21] followed 30 patients with morbid obesity and either CPAP or bilevel positive pressure ventilation (NIV) before and after bariatric surgery by RYGBP. After 1 year the authors noted a significant improvement of hypoxemia, hypercapnia (44.5 ± 5.7 mm Hg vs 40.6 ± 4.9 mm Hg), spirometry, and polysomnographic results. Treatment with positive airway pressure (CPAP or NIV) was required in only 14% of patients 1 year after surgery.

More recently, Lumachi and colleagues[22] described 11 obese subjects with a baseline average BMI of 52.3 kg/m^2, before and after laparoscopic RYGBP. Average weight loss was 39.6% of baseline value. Daytime oxygen saturation of hemoglobin estimated by pulsoximetry (Spo_2) improved markedly from 88.3 ± 3.9% at baseline to 96.2 ± 3.2% after maximal weight loss suggesting a marked improvement in alveolar ventilation. However, no data regarding $Paco_2$ or treatment of OHS or OSAS are provided.

Finally, an uncontrolled Italian study by De Cesare and colleagues[23] described 102 morbidly obese patients (range of BMI, 35–70.9 kg/m^2) undergoing "malabsorptive" biliodigestive surgery. Maximal weight loss occurred 12 to 24 months after surgery, and ranged from −45 to −64% of baseline after 3 to 5 years. Sixteen patients (15.7%) had OHS and 22 (21.7%) OSAHS. Postoperatively, no patient fulfilled criteria for OHS, and only two patients required CPAP for residual OSAS.

Bariatric surgery is associated with dramatic weight reduction but is also now considered as a "metabolic surgery," with a positive impact on control of hypertension and diabetes, and a decrease in morbidity and mortality.[24] In morbidly obese patients with OSAHS, in as much as NIV has a limited impact per se on cardiometabolic risk, bariatric surgery should be considered to address comorbidities.

In summary, although prospective randomized controlled studies are lacking, observational data clearly show that conventional medical treatment most often leads to at best a very modest weight loss; and bariatric surgery, when indicated, leads to substantial improvements in body weight and BMI, and improvements in AHI and alveolar ventilation, allowing in some cases (but not in all) interruption of CPAP or NIV. Clinicians must be aware of the time course of weight loss after bariatric surgery, with a maximal weight loss often reached 1 year after surgery and a possible relapse after a few years of follow-up. Also, objective measurements are important (ABG, sleep studies) because symptomatic improvements may not necessarily be corroborated by normalization of AHI or ABG. Because many patients demonstrate a reduction in AHI but still have a significant residual OSAHS, a frequently used option is a shift from NIV to CPAP, which is probably easier to tolerate and to set-up.

TRACHEOSTOMY IN OHS

Patients with OHS represent an increasing proportion of subjects treated by long-term home ventilation.[25–27] Although tracheostomy was the treatment of choice for patients with the pickwickian syndrome and severe upper airway obstruction before the report by Sullivan and colleagues[28] of successful management of OHS with nasal CPAP, tracheostomy in OHS has become exceptional since the advent of CPAP and NIV and is seldom reported. In Europe and the United States, home mechanical ventilation via tracheostomy concerns a small proportion of patients under home mechanical ventilation,[27,29–31] mainly pediatric and adult patients with primary or posttraumatic neuromuscular disorders[30,32–34] and to a lesser degree COPD.[31] Tracheostomy in patients with class III obesity (BMI>40 kg/m^2) is furthermore complicated by excess of subcutaneous tissue between the skin and the trachea. In our experience, patients with OHS who require a tracheostomy during an acute exacerbation are most often successfully weaned from their tracheostomy and shifted to NIV after a few weeks or months. There are, to the best of our knowledge, no recently published descriptions of patients with OHS under long-term home ventilation via tracheostomy, and invasive ventilation for this indication is anecdotal.

RESPIRATORY STIMULANTS FOR THE TREATMENT OF OHS

Certain pharmacologic agents have been considered as possible adjuncts or alternatives to treatment by CPAP or NIV in patients with OSAHS or OHS. Among these are doxapram hydrochloride, aminophylline and theophylline, medroxyprogesterone, and protryptiline. Doxapram led to anecdotic case reports in the late 1970s for chronic alveolar hypoventilation.[35] Before the CPAP and NIV era, medroxyprogesterone was tested for 1 month in 10 patients with the pickwickian syndrome and improved ABG, alveolar ventilation, and symptoms of cor pulmonale. A withdrawal and reinstitution of medroxyprogesterone supported its' role in these improvements.[36] No recent study has reproduced these results. A Cochrane review of 26 trials measuring the impact of 21 drugs on respiratory drive and OSAHS including acetazolamide, medroxyprogesterone, aminophylline, theophylline, protryptiline, and paroxetine concluded that there was insufficient evidence to recommend drug therapy as a treatment of OSAHS.[37] More recently, aminophylline was shown to increase minute ventilation, tidal volume (V_T), respiratory rate, and diaphragm contractility in awake canines,[38] and to increase minute ventilation, V_T, respiratory rate, and parasternal intercostal muscle activity (electromyogram) during hypoxia in humans,[39] confirming earlier studies of the impact of methylxanthines on respiratory drive.[40,41] The clinical relevance of these findings in the treatment of OHS remains undetermined.

Raurich and coworkers[42] showed that a high bicarbonate (HCO_3) blood content was associated with a blunted ventilatory response to CO_2 and a decreased occlusion pressure ($P_{0.1}$; another estimation of respiratory drive) in eight patients with OHS while on invasive mechanical ventilation. Acetazolamide reduced HCO_3 concentration by 8.4 ± 3.0 mmol/L, and increased ventilatory response to CO_2. Thus, acetazolamide may increase ventilatory drive in subjects with a high HCO_3 level but not enough to treat OHS.[43]

To conclude, impact of drugs, such as acetazolamide, methylxanthines, or medroxyprogesterone, on ABG and ventilatory drive in OHS has been documented, but none of these drugs are presently recommended as first- or second-line treatment of OHS because of the lack of appropriate clinical studies and their marginal impact.

LONG-TERM OXYGEN THERAPY FOR OHS

Hypoxemia results from two different mechanisms in OHS: alveolar hypoventilation, which by definition is associated with hypercapnia; and ventilation/perfusion (V/Q) mismatch, which may aggravate the consequences of alveolar hypoventilation on PaO_2 and SaO_2. OHS is most often associated with OSAHS. Alveolar hypoventilation results from a combination of factors, such as increased work of breathing, a possible decrease in the performance of inspiratory muscles (strength, endurance), decreased compliance of the respiratory system, and changes in ventilatory drive.[44] V/Q mismatch results from changes in lung volumes (mainly decreased functional residual capacity [FRC]) and thus a decrease in the difference between closing volume (CV) and FRC (Δ[FRC-CV]). During spontaneous breathing in the supine position, obese subjects breathe partially in their CV (ie, a variable proportion of alveoli do not expand during V_T breathing). These units, with a low V/Q ratio, cause hypoxemia through venous admixture (ie, a shunt effect). NIV and CPAP improve alveolar ventilation, either by unloading the respiratory muscles and resetting ventilatory response to CO_2 (NIV), or by decreasing upper airway resistance (related to OSAHS) and thus work of breathing (CPAP and NIV).[45–49] Both approaches improve hypoxemia and reduce V/Q mismatch by increasing FRC, and therefore Δ(FRC-CV).[46] Residual hypoxemia under CPAP[50] or NIV is, however, well described[48,51–53] and necessity of supplemental oxygen is actually an independent predictor of mortality in patients with OHS under NIV.[2,49] Recent best clinical practices recommendations for subjects with chronic alveolar hypoventilation and NIV recommend supplementation with oxygen in patients with an awake SpO_2 less than 88% or when pressure support and respiratory rate have been optimized but SpO_2 remains less than 90% for 5 minutes or more.[54] These recommendations are, however, based on expert opinion and do not stem from randomized clinical trials.

There is no clear rationale for long-term oxygen therapy (LTOT) without either CPAP or NIV in OHS, because LTOT does not decrease work of breathing and thus does not improve alveolar ventilation, has no effect on V/Q mismatch and alveolar recruitment, and may prolong obstructive hypopnea or apnea.[53] Indeed, impact of LTOT alone has never been studied in patients with OHS. Moreover, OHS has never been viewed as an indication for LTOT in large cohorts of patients with chronic respiratory failure. This contrasts with recently published data by Carrillo and colleagues[55] reporting that 39% of patients with OHS admitted to an intensive care unit for acute hypercapnic respiratory failure were in fact previously treated with domiciliary oxygen therapy, whereas only 9% were under NIV. This suggests that the relevance of LTOT in OHS remains unclear for many clinicians in routine practice.

Oxygen therapy may in fact have a deleterious impact in OHS. A high inspired fraction of oxygen (100%) has been shown to increase transcutaneous CO_2 values and dead space to V_T ratio (V_D/V_T) while decreasing minute ventilation in subjects with OHS.[56] Short-term (20 minutes) O_2 supplementation during wakefulness worsened hypoventilation and acidemia in patients with OHS even with moderate O_2 concentrations (28%–50%).[57] In an earlier observation by Masa and colleagues,[58] 11 obese patients

(42.9 ± 8 kg/m^2) with nocturnal hypoventilation (mean PtcCO$_2$, 52 ± 10 mm Hg) were treated sequentially by home nocturnal oxygen supplementation for 15 nights followed by an equivalent period with nocturnal NIV. Oxygen tended to worsen nocturnal hypoventilation, aggravated morning headaches and morning obtundation, and decreased sleep efficiency compared with room air or NIV. Thus, even in the absence of randomized clinical trials, the limited available evidence shows that LTOT alone is inappropriate in OHS as single therapy.

Reports suggest that up to 69% of patients with OHS receive supplemental nocturnal oxygen with their CPAP or NIV. Thus, supplemental oxygen is often added to NIV in patients who do not necessarily qualify for LTOT (based on daytime ABG) but who exhibit persistent nocturnal desaturation despite positive pressure therapy; several arbitrarily thresholds of oxygen desaturation are reported in the literature.

In summary, (1) oxygen therapy (nocturnal and/or diurnal) without CPAP or NIV is not recommended in patients with stable OHS; (2) current evidence does not clearly support the prescription of supplemental oxygen during adequately titrated nocturnal positive pressure therapy in patients with persistent desaturation who are not eligible for LTOT based on their daytime ABG (Pao$_2$ <7.3 kPa/55 mm Hg or <8 kPa/60 mm Hg with pulmonary hypertension, signs of cor pulmonale, or right heart failure); and (3) in patients with severe chronic hypoxemia, supplemental oxygen is needed but its titration must be performed with caution.

SUMMARY

Although NIV is an efficient symptomatic treatment of OHS, a multidisciplinary management of OHS is important to maximize the impact of treatment as much as possible on the cause of OHS: obesity. Rehabilitation programs offer the possibility of adapted exercise programs, increasing exercise capacity, and decreasing dyspnea. Medical and supportive management of weight loss often has limited results, but bariatric surgery can induce significant weight loss in selected individuals, contributing to an improvement in AHI and hypoventilation. A few drugs have been shown to have a modest effect on respiratory drive in OHS, but their impact is marginal and no medication is presently recommended for the treatment of OHS. LTOT must not be considered as an alternative to positive pressure therapy (CPAP or NIV), and may have deleterious effects. However, oxygen supplementation may be indicated after optimal titration of NIV. The benefit in terms of survival, HRQL, and prevention of secondary pulmonary hypertension of nocturnal oxygen supplementation for patients having a daytime Pao$_2$ higher than 8 kPa (60 mm Hg) has yet to be established through randomized trials.

REFERENCES

1. Borel JC, Burel B, Tamisier R, et al. Comorbidities and mortality in hypercapnic obese under domiciliary noninvasive ventilation. PLoS One 2013;8(1): e52006.
2. Budweiser S, Heidtkamp F, Jorres RA, et al. Predictive significance of the six-minute walk distance for long-term survival in chronic hypercapnic respiratory failure. Respiration 2008;75(4):418–26.
3. Gungor G, Karakurt Z, Adiguzel N, et al. The 6-minute walk test in chronic respiratory failure: does observed or predicted walk distance better reflect patient functional status? Respir Care 2013;58(5): 850–7.
4. Murphy PB, Davidson C, Hind MD, et al. Volume targeted versus pressure support non-invasive ventilation in patients with super obesity and chronic respiratory failure: a randomised controlled trial. Thorax 2012;67(8):727–34.
5. West SD, Kohler M, Nicoll DJ, et al. The effect of continuous positive airway pressure treatment on physical activity in patients with obstructive sleep apnoea: a randomised controlled trial. Sleep Med 2009;10(9):1056–8.
6. Duiverman ML, Wempe JB, Bladder G, et al. Nocturnal non-invasive ventilation in addition to rehabilitation in hypercapnic patients with COPD. Thorax 2008;63(12):1052–7.
7. Garrod R, Mikelsons C, Paul EA, et al. Randomized controlled trial of domiciliary noninvasive positive pressure ventilation and physical training in severe chronic obstructive pulmonary disease. Am J Respir Crit Care Med 2000;162(4 Pt 1):1335–41.
8. Baghai-Ravary R, Quint JK, Goldring JJ, et al. Determinants and impact of fatigue in patients with chronic obstructive pulmonary disease. Respir Med 2009;103(2):216–23.
9. Jennum P, Kjellberg J. Health, social and economical consequences of sleep-disordered breathing: a controlled national study. Thorax 2011;66(7): 560–6.
10. Jordan KE, Ali M, Shneerson JM. Attitudes of patients towards a hospital-based rehabilitation service for obesity hypoventilation syndrome. Thorax 2009;64(11):1007.
11. Holland AE, Wadell K, Spruit MA. How to adapt the pulmonary rehabilitation programme to patients with chronic respiratory disease other than COPD. Eur Respir Rev 2013;22(130):577–86.

12. Schonhofer B, Rosenbluh J, Voshaar T, et al. Ergometry separates sleep apnea syndrome from obesity-hypoventilation after therapy positive pressure ventilation therapy. Pneumologie 1997;51(12): 1115–9 [in German].

13. Spruit MA, Singh SJ, Garvey C, et al. An official American Thoracic Society/European Respiratory Society statement: key concepts and advances in pulmonary rehabilitation. Am J Respir Crit Care Med 2013;188(8):e13–64.

14. Dreher M, Kabitz HJ, Burgardt V, et al. Proportional assist ventilation improves exercise capacity in patients with obesity. Respiration 2010;80(2): 106–11.

15. Villiot-Danger JC, Villiot-Danger E, Borel JC, et al. Respiratory muscle endurance training in obese patients. Int J Obes (Lond) 2011;35(5):692–9.

16. Dobbin CJ, Milross MA, Piper AJ, et al. Sequential use of oxygen and bi-level ventilation for respiratory failure in cystic fibrosis. J Cyst Fibros 2004; 3(4):237–42.

17. Sjostrom L, Narbro K, Sjostrom CD, et al. Effects of bariatric surgery on mortality in Swedish obese subjects. N Engl J Med 2007;357(8):741–52.

18. Flum DR, Belle SH, King WC, et al. Perioperative safety in the longitudinal assessment of bariatric surgery. N Engl J Med 2009;361(5):445–54.

19. Sugerman HJ, Fairman RP, Sood RK, et al. Long-term effects of gastric surgery for treating respiratory insufficiency of obesity. Am J Clin Nutr 1992; 55(Suppl 2):597S–601S.

20. Boone KA, Cullen JJ, Mason EE, et al. Impact of vertical banded gastroplasty on respiratory insufficiency of severe obesity. Obes Surg 1996;6(6): 454–8.

21. Marti-Valeri C, Sabate A, Masdevall C, et al. Improvement of associated respiratory problems in morbidly obese patients after open Roux-en-Y gastric bypass. Obes Surg 2007;17(8):1102–10.

22. Lumachi F, Marzano B, Fanti G, et al. Hypoxemia and hypoventilation syndrome improvement after laparoscopic bariatric surgery in patients with morbid obesity. In Vivo 2010;24(3):329–31.

23. De Cesare A, Cangemi B, Fiori E, et al. Early and long-term clinical outcomes of bilio-intestinal diversion in morbidly obese patients. Surg Today 2014. Feb 12. [Epub ahead of print].

24. Ashrafian H, le Roux CW, Rowland SP, et al. Metabolic surgery and obstructive sleep apnoea: the protective effects of bariatric procedures. Thorax 2012;67(5):442–9.

25. Chiner E, Llombart M, Martinez-Garcia MA, et al. Noninvasive mechanical ventilation in Valencia, Spain: from theory to practice. Arch Bronconeumol 2009;45(3):118–22 [in Spanish].

26. Janssens JP, Derivaz S, Breitenstein E, et al. Changing patterns in long-term noninvasive ventilation: a 7-year prospective study in the Geneva Lake area. Chest 2003;123(1):67–79.

27. Laub M, Midgren B. Survival of patients on home mechanical ventilation: a nationwide prospective study. Respir Med 2007;101(6):1074–8.

28. Sullivan CE, Issa FG, Berthon-Jones M, et al. Reversal of obstructive sleep apnoea by continuous positive airway pressure applied through the nares. Lancet 1981;1(8225):862–5.

29. Chatwin M, Heather S, Hanak A, et al. Analysis of home support and ventilator malfunction in 1,211 ventilator-dependent patients. Eur Respir J 2010; 35(2):310–6.

30. Lloyd-Owen SJ, Donaldson GC, Ambrosino N, et al. Patterns of home mechanical ventilation use in Europe: results from the Eurovent survey. Eur Respir J 2005;25(6):1025–31.

31. Marchese S, Lo Coco D, Lo Coco A. Outcome and attitudes toward home tracheostomy ventilation of consecutive patients: a 10-year experience. Respir Med 2008;102(3):430–6.

32. Divo MJ, Murray S, Cortopassi F, et al. Prolonged mechanical ventilation in Massachusetts: the 2006 prevalence survey. Respir Care 2010; 55(12):1693–8.

33. Kamm M, Burger R, Rimensberger P, et al. Survey of children supported by long-term mechanical ventilation in Switzerland. Swiss Med Wkly 2001; 131(19–20):261–6.

34. Unroe M, Kahn JM, Carson SS, et al. One-year trajectories of care and resource utilization for recipients of prolonged mechanical ventilation: a cohort study. Ann Intern Med 2010;153(3):167–75.

35. Houser WC, Schlueter DP. Prolonged doxapram infusion in obesity-hypoventilation syndrome. JAMA 1978;239(4):340–1.

36. Sutton FD Jr, Zwillich CW, Creagh CE, et al. Progesterone for outpatient treatment of Pickwickian syndrome. Ann Intern Med 1975;83(4):476–9.

37. Smith I, Lasserson TJ, Wright J. Drug therapy for obstructive sleep apnoea in adults. Cochrane Database Syst Rev 2006;(2):CD003002.

38. Jagers JV, Hawes HG, Easton PA. Aminophylline increases ventilation and diaphragm contractility in awake canines. Respir Physiol Neurobiol 2009; 167(3):273–80.

39. Nishii Y, Okada Y, Yokoba M, et al. Aminophylline increases parasternal intercostal muscle activity during hypoxia in humans. Respir Physiol Neurobiol 2008;161(1):69–75.

40. Gorini M, Duranti R, Misuri G, et al. Aminophylline and respiratory muscle interaction in normal humans. Am J Respir Crit Care Med 1994;149(5):1227–34.

41. Javaheri S, Guerra L. Lung function, hypoxic and hypercapnic ventilatory responses, and respiratory muscle strength in normal subjects taking oral theophylline. Thorax 1990;45(10):743–7.

42. Raurich JM, Rialp G, Ibanez J, et al. Hypercapnic respiratory failure in obesity-hypoventilation syndrome: CO(2) response and acetazolamide treatment effects. Respir Care 2010;55(11):1442–8.

43. Powers MA. Obesity hypoventilation syndrome: bicarbonate concentration and acetazolamide. Respir Care 2010;55(11):1504–5.

44. Chouri-Pontarollo N, Borel JC, Tamisier R, et al. Impaired objective daytime vigilance in obesity-hypoventilation syndrome: impact of noninvasive ventilation. Chest 2007;131(1):148–55.

45. Borel JC, Tamisier R, Gonzalez-Bermejo J, et al. Noninvasive ventilation in mild obesity hypoventilation syndrome: a randomized controlled trial. Chest 2012;141(3):692–702.

46. Heinemann F, Budweiser S, Dobroschke J, et al. Non-invasive positive pressure ventilation improves lung volumes in the obesity hypoventilation syndrome. Respir Med 2007;101(6):1229–35.

47. Masa JF, Celli BR, Riesco JA, et al. The obesity hypoventilation syndrome can be treated with noninvasive mechanical ventilation. Chest 2001;119(4): 1102–7.

48. Perez de Llano LA, Golpe R, Ortiz Piquer M, et al. Short-term and long-term effects of nasal intermittent positive pressure ventilation in patients with obesity-hypoventilation syndrome. Chest 2005; 128(2):587–94.

49. Priou P, Hamel JF, Person C, et al. Long-term outcome of noninvasive positive pressure ventilation for obesity hypoventilation syndrome. Chest 2010;138(1):84–90.

50. Mokhlesi B. Positive airway pressure titration in obesity hypoventilation syndrome: continuous positive airway pressure or bilevel positive airway pressure. Chest 2007;131(6):1624–6.

51. Banerjee D, Yee BJ, Piper AJ, et al. Obesity hypoventilation syndrome: hypoxemia during continuous positive airway pressure. Chest 2007;131(6): 1678–84.

52. Cuvelier A, Muir JF. Acute and chronic respiratory failure in patients with obesity-hypoventilation syndrome: a new challenge for noninvasive ventilation. Chest 2005;128(2):483–5.

53. Mokhlesi B, Tulaimat A, Parthasarathy S. Oxygen for obesity hypoventilation syndrome: a double-edged sword? Chest 2011;139(5):975–7.

54. Berry RB, Chediak A, Brown LK, et al. Best clinical practices for the sleep center adjustment of noninvasive positive pressure ventilation (NPPV) in stable chronic alveolar hypoventilation syndromes. J Clin Sleep Med 2010;6(5):491–509.

55. Carrillo A, Ferrer M, Gonzalez-Diaz G, et al. Noninvasive ventilation in acute hypercapnic respiratory failure caused by obesity hypoventilation syndrome and chronic obstructive pulmonary disease. Am J Respir Crit Care Med 2012;186(12): 1279–85.

56. Wijesinghe M, Williams M, Perrin K, et al. The effect of supplemental oxygen on hypercapnia in subjects with obesity-associated hypoventilation: a randomized, crossover, clinical study. Chest 2011;139(5):1018–24.

57. Hollier CA, Harmer AR, Maxwell LJ, et al. Moderate concentrations of supplemental oxygen worsen hypercapnia in obesity hypoventilation syndrome: a randomised crossover study. Thorax 2014;69(4): 346–53.

58. Masa JF, Celli BR, Riesco JA, et al. Noninvasive positive pressure ventilation and not oxygen may prevent overt ventilatory failure in patients with chest wall diseases. Chest 1997;112(1):207–13.

Pulmonary Overlap Syndromes, with a Focus on COPD and ILD

Katherine A. Dudley, MD[a], Robert L. Owens, MD[b,*], Atul Malhotra, MD[c]

KEYWORDS

- Overlap syndrome • Sleep • Chronic obstructive pulmonary disease • Idiopathic pulmonary fibrosis
- Obstructive sleep apnea

KEY POINTS

- Overlap syndrome refers to the coexistence of chronic lung disease and obstructive sleep apnea (OSA) in the same patient. To date, overlap syndromes have been poorly studied for a variety of reasons.
- One difficulty is that each of the underlying disorders in an overlap syndrome occurs along a spectrum of disease severity. Thus, patients with an overlap syndrome are heterogeneous, and the goals of therapy may differ in different patients.
- However, the importance of overlap syndromes is highlighted by recent data demonstrating increased morbidity and mortality in patients with the overlap of both chronic obstructive pulmonary disease (COPD) and OSA compared with either underlying disorder alone.
- Unrecognized OSA may also contribute to symptoms of sleepiness/fatigue in patients with chronic lung disease. Clinicians should be mindful of the possibility of overlap syndromes in these patients.

First described in the 1980s by pulmonologist David Flenley,[1] *overlap* syndromes (OVSs) refer to the coexistence of chronic lung disease and obstructive sleep apnea (OSA). Although it could refer to any of the lung diseases and OSA, *the* OVS is usually reserved for the coexistence of OSA and chronic obstructive pulmonary disease (COPD), which Flenley thought to have unique adverse health consequences distinct from either condition alone. Given the high prevalence of each disorder alone, OVS is also likely to be common and clinically relevant. However, although OVS has been described in the literature for nearly 30 years, the lack of standard diagnostic criteria for the syndrome has limited rigorous discussion of diagnosis, prevalence, pathophysiology, treatment,

and outcomes. These challenges are explored in more detail later and throughout this review. Importantly, several recent studies suggest that OVS does, as Flenley thought, have worse outcomes than either disease in isolation. These findings have highlighted the urgent need for further study of both *the* OVS and all overlaps between OSA and chronic lung disease.

CLINICAL AND RESEARCH CHALLENGES OF THE OVS

OVSs are poorly understood for many reasons. Using *the* OVS as a prototype:

1. The diagnosis of OVS is nebulous, as both OSA and COPD are heterogeneous disorders.

a Harvard Combined Program of Pulmonary and Critical Care and Division of Sleep and Circadian Disorders at Brigham and Women's Hospital, 221 Longwood Avenue, Boston, MA 02115, USA; b Divisions of Pulmonary and Critical Care and Sleep and Circadian Disorders, Brigham and Women's Hospital, 221 Longwood Avenue, Boston, MA 02115, USA; c University of California, San Diego, San Diego, CA
* Corresponding author.
E-mail address: rowens@partners.org

Sleep Med Clin 9 (2014) 365–379
http://dx.doi.org/10.1016/j.jsmc.2014.05.008
1556-407X/14/$ – see front matter © 2014 Elsevier Inc. All rights reserved.

COPD and OSA both have wide ranges of severity, in terms of both objective measurements of disease (eg, forced expiratory volume in 1 second [FEV_1], and apnea-hypopnea index [AHI]) and patient-reported symptoms (eg, dyspnea and daytime tiredness). OVS is defined by the presence of both conditions regardless of the relative burden of one or the other. Therefore, patients with OVS may represent a very heterogeneous population, falling into one of many potential categories: mild COPD with mild OSA, mild COPD with severe OSA, severe COPD with mild OSA, severe COPD with severe OSA, and so forth. Prognosis and treatment, therefore, could be considerably different depending on the relative impact of each condition. Although it is a minor point, there is not a single *International Classification of Diseases, Ninth Revision* code for OVS, which impedes even epidemiologic research.

2. The diagnosis of OSA in the setting of hypoxemic lung disease is uncertain. The definition of OSA includes hypopneas and reductions in airflow with associated desaturation, which is more likely to occur in those with chronic lung disease. The AHI, used to grade OSA severity, does not differentiate between apneas and hypopneas. Thus, a patient with severe COPD might have the same AHI consistent with severe OSA (based on a large number of hypopneas) as another patient with a very collapsible upper airway without lung disease (who predominantly has apneas). In addition, a 10-minute prolonged desaturation caused by hypoventilation may be scored as a single hypopnea because the event duration has minimal effect on the definitions used. More rigorous definitions of OSA might be useful, such as the apnea index or scoring based on airflow alone and arousals independent of oxygen desaturation.

3. The interactions of COPD and OSA are not understood. Thus, it is unknown at a pathophysiologic level whether each disorder might predispose to the other disease. As discussed earlier, the baseline hypoxemia of COPD likely predisposes to a diagnosis of OSA. But other links are possible; for example, the changes in lung volumes that occur with COPD might impact upper airway collapsibility. How COPD and OSA interact to cause the increased morbidity and mortality attributable to OVS is not known. Is it simply from more prolonged hypoxemia or hypercapnia than either disorder alone? Or are poor outcomes caused by the indirect effects of the disorders, such as cardiovascular disease?

4. Thus, the goals of therapy in OVS are poorly defined. For a patient with severe OSA with many apneas, the goal of therapy may be to support patency of the upper airway and eliminate apneic events. For a patient with evidence of hypoventilation, the goal may be to improve nocturnal gas exchange and hypercarbia. Maybe the best approach would be intensive modification of cardiovascular risk factors (eg, blood pressure, cholesterol modification). These uncertainties contribute to the confusion as to the ideal therapy to use.

5. The optimal treatment of OVS is unknown. Few large clinical trials have been undertaken, and no large studies have compared long-term outcomes between randomized therapies. Although continuous positive airway pressure (CPAP) is the most commonly applied therapy, some groups have used bilevel positive airway pressure, which provides a higher pressure during inspiration than during expiration. Bilevel may have benefits over CPAP for some patients, particularly among patients with severe COPD whereby it may aid with nocturnal ventilation and resting of respiratory muscles. Finally, the role of oxygen therapy, another treatment used clinically, has not been fully explored in this population. The role of medical therapy aimed at limiting cardiovascular events has also not been explored.

6. An additional under-recognized consideration is that sleep is poor in chronic lung diseases, independent of upper airway collapse. Many studies have highlighted the high prevalence of sleep complaints among patients with chronic lung diseases. There are many reasons behind this finding, ranging from cough interfering with sleep, increased anxiety and insomnia, side effects of medications (eg, chronic glucocorticoids, beta agonists), and frequent arousals. Although treatment of OVS with CPAP may improve upper airway patency, CPAP will not address many of the nonrespiratory problems that plague sleep in this population. Thus, CPAP adherence may be challenged in ways that are unique compared with those without chronic lung disease.

These points are illustrated as the authors discuss what is known about OVSs, focusing on OSA and idiopathic pulmonary fibrosis (IPF), perhaps the most common of the interstitial lung diseases (ILDs).

COPD AND OSA

Throughout this section, *OVS* refers exclusively to those with COPD and OSA.

COPD

COPD is a progressive lung disease characterized by irreversible airway obstruction (FEV_1/forced vital capacity [FVC]<70%). This disease can involve the small airways, pulmonary parenchyma, or both. COPD results from an inflammatory response that can result in chronic sputum production (chronic bronchitis) as well as the destruction of alveolar walls distal to the terminal bronchioles, leading to enlargement of the airspaces (emphysema). Although tobacco use is strongly associated with the development of COPD, it is not the only risk factor. In developing countries, exposure to indoor air pollution plays a critical role, in particular as a result of fuels burned for cooking and heating. Occupational causes are also well described, such as irritants and fumes. Estimates are now that most COPD worldwide is non–smoking related, emphasizing caution about labeling the disease as self-inflicted. COPD may present as dyspnea, wheezing, cough, sputum production, poor exercise tolerance, hypoxic and/or hypercarbic respiratory failure, and right heart failure (cor pulmonale). There are Global Initiative for Chronic Obstructive Lung Disease (GOLD)–defined stages of disease severity based on pulmonary function testing (the FEV_1) and symptoms. In the United States, more than 5% of the population (at least 13.7 million people) is burdened by COPD,[2,3] which is a leading cause of morbidity. Worldwide, about 10% of the population is affected.[4] Although medications may improve symptomatic control of the disease and slow progression, the health-related consequences of COPD remain high.[3] As of 2011, COPD was the third leading cause of death in the United States.[5] Annual expenditures for the disease are approaching $40 billion when direct and indirect costs are considered.[6]

Although COPD is often considered a respiratory condition, the impact on other organ systems and overall health is increasingly well recognized. The most recent GOLD definition of the disease highlights COPD as a systemic process with "significant extrapulmonary effects that may contribute to the severity in individual patients."[7] Indeed, depression, skeletal-muscle myopathy, anemia, and osteoporosis are all common in COPD. Similarly, as is discussed later, sleep disturbance and its consequences could be thought of as one of these extrapulmonary manifestations. COPD is also associated with adverse cardiac outcomes, which may be of particularly importance when thinking about the overlap with OSA, which also has cardiovascular consequences.[8–12] Even after consideration of shared risk factors, such as cigarette smoking, COPD is associated with higher rates of coronary artery disease, congestive heart failure, and arrhythmias.[13,14] Additional mechanisms by which COPD may play a role in cardiovascular disease include increased oxidative stress, inflammation, and increased platelet activation.

Of particular interest in the current discussion, COPD is a heterogeneous disorder, with variable amounts of airway and parenchymal disease. Most patients have a predominance of one phenotype, though there is usually some overlap. In the past, patients with chronic bronchitis were described as *blue bloaters*, referring to hypoxemia, polycythemia, and cor pulmonale that often accompanies patients with this form of COPD. *Pink puffers* were those with an emphysematous phenotype of COPD, often with muscle wasting and hyperinflation but without oxygen desaturation. The GOLD criteria are designed to be inclusive to maximize disease recognition and prompt treatment and, therefore, do not highlight these distinctions. However, there may be critical differences in the pathophysiology among different phenotypes that are important when considering OVS.

Sleep and COPD

More than three-quarters of patients with COPD report bothersome nocturnal symptoms, such as dyspnea.[15,16] Patients who report cough and wheeze during the day are more likely to have sleep disturbances than those who do not.[17] Patients report trouble falling asleep, frequent awakening, difficultly returning to sleep, and nonrestorative sleep. In a survey of patients with COPD, more than 60% had experienced at least one sleep symptom in the preceding 28 days.[15] Rates of clinical insomnia are high among patients with COPD, present in more than one-fourth.[18] As compared with controls, COPD confers an increased risk of insomnia nearly twice that of non-COPD patients.[19] These sleep disturbances are chronic, persisting over many years.[20]

Sleep complaints increase with more severe disease. Although mild obstructive lung disease is associated with preserved sleep quality,[21] a more severe obstructive disease is associated with increased sleep complaints.[22] Severe disease negatively impacts several objective sleep parameters, such as total sleep time, sleep efficiency, rapid eye movement (REM) sleep,[23] as well as sleep-onset latency, arousals, and sleep-stage transitions.[24–27]

The mechanisms behind the sleep disturbances are likely multifactorial. Symptoms such as cough and wheezing may play a role as noted earlier.[28,29]

Recent work has also highlighted nonrespiratory factors that also perturb sleep among patients with COPD.[30] For example, restless leg syndrome has been found in up to one-third of patients with COPD, and periodic limb movements are associated with worse insomnia.[31] As a result of all of these factors, the use of medications to aid sleep is common, especially sedative hypnotics, which are used by 25% of patients with COPD.[17] Although data are sparse, these medications could theoretically worsen hypoxemia/hypercapnia, though this may not be true for all patients.[32–35]

Changes in Respiration During Sleep with COPD and Nocturnal Oxygen Desaturation

Nocturnal oxygen desaturation (NOD) in chronic lung disease is the result of the normal changes that occur in ventilation with sleep. Put another way, sleep is a stress test for those patients with chronic lung disease that leads to nocturnal hypoxemia and hypercapnia. Understanding the normal changes in respiration that occur with sleep is key to understanding NOD.

Normal Changes in Respiration During Sleep

Sleep is divided into different stages based on electroencephalography waveforms, muscle tone, eye movement, and breathing pattern, with the main distinction being between non-REM sleep and REM sleep. The main respiratory changes that occur during sleep are a decrease in ventilation (largely a decrease in tidal volume without a compensatory increase in respiratory rate) and decreased accessory muscle activity. The changes in respiration are most pronounced in REM sleep, which is notable for skeletal muscle atonia (with the exception of certain muscles, including the diaphragm); in addition to decreased ventilation, the breathing pattern becomes very irregular (especially during bursts of REMs). The decrease in respiratory drive reflects both a decrease in metabolic rate, which results in less carbon dioxide (CO_2) production and, thus, requirement for elimination, and an increase in the CO_2 set point.[36] The reduction in minute ventilation is further pronounced during REM, when ventilation may be 40% less compared with wakefulness.[37,38] In addition to the decrease in the respiratory set point, there is decreased responsiveness to hypercapnia and hypoxia compared with wakefulness.[39–41] Finally, upper airway resistance increases during sleep, even in those without OSA.[42] An overview of the changes is outlined in **Fig. 1**.

Sleep and Breathing with COPD

All of the aforementioned changes are physiologic changes that occur from wakefulness to sleep. However, in the presence of lung disease, the consequences may be dramatic and lead to oxygen desaturation. First, these patients may already have borderline hypoxemia, which puts them on the steep part of the oxygen hemoglobin binding curve; that is, small changes in Pao_2 lead to a decrease in oxygen saturation. Second, patients with COPD have increased minute ventilation for a variety of reasons and frequently rely on accessory muscles to aid ventilation. As a result, ventilation can decrease dramatically during sleep and

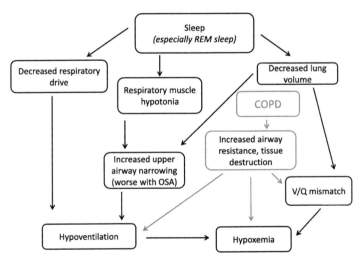

Fig. 1. The normal physiologic changes that occur with sleep. With sleep onset, respiratory drive is decreased, and there is respiratory muscle hypotonia and a decrease in lung volumes. Even without OSA, the result is hypoventilation compared with wakefulness. Particularly with OSA and COPD, there are further pathophysiologic changes that lead to greater hypoventilation and hypoxemia.

particularly in REM sleep when muscle activity decreases. Furthermore, patients with COPD may have chest hyperinflation, which stretches the diaphragm and impairs contractile function.[43]

NOD is perhaps the most common sleep abnormality attributed to COPD, occurring in anywhere from one-quarter to three-quarters of patients with an awake oxygen saturation greater than 90% to 95%.[44–46] During sleep, desaturations are frequent among patients with an FEV_1/FVC less than 65%[21]; increasing severity of obstructive disease is associated with more severe desaturations during sleep. Among those with severe obstructive lung disease ($FEV_1<30\%$), a 20% decrease of oxygen saturation can be seen during non-REM sleep and an impressive decline of 40% during REM.[37] There is substantial variation in reported NOD rates, in part caused by the heterogeneous nature of COPD as well as the definition of NOD, which may be based either on nadir levels or the duration of low oxygen tension.

COPD and OSA: the OVS

OSA is a common disorder, characterized by partial or complete collapse of the upper airway during sleep, resulting in intermittent hypoxia and arousals. The repetitive nature of these breathing events results in fragmented and nonrestorative sleep. Among middle-aged men (50–70 years old), the prevalence of moderate to severe OSA is predicted to be as high as 17% and slightly lower but still concerning at 9% among middle-aged women.[47] OSA is associated with an increased risk of serious neurocognitive and cardiovascular consequences, including hypertension, congestive heart failure, and stroke.[48–51] CPAP is the gold standard treatment of OSA and consists of a mask worn during sleep connected to a machine that delivers pressurized air, thereby splinting open the airway during sleep. Although CPAP is efficacious in treating OSA in almost all cases, its effectiveness is limited by patient adherence. Although adherence rates may be improved through intensive support and behavioral therapy, the real-world nonadherence rates may approach 50%. In the context of OVS, these facts illustrate the potentially large number of patients with OSA at risk for OVS, that both OSA and COPD have substantial cardiovascular morbidity and mortality, and that positive airway pressure is unlikely to be accepted by many patients.

Diagnosing OSA Among Those Patients with COPD

OSA is diagnosed through polysomnography, with apneas and hypopneas recorded during sleep. The tendency toward oxygen desaturation described earlier in those patients with chronic lung disease impacts the diagnosis of OSA. Although the designation of apneas is straightforward and independent of oxygen desaturation, hypopneas are based on flow limitation of at least 30% and require either an accompanying 3% or greater oxygen desaturation or an arousal. Based on the sigmoidal shape of the oxygen-hemoglobin desaturation curve, any small change in Pao_2 that occurs during sleep will be reflected as a larger (and therefore scorable as a hypopnea) change in oxygen saturation. Put another way, 2 patients with the same upper airway tendency to collapse, but one healthy and the other with chronic lung disease, might have very different apnea-hypopnea indices. A similar observation that makes the same point is that the AHI improves with descent from altitude, largely because of a decrease in the number of hypopneas.[52] Nevertheless, there are no current alternative scoring criteria or guidelines for OSA diagnosis in the setting of chronic lung disease.

Among patients with COPD, there are clues to suggest OSA beyond the classic symptoms of snoring, witnessed apneas, and daytime sleepiness. For example, headaches with the initiation of nocturnal supplemental oxygen suggest coexistent OSA (caused by increased hypercapnia). Hypercapnia, despite relatively preserved pulmonary function tests, may also signal the presence of sleep-disordered breathing and prompt evaluation. Indeed, based on findings from one cohort, FEV_1 was severely decreased among patients with COPD only with hypercapnia but only moderately reduced in patients who had both COPD and OSA. Despite this difference in pulmonary function tests, daytime $Paco_2$ was higher among those with OVS compared with COPD only.[53,54] Additionally, obesity is more common among hypercarbic patients with COPD who have OSA as compared with COPD only.[54] For comparison, the characteristics of COPD alone, OSA alone, and OVS from one cohort are outlined in **Table 1**.

The American Thoracic Society/European Respiratory Society's guidelines also highlight the role of referring for overnight testing among those with mild COPD and evidence of pulmonary hypertension. Although only 16% of patients with OSA have been observed to have pulmonary hypertension, this number jumps to 86% for those with OVS.[55] This is an intriguing finding, given that traditional markers of OSA severity and nocturnal hypoxia in COPD are not predictive of pulmonary hypertension. However, time spent with oxygen saturation less than 90% is high among patients with OVS, even without a severe obstructive pattern on spirometry.

Table 1
Characteristics and physiologic measures of patients with COPD only, OSA only, and OVS

	COPD Group (n = 32)	Overlap Group (n = 29)	Pure OSA Group (n = 152)
Age (y)	60.1 ± 10.4	57.2 ± 9.5	48.9 ± 12.9
Weight (kg)	87.6 ± 17.5	102.2 ± 20.6	106.8 ± 28.8
BMI (kg/m^2)	31 ± 7	36 ± 6	39 ± 10
FVC (% predicted)	60 ± 19	72 ± 17	89 ± 21
FEV$_1$ (% predicted)	47 ± 16	63 ± 16	89 ± 20
FEV$_1$/FVC (%)	59 ± 9	67 ± 5	87 ± 9
P$_{ao2}$ (mm Hg)	69 ± 10	70 ± 11	79 ± 12
P$_{aco2}$ (mm Hg)	40 ± 5	45 ± 5	39 ± 4
AHI (events/h)	6 ± 5	40 ± 20	42 ± 23
Time S$_{pO2}$ <90% (%)	16 ± 28	48 ± 28	30 ± 28

Overlap refers to both COPD and OSA.
  Abbreviations: BMI, body mass index; S$_{pO2}$, oxygen saturation.
  Values are mean ± SD.
  Adapted from Resta O, Foschino Barbaro MP, Brindicci C, et al. Hypercapnia in overlap syndrome: possible determinant factors. Sleep Breath 2002;6(1):14; with permission.

Prevalence and Epidemiology of OVS

In general, small studies from the early 1990s suggested that severe COPD was a risk factor for OSA.[56] For example, one early study found greater than 80% prevalence of OSA among patients with COPD and excessive daytime sleepiness referred for evaluation.[12] In certain populations, too, such as Veterans Administration patients, the coexistence of OSA and COPD was high (29%) among patients who had polysomnogram and spirometry data available.[57]

More recently, larger epidemiology studies including a more broad range of subjects, such as the Sleep Heart Health Study and Multinational Monitoring of Trends and Determinants in Cardiovascular Disease, have not demonstrated an increased risk of OSA among those with obstructive lung disease, at least among those with mild obstructive lung disease.[21,58] In these large cohorts, the prevalence of OSA was 11% to 14%, which was similar in those with or without obstructive lung disease.[21,58] Thus, it seems likely that there is little connection among those with mild COPD; whether more severe COPD can contribute to OSA is not clear.

Although the answer is not yet known, proposed mechanisms of OSA risk in severe COPD include the following: fluid shifts in those with cor pulmonale from lower extremity edema to the neck,[59] a generalized myopathy from COPD alone that affects the upper airway muscles,[60] or a steroid-induced myopathy from systemic or inhaled corticosteroids. All of these changes would increase upper airway collapsibility.

Clinical Consequences of OSA and COPD

The large aforementioned cohort studies did highlight that among those with obstructive lung disease and OSA, the nocturnal desaturations and sleep disturbances are greater (both oxygen saturation nadir and duration of hypoxemia) than would be expected for either disease alone.[21] Whether causal or not, more recent reports have suggested an increased mortality in OVS compared with COPD and OSA alone and have increased awareness about OVSs. First, Marin and colleagues[61] found decreased survival among patients with OVS compared with either COPD or OSA alone (**Fig. 2**). There were differences in death from any cause and cardiovascular causes when patients with OVS using CPAP were compared with those not on CPAP. No differences were seen between COPD only and patients with OVS using CPAP.[61] That patients with OVS using CPAP have reduced mortality compared with OVS without CPAP has now also been reported in other cohorts[62–64] Jaoude and colleagues[64] found that CPAP only improved outcomes from OVS in those patients who were also hypercapnic. Further exploring the observed therapeutic benefit of CPAP, Stanchina and colleagues[63] found that greater time on CPAP was associated with reduced mortality in patients with OVS.

Although the improvement with CPAP seems dramatic, these are not randomized data; these were cohort studies in which subjects chose to adhere to or abandon CPAP therapy. Patients who did not adhere to CPAP may have been those with more COPD/less OSA; had more respiratory

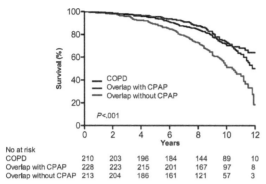

No at risk						
COPD	210	203	196	184	144	89	10
Overlap with CPAP	228	223	215	201	167	97	8
Overlap without CPAP	213	204	186	161	121	57	3

Fig. 2. Kaplan-Meier survival curves for patients with COPD. Patients with OVS on CPAP, and patients with OVS not on CPAP. Treatment with CPAP seems to prevent against the excess mortality in patients with OVS. Importantly, these data are observational. (*Adapted from* Marin JM, Soriano JB, Carrizo SJ, et al. Outcomes in patients with chronic obstructive pulmonary disease and obstructive sleep apnea: the overlap syndrome. Am J Respir Crit Care Med 2010;182(3):328; with permission.)

symptoms, such as dyspnea or sputum that limit CPAP use; or were less likely to adhere to other medication therapy, which is also important for limiting poor outcomes (eg, statin therapy). Nevertheless, these findings highlight the need to focus more resources on the care and understanding of these patients.

It is assumed, but not known, that the worse outcomes in OVS are caused by excess cardiovascular events. As discussed earlier, both COPD and OSA increase cardiovascular risk. Some data support this potential mechanism, suggesting that OSA can augment vascular changes among patients with COPD, such as arterial stiffness.[65] Sharma and colleagues[66] found that patients with OSA have more extensive remodeling of the right ventricle seen on cardiac magnetic resonance compared with those with COPD alone; the extent of right ventricle remodeling was correlated with the oxygen desaturation index.

Treatment of OVS

Treatment of OVS may be thought of as addressing the underlying COPD, OSA, or both. Although the specific goals of treatment remain poorly defined, most clinicians strive to eliminate sleep-disordered breathing and eliminate NOD. What to target for ideal oxygen saturation, however, remains unclear, as does the impact of normalizing hypercarbia. The most commonly applied therapy is CPAP.

Before CPAP is applied, however, it is critical to consider the use of therapies that target the

underlying COPD, such as bronchodilators and antiinflammatories. Therapies aimed at COPD alone can improve nocturnal oxygen saturation as well as decrease symptoms. Ipratropium and tiotropium, cholinergic bronchodilators, long-acting beta-agonists, and oral steroids all have data to support improvements in oxygen saturation during sleep.[67–70] Some of these agents, such as ipratropium, have also been shown to improve sleep quality and increase REM and total sleep time, although, surprisingly, tiotropium did not.[67,68,70] Although the mechanism of these improvements has yet to be teased out, these studies suggest that optimizing COPD treatment can play a key role in the degree of nocturnal oxygen saturation. The impact on upper airway patency is unknown; some have hypothesized that (inhaled) steroids might predispose the upper airway to myopathy and increased collapsibility. However, at least in asthmatic patients receiving high-dose inhaled corticosteroids, there was no increase in collapsibility.[71]

Nocturnal oxygen is a mainstay of therapy for hypoxemia in COPD with demonstrated mortality benefits.[72,73] Among patients with OSA, nocturnal oxygen therapy alone may improve hypoxemia; however, arousals, sleep architecture, and daytime symptoms, such as sleepiness, are not impacted,[74] pointing to the potential impact of sleep fragmentation caused by arousals triggered by airway obstruction, which is not addressed by oxygen therapy. Thus, supplemental oxygen alone for OSA seems unlikely to be of benefit.

CPAP and Lung Function in COPD

There are a few studies that have assessed treatment with CPAP in patients with OVS. Small studies have demonstrated improvements in daytime oxygen saturation and degree of hypercarbia with nocturnal CPAP use.[75,76] Improvements in FEV_1, echocardiogram estimates of mean pulmonary artery pressure, Pao_2, and $Paco_2$ have been documented.[75,77,78] Other studies have found a decline in lung function among patients with OVS who were adherent to CPAP therapy.[79] Differences in study design, and subject characteristics make it difficult to generalize or reconcile the findings from these studies. It has been hypothesized that improvements in gas exchange may reflect improvement in daytime lung function, although the mechanism remains unclear and controversial. The prevention of repetitive upper airway collapse in an animal model seemed to improve lower airway resistance.[80] Off-loading of respiratory muscles during sleep through CPAP may also be important, contributing to decreased oxygen consumption, CO_2 production, and reducing sleep hypoventilation. After CPAP initiation, fewer COPD-related hospital admissions are seen in some populations.[63,81]

As discussed earlier, recent papers suggest that the treatment of OVS with CPAP is associated with reduced mortality. First, in the Brazilian cohort, 5-year survival with CPAP was 71%, as compared with 26% among patients using oxygen alone.[62] This cohort included more than 600 patients who required long-term oxygen therapy for hypoxemic COPD and had at least moderate OSA. Patients with OSA were prescribed CPAP, and those who were nonadherent to CPAP continued to use oxygen for COPD. Similarly, the findings from a Spanish cohort of patients with OVS also suggested a benefit, lowering the mortality risk to that of COPD alone.[61] The striking improvement in both cohorts supports a beneficial role of CPAP as well as highlighting the very poor outcomes in those with OVS. Again, patients in both studies were not randomized but were self-selected based on adherence to CPAP (or were not able to afford CPAP therapy). That is, these are observational studies comparing patients with OVS who are and are not adherent to CPAP. Although these studies do not elicit the mechanism for the reduced mortality, if caused by CPAP, this may be through the reduction in cardiac risk factors. Indeed, CRP levels, a nonspecific marker of inflammation, were significantly reduced in patients with OVS using CPAP as compared with pretreatment.[82]

Noninvasive ventilation (NIV), such as bilevel positive airway pressure, is an attractive treatment modality in this population. Even in the absence of OSA, nocturnal NIV is often applied for patients with more severe COPD to off-load respiratory muscles, supplement ventilation, decrease hypercapnia, and reduce hypoxemia. Studies in this area have generally been small, nonrandomized, and in patients with stable disease. Taken together, these studies did not demonstrate any improvements in lung function, gas, exchange, sleep efficiency, or mortality according to a 2003 meta-analysis.[83] Since that time, however, 2 areas of investigation deserve to be highlighted. Among patients with OVS with stable hypercapnic COPD (patients with OSA were excluded), one moderately large randomized trial demonstrated a mortality benefit with NIV use, though NIV was accompanied by a decrease in quality of life.[84] A mortality benefit compared with historical controls has also been seen using very high ventilation settings.[85] These investigators argue that so-called high-intensity noninvasive positive pressure ventilation (with very high driving pressures, for example, inspiratory pressures of 28 cm of H_2O and respiratory rate of more than 20 breaths per minute) among patients with COPD does not seem to impact sleep quality and may have some benefits, such as improvement in gas exchange and lung function.[86–88]

Weight loss is beneficial among patients with OSA and obesity.[89] Among patients with COPD alone, however, weight loss is often a concerning finding, stemming from pulmonary cachexia, infection, malignancy, or deconditioning. The role of weight loss among patients with OVS has not been examined; however, it is probably safe for obese patients with OVS to target weight loss.[90] Although purely speculative, given the high rates of cardiovascular disease in OSA and COPD, it may also make sense to consider cardioprotective therapies (eg, aspirin, statin) as the primary prevention in patients with OVS.

Based on all of the aforementioned information, the authors propose the diagnostic and treatment algorithm in **Fig. 3**.

OSA AND ILD, WITH EMPHASIS ON IPF
ILD/IPF Background

ILD may refer to several heterogeneous conditions, such as IPF; sarcoidosis; autoimmune-related pulmonary disorders, such as systemic sclerosis and hypersensitivity pneumonitis; or secondary to an environmental or drug exposure, such as amiodarone. The common features of the ILDs are (1) that these are distinct from obstructive lung diseases (such as COPD) and demonstrate restrictive physiology and (2) that the anatomic basis of the disease is usually the interstitium (the alveolar epithelium, pulmonary capillary endothelium, basement membrane, perivascular, and perilymphatic tissues). The focus of the authors' discussion is primarily among patients with IPF.

IPF is a restrictive lung disease of unknown cause. It is characterized by chronic, progressive lung fibrosis of unknown cause.[91] It is an irreversible process, with an unpredictable course. Progression can vary markedly on an individual basis, from slow chronic decline to a rapid acceleration of disease; acute exacerbations may also punctuate the disease course. Prognosis is generally very poor, and there are no known effective medical treatments. Despite ongoing research, the cause of the disease remains poorly understood. Histologically, IPF correlates with the pattern of usual interstitial pneumonitis; the terms are sometimes used synonymously.

As compared with COPD, IPF is a rare condition, affecting approximately 14 to 28 per 100,000

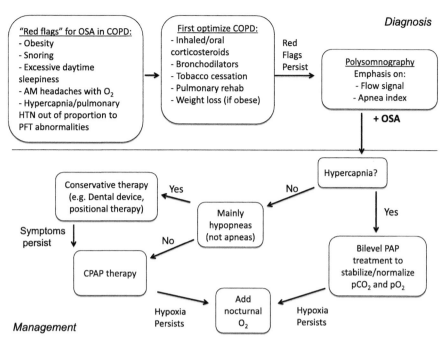

Fig. 3. Management algorithm for patients with COPD. Patients with COPD should be assessed for any red flags that might suggest the presence of concurrent OSA. If present, COPD should be optimized before undergoing polysomnography. Attention should be paid to the flow signal and apnea index when assessing the severity of OSA. If hypercapnia is present, patients can begin on bilevel positive airway pressure (PAP). If flow limitation is present without significant apneas, conservative therapy, such as a mandibular advancement device, weight loss, and positional therapy, should be considered. If apneas predominate, CPAP should be started. Supplemental oxygen should be added if hypoxemia persists. HTN, hypertension; PFT, pulmonary function tests.

people in the United States.[92] It is more common in older individuals and mens.[93] The relatively low prevalence of IPF means that, as compared with COPD, the prevalence of coexisting OSA and IPF (or any ILD) is presumably also rare. However, OSA and IPF might be worth studying if (1) IPF predisposes to OSA, (2) symptoms traditionally ascribed to IPF (eg, fatigue) are actually caused by OSA and can be successfully treated with OSA treatment, and (3) treatment of OSA in these patients improves outcomes.

Sleep in IPF

Poor sleep is common among patients with IPF. Global measures of sleep quality and excessive daytime sleepiness are significantly different as compared with controls, with patients with IPF complaining of poor sleep and excessive daytime sleepiness.[94] Insomnia is also a frequent occurrence, found in almost one-half of patients with IPF, which may contribute to the high rates of daytime symptoms.[95] When sleep is objectively assessed by polysomnography, as compared with controls, patients with IPF have increased sleep fragmentation and stage I sleep.[96–98] Total sleep

time, sleep efficiency, and REM sleep are all reduced.[96–98]

The mechanisms for these sleep abnormalities remain incompletely understood, though are likely to be multifactorial. Disruption from cough has been frequently cited as one factor that contributes to sleep disturbance and the inability to sleep.[95,99–101] The effect of medications, such as corticosteroids, which are still used empirically given the lack of other treatment options, may further contribute to some of the sleep abnormalities reported by patients with IPF. Nearly two-thirds of patients in one series were on prednisone,[94] which may interfere with sleep when used at high doses. Patients with IPF are often additionally burdened by depression and other mood disorders, which are often characterized by sleep disturbances and changes in energy level; the medications used to treat these disorders may also impact sleep and daytime function.

Respiration During Sleep in IPF

The pathologic changes in pulmonary fibrosis are decreased lung compliance and increased ventilation/perfusion mismatch. These changes will increase minute ventilation and the work of breathing. As a result, patients with IPF exhibit rapid, shallow breathing during wakefulness.[98] During sleep, the tachypnea persists; as compared with normal controls, there is no decrease in respiratory rate, although tidal volume decreases.[98] Thus, similar to COPD as discussed earlier, among patients with ILD, sleep may serve as a stressor to the respiratory system. Oxygen desaturation is frequently more profound than during wakefulness. The importance of evaluating nighttime respiratory patterns has been recently highlighted, as it may have prognostic value in assessing mortality in ILD.[102] Specifically, among patients with newly diagnosed IPF, the degree of nocturnal desaturation was greater than seen during exercise and was predictive of survival,[103–105] possibly mediated through worsening pulmonary artery hypertension.[103]

ILD and Sleep-Disordered Breathing

The prevalence of sleep-disordered breathing is reported to be extraordinarily high among patients with ILD. Symptoms such as fatigue, commonly reported in patients with IPF, may be attributable to this.[98] In published series, the incidence of OSA ranges from more than two-thirds to nearly 90%.[106–108] **Fig. 4** outlines the symptoms that are commonly reported in IPF and how they may overlap with OSA. The nature of OSA in these populations remains incompletely characterized, such as whether events are caused by airway collapse and flow limitation or oxygen desaturations. Among patients with IPF, AHI is not strongly correlated with the body mass index, again suggesting that other mechanisms, aside from obesity, may be contributing to the diagnosis of OSA in this population.[108] Indeed, as compared with controls, patients with IPF spend more time with an oxygen saturation less than 90%, even when the AHI is similar. These observations raise the possibility

that the lower baseline oxygen saturation and increased tendency toward desaturation are overestimating the collapsibility of the upper airway. The 2009 study by Lancaster and colleagues[108] is helpful in this regard. First, their subjects with mild OSA had a mean AHI of 10.7 events per hour, of which less than 1 event per hour was apnea. Additionally, approximately half of the hypopneas were scored based on a 3% oxygen desaturation (rather than arousal). In those with moderate to severe OSA, the average AHI was 39.4 events per hour. But again, the apnea index was only 7.1 events per hour; nearly half of all hypopneas were scored based on oxygen desaturation.

In support of a mechanistic link between IPF and OSA, some investigators have invoked so-called tracheal traction, the link between lung volumes and the upper airway.[109,110] Briefly, in patients without lung disease, a decrease in lung volumes leads to increased upper airway resistance, increased collapsibility, and worse OSA severity.[111,112] However, whether this relationship still holds when compliance of the lung is altered is not clear; no formal measurement of airway resistance or collapsibility has been made in patients with IPF to test this hypothesis. Again, in the study by Lancaster and colleagues,[108] total lung capacity did not seem to predict OSA.

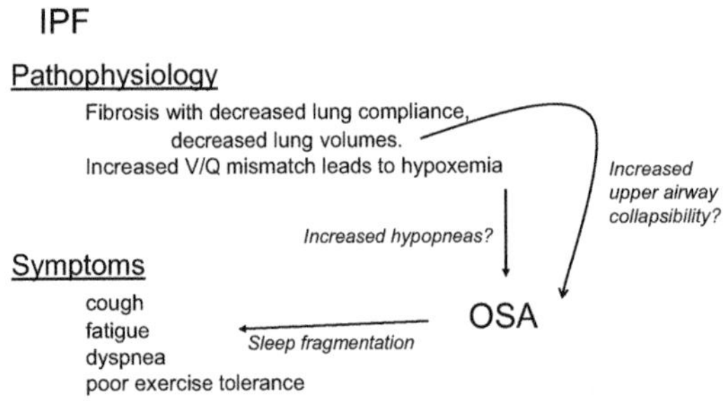

Treatment

There are no proven therapies that target the underlying disease process in IPF. Oxygen therapy is widely used as supportive care. Studies suggest that oxygen therapy can be associated with improvements in exercise performance.[113,114] However, no studies have demonstrated a mortality benefit[115] or improvement in exertional dyspnea,[116] as rapid shallow breathing persists despite addressing hypoxemia.

Treatment with CPAP among patients with IPF with at least moderate OSA results in gains in sleep-related quality-of-life measures, though adherence to CPAP may be challenging in light of chronic cough and other barriers.[117] There are no studies that have explored the impact of CPAP on outcomes in IPF, such as disease progression or mortality. Taken together, OSA may be common in IPF; treatment with CPAP may improve OSA symptoms.

Other OVS: Beyond COPD and IPF

From the earlier discussion, it is clear that there are many research and clinical questions that remain for OVS, even for *the* OVS, which is relatively common. Even less is known about the prevalence,

Fig. 4. Links between IPF and OSA. Many symptoms and findings among by patients with IPF overlap with those of OSA, including daytime fatigue, poor sleep, and nocturnal hypoxia. Similarly, the pathophysiologic changes of IPF may contribute to OSA.

consequences, and best management of OSA among other chronic lung diseases. However, there are some pearls that the sleep physician should know regarding other lung diseases.

Sarcoidosis is a chronic condition of unknown cause characterized by the formation of granulomas in many organs, most commonly the lung. Lung disease may range from mild to severe and fibrosing in nature. Steroids are often given in more severe disease. Fatigue and excessive daytime sleepiness are more common among patients with sarcoid as compared with controls.[118–120] Consideration of OSA among these patients is, therefore, important, particularly among those with abnormal lung function.[118] There remains a population of patients, however, with hypersomnolence unrelated to OSA. Relevant for sleep medicine physicians, fatigue improves with stimulant therapy (armodafinil).[121] This improvement may serve as a paradigm for patients with chronic lung disease and fatigue to receive empiric therapy.

Although most of the data are in pediatric populations, OSA seems to be more common among patients with sickle cell anemia as compared with controls.[122–124] OSA among patients with sickle cell disease is accompanied by more severe nocturnal desaturations and hypercarbia.[123] Although larger studies are needed to better describe the relationship, OSA, through nocturnal hypoxia, may serve as a trigger for vasoocclusive sickle events.[125] This relationship highlights the potential importance of recognizing and treating OSA among those with sickle cell disease.

Cystic fibrosis (CF) is a systemic disease characterized by abnormal chloride channel function. Obstructive lung disease, bronchiectasis, and repeated pulmonary infections caused by tenacious sputum are common among patients with CF. Sleep apnea is common (in up to 70% of children with CF).[126] OSA presents at an early age as compared with controls, as young as preschool age.[126] NOD is also common among patients with CF, particularly those with awake oxygen saturation less than 94%.[127]

SUMMARY

The combination of chronic lung disease and OSA in a single patient is still, as yet, poorly understood. Many research and clinical questions remain, including how best to quantify upper airway collapsibility and sleep fragmentation in patients already at risk for hypoxemia caused by chronic lung disease. These questions must be answered given the high prevalence of the OVS, COPD and OSA, and observational cohort studies that show very high mortality without OSA treatment.

Other chronic lung diseases, such as IPF, are much less common; yet diagnosis and treatment of OSA may be important. Within these patient populations, there are few or no therapies available to target the underlying disease and its consequences. Recognition and treatment of OSA, therefore, could offer key benefits, such as improvements in quality of life or fatigue level.

REFERENCES

1. Flenley DC. Sleep in chronic obstructive lung disease. Clin Chest Med 1985;6(4):651–61.
2. Pauwels RA, Buist AS, Calverley PM, et al, GOLD Scientific Committee. Global strategy for the diagnosis, management, and prevention of chronic obstructive pulmonary disease. NHLBI/WHO Global Initiative for Chronic Obstructive Lung Disease (GOLD) workshop summary. Am J Respir Crit Care Med 2001;163(5):1256–76.
3. Ford ES, Croft JB, Mannino DM, et al. COPD surveillance–United States, 1999-2011. Chest 2013; 144(1):284–305.
4. Buist AS, McBurnie MA, Vollmer WM, et al. International variation in the prevalence of COPD (the BOLD study): a population-based prevalence study. Lancet 2007;370(9589):741–50.
5. Hoyert DL, Xu J. Deaths: preliminary data for 2011. Natl Vital Stat Rep 2012;61(6):1–65. Hyattsville, MD: National Center for Health Statistics. 2012.
6. Foster TS, Miller JD, Marton JP, et al. Assessment of the economic burden of COPD in the U.S.: a review and synthesis of the literature. COPD 2006; 3(4):211–8.
7. Rabe KF, Hurd S, Anzueto A, et al. Global strategy for the diagnosis, management, and prevention of chronic obstructive pulmonary disease: GOLD executive summary. Am J Respir Crit Care Med 2007;176(6):532–55.
8. Shepard JW Jr, Schweitzer PK, Keller CA, et al. Myocardial stress. Exercise versus sleep in patients with COPD. Chest 1984;86(3):366–74.
9. Fletcher EC, Luckett RA, Miller T, et al. Exercise hemodynamics and gas exchange in patients with chronic obstruction pulmonary disease, sleep desaturation, and a daytime PaO2 above 60 mm hg. Am Rev Respir Dis 1989;140(5):1237–45.
10. Fletcher EC, Luckett RA, Miller T, et al. Pulmonary vascular hemodynamics in chronic lung disease patients with and without oxyhemoglobin desaturation during sleep. Chest 1989;95(4):757–64.
11. Boysen PG, Block AJ, Wynne JW, et al. Nocturnal pulmonary hypertension in patients with chronic obstructive pulmonary disease. Chest 1979;76(5):536–42.
12. Guilleminault C, Cummiskey J, Motta J. Chronic obstructive airflow disease and sleep studies. Am Rev Respir Dis 1980;122(3):397–406.

13. Cheong TH, Magder S, Shapiro S, et al. Cardiac arrhythmias during exercise in severe chronic obstructive pulmonary disease. Chest 1990;97(4): 793–7.

14. Slutsky R, Hooper W, Ackerman W, et al. Evaluation of left ventricular function in chronic pulmonary disease by exercise gated equilibrium radionuclide angiography. Am Heart J 1981;101(4):414–20.

15. Price D, Small M, Milligan G, et al. Impact of night-time symptoms in COPD: a real-world study in five European countries. Int J Chron Obstruct Pulmon Dis 2013;8:595–603.

16. Agusti A, Hedner J, Marin JM, et al. Night-time symptoms: a forgotten dimension of COPD. Eur Respir Rev 2011;20(121):183–94.

17. Klink ME, Dodge R, Quan SF. The relation of sleep complaints to respiratory symptoms in a general population. Chest 1994;105(1):151–4.

18. Budhiraja P, Budhiraja R, Goodwin JL, et al. Incidence of restless legs syndrome and its correlates. J Clin Sleep Med 2012;8(2):119–24.

19. Budhiraja R, Roth T, Hudgel DW, et al. Prevalence and polysomnographic correlates of insomnia co-morbid with medical disorders. Sleep 2011;34(7): 859–67.

20. Dodge R, Cline MG, Quan SF. The natural history of insomnia and its relationship to respiratory symptoms. Arch Intern Med 1995;155(16):1797–800.

21. Sanders MH, Newman AB, Haggerty CL, et al. Sleep and sleep-disordered breathing in adults with predominantly mild obstructive airway disease. Am J Respir Crit Care Med 2003;167(1): 7–14.

22. Krachman S, Minai OA, Scharf SM. Sleep abnormalities and treatment in emphysema. Proc Am Thorac Soc 2008;5(4):536–42.

23. Valipour A, Lavie P, Lothaller H, et al. Sleep profile and symptoms of sleep disorders in patients with stable mild to moderate chronic obstructive pulmonary disease. Sleep Med 2011;12(4):367–72.

24. McSharry DG, Ryan S, Calverley P, et al. Sleep quality in chronic obstructive pulmonary disease. Respirology 2012;17(7):1119–24.

25. Manni R, Cerveri I, Bruschi C, et al. Sleep and oxyhemoglobin desaturation patterns in chronic obstructive pulmonary diseases. Eur Neurol 1988; 28(5):275–8.

26. Fleetham J, West P, Mezon B, et al. Sleep, arousals, and oxygen desaturation in chronic obstructive pulmonary disease. the effect of oxygen therapy. Am Rev Respir Dis 1982;126(3): 429–33.

27. Brezinova V, Catterall JR, Douglas NJ, et al. Night sleep of patients with chronic ventilatory failure and age matched controls: number and duration of the EEG episodes of intervening wakefulness and drowsiness. Sleep 1982;5(2):123–30.

28. Kwon JS, Wolfe LF, Lu BS, et al. Hyperinflation is associated with lower sleep efficiency in COPD with co-existent obstructive sleep apnea. COPD 2009;6(6):441–5.

29. Krachman SL, Chatila W, Martin UJ, et al. Physiologic correlates of sleep quality in severe emphysema. COPD 2011;8(3):182–8.

30. Hynninen MJ, Pallesen S, Hardie J, et al. Insomnia symptoms, objectively measured sleep, and disease severity in chronic obstructive pulmonary disease outpatients. Sleep Med 2013;14(12): 1328–33.

31. Lo Coco D, Mattaliano A, Lo Coco A, et al. Increased frequency of restless legs syndrome in chronic obstructive pulmonary disease patients. Sleep Med 2009;10(5):572–6.

32. Timms RM, Dawson A, Hajdukovic RM, et al. Effect of triazolam on sleep and arterial oxygen saturation in patients with chronic obstructive pulmonary disease. Arch Intern Med 1988;148(10):2159–63.

33. Steens RD, Pouliot Z, Millar TW, et al. Effects of zolpidem and triazolam on sleep and respiration in mild to moderate chronic obstructive pulmonary disease. Sleep 1993;16(4):318–26.

34. Stege G, Heijdra YF, van den Elshout FJ, et al. Temazepam 10mg does not affect breathing and gas exchange in patients with severe normocapnic COPD. Respir Med 2010;104(4):518–24.

35. Ekstrom MP, Bornefalk-Hermansson A, Abernethy AP, et al. Safety of benzodiazepines and opioids in very severe respiratory disease: national prospective study. BMJ 2014;348:g445.

36. Douglas NJ, White DP, Pickett CK, et al. Respiration during sleep in normal man. Thorax 1982; 37(11):840–4.

37. Becker HF, Piper AJ, Flynn WE, et al. Breathing during sleep in patients with nocturnal desaturation. Am J Respir Crit Care Med 1999;159(1):112–8.

38. Catterall JR, Douglas NJ, Calverley PM, et al. Transient hypoxemia during sleep in chronic obstructive pulmonary disease is not a sleep apnea syndrome. Am Rev Respir Dis 1983;128(1):24–9.

39. Douglas NJ, White DP, Weil JV, et al. Hypoxic ventilatory response decreases during sleep in normal men. Am Rev Respir Dis 1982;125(3):286–9.

40. Douglas NJ, White DP, Weil JV, et al. Hypercapnic ventilatory response in sleeping adults. Am Rev Respir Dis 1982;126(5):758–62.

41. Douglas NJ. Control of ventilation during sleep. Clin Chest Med 1985;6(4):563–75.

42. Hudgel DW, Martin RJ, Johnson B, et al. Mechanics of the respiratory system and breathing pattern during sleep in normal humans. J Appl Physiol Respir Environ Exerc Physiol 1984;56(1): 133–7.

43. Ottenheijm CA, Heunks LM, Sieck GC, et al. Diaphragm dysfunction in chronic obstructive

pulmonary disease. Am J Respir Crit Care Med 2005;172(2):200–5.

44. Chaouat A, Weitzenblum E, Kessler R, et al. Sleep-related O2 desaturation and daytime pulmonary haemodynamics in COPD patients with mild hypoxaemia. Eur Respir J 1997;10(8):1730–5.

45. Fletcher EC, Miller J, Divine GW, et al. Nocturnal oxyhemoglobin desaturation in COPD patients with arterial oxygen tensions above 60 mm hg. Chest 1987;92(4):604–8.

46. Lewis CA, Fergusson W, Eaton T, et al. Isolated nocturnal desaturation in COPD: prevalence and impact on quality of life and sleep. Thorax 2009; 64(2):133–8.

47. Peppard PE, Young T, Barnet JH, et al. Increased prevalence of sleep-disordered breathing in adults. Am J Epidemiol 2013;177(9):1006–14.

48. Yaggi HK, Concato J, Kernan WN, et al. Obstructive sleep apnea as a risk factor for stroke and death. N Engl J Med 2005;353(19):2034–41.

49. Kendzerska T, Mollayeva T, Gershon AS, et al. Untreated obstructive sleep apnea and the risk for serious long-term adverse outcomes: a systematic review. Sleep Med Rev 2014;18(1):49–59.

50. Shahar E, Whitney CW, Redline S, et al. Sleep-disordered breathing and cardiovascular disease: cross-sectional results of the sleep heart health study. Am J Respir Crit Care Med 2001;163(1): 19–25.

51. Findley LJ, Barth JT, Powers DC, et al. Cognitive impairment in patients with obstructive sleep apnea and associated hypoxemia. Chest 1986; 90(5):686–90.

52. Patz D, Spoon M, Corbin R, et al. The effect of altitude descent on obstructive sleep apnea. Chest 2006;130(6):1744–50.

53. Sharma B, Feinsilver S, Owens RL, et al. Obstructive airway disease and obstructive sleep apnea: effect of pulmonary function. Lung 2011;189(1): 37–41.

54. Resta O, Foschino Barbaro MP, Brindicci C, et al. Hypercapnia in overlap syndrome: possible determinant factors. Sleep Breath 2002;6(1):11–8.

55. Hawrylkiewicz I, Palasiewicz G, Plywaczewski R, et al. Pulmonary hypertension in patients with pure obstructive sleep apnea. Pol Arch Med Wewn 2004;111(4):449–54.

56. Chaouat A, Weitzenblum E, Krieger J, et al. Association of chronic obstructive pulmonary disease and sleep apnea syndrome. Am J Respir Crit Care Med 1995;151(1):82–6.

57. Lopez-Acevedo MN, Torres-Palacios A, Elena Ocasio-Tascon M, et al. Overlap syndrome: an indication for sleep studies?: a pilot study. Sleep Breath 2009;13(4):409–13.

58. Bednarek M, Plywaczewski R, Jonczak L, et al. There is no relationship between chronic obstructive pulmonary disease and obstructive sleep apnea syndrome: a population study. Respiration 2005;72(2):142–9.

59. White LH, Motwani S, Kasai T, et al. Effect of rostral fluid shift on pharyngeal resistance in men with and without obstructive sleep apnea. Respir Physiol Neurobiol 2014;192:17–22.

60. Agusti AG, Noguera A, Sauleda J, et al. Systemic effects of chronic obstructive pulmonary disease. Eur Respir J 2003;21(2):347–60.

61. Marin JM, Soriano JB, Carrizo SJ, et al. Outcomes in patients with chronic obstructive pulmonary disease and obstructive sleep apnea: the overlap syndrome. Am J Respir Crit Care Med 2010;182(3): 325–31.

62. Machado MC, Vollmer WM, Togeiro SM, et al. CPAP and survival in moderate-to-severe obstructive sleep apnoea syndrome and hypoxaemic COPD. Eur Respir J 2010;35(1):132–7.

63. Stanchina ML, Welicky LM, Donat W, et al. Impact of CPAP use and age on mortality in patients with combined COPD and obstructive sleep apnea: the overlap syndrome. J Clin Sleep Med 2013; 9(8):767–72.

64. Jaoude P, Kufel T, El-Solh AA. Survival benefit of CPAP favors hypercapnic patients with the overlap syndrome. Lung 2014;192(2):251–8.

65. Shiina K, Tomiyama H, Takata Y, et al. Overlap syndrome: additive effects of COPD on the cardiovascular damages in patients with OSA. Respir Med 2012;106(9):1335–41.

66. Sharma B, Neilan TG, Kwong RY, et al. Evaluation of right ventricular remodeling using cardiac magnetic resonance imaging in co-existent chronic obstructive pulmonary disease and obstructive sleep apnea. COPD 2013;10(1):4–10.

67. Martin RJ, Bartelson BL, Smith P, et al. Effect of ipratropium bromide treatment on oxygen saturation and sleep quality in COPD. Chest 1999;115(5):1338–45.

68. McNicholas WT, Calverley PM, Lee A, et al, Tiotropium Sleep Study in COPD Investigators. Long-acting inhaled anticholinergic therapy improves sleeping oxygen saturation in COPD. Eur Respir J 2004;23(6):825–31.

69. Ryan S, Doherty LS, Rock C, et al. Effects of salmeterol on sleeping oxygen saturation in chronic obstructive pulmonary disease. Respiration 2010; 79(6):475–81.

70. Sposato B, Mariotta S, Palmiero G, et al. Oral corticosteroids can improve nocturnal isolated hypoxemia in stable COPD patients with diurnal PaO2 > 60 mm Hg. Eur Rev Med Pharmacol Sci 2007;11(6):365–72.

71. Teodorescu M, Xie A, Sorkness CA, et al. Effects of inhaled fluticasone on upper airway during sleep and wakefulness in asthma: a pilot study. J Clin Sleep Med 2014;10(2):183–93.

72. Continuous or nocturnal oxygen therapy in hypoxemic chronic obstructive lung disease: a clinical trial. Nocturnal oxygen therapy trial group. Ann Intern Med 1980;93(3):391–8.

73. Long term domiciliary oxygen therapy in chronic hypoxic cor pulmonale complicating chronic bronchitis and emphysema. Report of the medical research council working party. Lancet 1981; 1(8222):681–6.

74. Loredo JS, Ancoli-Israel S, Kim EJ, et al. Effect of continuous positive airway pressure versus supplemental oxygen on sleep quality in obstructive sleep apnea: a placebo-CPAP-controlled study. Sleep 2006;29(4):564–71.

75. Mansfield D, Naughton MT. Effects of continuous positive airway pressure on lung function in patients with chronic obstructive pulmonary disease and sleep disordered breathing. Respirology 1999;4(4):365–70.

76. Sforza E, Krieger J, Weitzenblum E, et al. Long-term effects of treatment with nasal continuous positive airway pressure on daytime lung function and pulmonary hemodynamics in patients with obstructive sleep apnea. Am Rev Respir Dis 1990;141(4 Pt 1):866–70.

77. de Miguel J, Cabello J, Sanchez-Alarcos JM, et al. Long-term effects of treatment with nasal continuous positive airway pressure on lung function in patients with overlap syndrome. Sleep Breath 2002;6(1):3–10.

78. Toraldo DM, De Nuccio F, Nicolardi G. Fixed-pressure nCPAP in patients with obstructive sleep apnea (OSA) syndrome and chronic obstructive pulmonary disease (COPD): a 24-month follow-up study. Sleep Breath 2010;14(2):115–23.

79. O'Brien A, Whitman K. Lack of benefit of continuous positive airway pressure on lung function in patients with overlap syndrome. Lung 2005;183(6):389–404.

80. Nadel JA, Widdicombe JG. Reflex effects of upper airway irritation on total lung resistance and blood pressure. J Appl Physiol 1962;17:861–5.

81. Peker Y, Hedner J, Johansson A, et al. Reduced hospitalization with cardiovascular and pulmonary disease in obstructive sleep apnea patients on nasal CPAP treatment. Sleep 1997;20(8):645–53.

82. Nural S, Gunay E, Halici B, et al. Inflammatory processes and effects of continuous positive airway pressure (CPAP) in overlap syndrome. Inflammation 2013;36(1):66–74.

83. Wijkstra PJ, Lacasse Y, Guyatt GH, et al. A meta-analysis of nocturnal noninvasive positive pressure ventilation in patients with stable COPD. Chest 2003;124(1):337–43.

84. McEvoy RD, Pierce RJ, Hillman D, et al. Nocturnal non-invasive nasal ventilation in stable hypercapnic COPD: a randomised controlled trial. Thorax 2009;64(7):561–6.

85. Windisch W, Haenel M, Storre JH, et al. High-intensity non-invasive positive pressure ventilation for stable hypercapnic COPD. Int J Med Sci 2009; 6(2):72–6.

86. Dreher M, Ekkernkamp E, Walterspacher S, et al. Noninvasive ventilation in COPD: impact of inspiratory pressure levels on sleep quality. Chest 2011; 140(4):939–45.

87. Windisch W, Kostic S, Dreher M, et al. Outcome of patients with stable COPD receiving controlled noninvasive positive pressure ventilation aimed at a maximal reduction of pa(CO2). Chest 2005; 128(2):657–62.

88. Windisch W, Dreher M, Storre JH, et al. Nocturnal non-invasive positive pressure ventilation: physiological effects on spontaneous breathing. Respir Physiol Neurobiol 2006;150(2–3):251–60.

89. Poulain M, Doucet M, Major GC, et al. The effect of obesity on chronic respiratory diseases: pathophysiology and therapeutic strategies. CMAJ 2006;174(9):1293–9.

90. Sood A, Petersen H, Meek P, et al. Spirometry and health status worsen with weight gain in obese smokers but improve in normal-weight smokers. Am J Respir Crit Care Med 2014;189(3):274–81.

91. Raghu G. Idiopathic pulmonary fibrosis: guidelines for diagnosis and clinical management have advanced from consensus-based in 2000 to evidence-based in 2011. Eur Respir J 2011;37(4):743–6.

92. Nalysnyk L, Cid-Ruzafa J, Rotella P, et al. Incidence and prevalence of idiopathic pulmonary fibrosis: review of the literature. Eur Respir Rev 2012;21(126):355–61.

93. Raghu G, Weycker D, Edelsberg J, et al. Incidence and prevalence of idiopathic pulmonary fibrosis. Am J Respir Crit Care Med 2006;174(7):810–6.

94. Krishnan V, McCormack MC, Mathai SC, et al. Sleep quality and health-related quality of life in idiopathic pulmonary fibrosis. Chest 2008;134(4): 693–8.

95. Bajwah S, Higginson IJ, Ross JR, et al. The palliative care needs for fibrotic interstitial lung disease: a qualitative study of patients, informal caregivers and health professionals. Palliat Med 2013;27(9): 869–76.

96. Perez-Padilla R, West P, Lertzman M, et al. Breathing during sleep in patients with interstitial lung disease. Am Rev Respir Dis 1985;132(2):224–9.

97. Bye PT, Issa F, Berthon-Jones M, et al. Studies of oxygenation during sleep in patients with interstitial lung disease. Am Rev Respir Dis 1984;129(1):27–32.

98. Mermigkis C, Stagaki E, Amfilochiou A, et al. Sleep quality and associated daytime consequences in patients with idiopathic pulmonary fibrosis. Med Princ Pract 2009;18(1):10–5.

99. Swigris JJ, Stewart AL, Gould MK, et al. Patients' perspectives on how idiopathic pulmonary fibrosis

affects the quality of their lives. Health Qual Life Outcomes 2005;3:61.

100. Mermigkis C, Mermigkis D, Varouchakis G, et al. CPAP treatment in patients with idiopathic pulmonary fibrosis and obstructive sleep apnea–therapeutic difficulties and dilemmas. Sleep Breath 2012;16(1):1–3.

101. Rasche K, Orth M. Sleep and breathing in idiopathic pulmonary fibrosis. J Physiol Pharmacol 2009;60(Suppl 5):13–4.

102. Corte TJ, Wort SJ, Talbot S, et al. Elevated nocturnal desaturation index predicts mortality in interstitial lung disease. Sarcoidosis Vasc Diffuse Lung Dis 2012;29(1):41–50.

103. Kolilekas L, Manali E, Vlami KA, et al. Sleep oxygen desaturation predicts survival in idiopathic pulmonary fibrosis. J Clin Sleep Med 2013;9(6): 593–601.

104. Lettieri CJ, Nathan SD, Browning RF, et al. The distance-saturation product predicts mortality in idiopathic pulmonary fibrosis. Respir Med 2006; 100(10):1734–41.

105. Triantafillidou C, Manali E, Lyberopoulos P, et al. The role of cardiopulmonary exercise test in IPF prognosis. Pulm Med 2013;2013:514817.

106. Pihtili A, Bingol Z, Kiyan E, et al. Obstructive sleep apnea is common in patients with interstitial lung disease. Sleep Breath 2013;17(4):1281–8.

107. Mermigkis C, Stagaki E, Tryfon S, et al. How common is sleep-disordered breathing in patients with idiopathic pulmonary fibrosis? Sleep Breath 2010;14(4):387–90.

108. Lancaster LH, Mason WR, Parnell JA, et al. Obstructive sleep apnea is common in idiopathic pulmonary fibrosis. Chest 2009;136(3):772–8.

109. Van de Graaff WB. Thoracic influence on upper airway patency. J Appl Physiol (1985) 1988;65(5): 2124–31.

110. Ruhle KH. Commentary on how common is sleep-disordered breathing in patients with idiopathic pulmonary fibrosis? Mermigkis C. et al. Sleep Breath 2010;14(4):289.

111. Heinzer RC, Stanchina ML, Malhotra A, et al. Effect of increased lung volume on sleep disordered breathing in patients with sleep apnoea. Thorax 2006;61(5):435–9.

112. Owens RL, Malhotra A, Eckert DJ, et al. The influence of end-expiratory lung volume on measurements of pharyngeal collapsibility. J Appl Physiol (1985) 2010;108(2):445–51.

113. Harris-Eze AO, Sridhar G, Clemens RE, et al. Oxygen improves maximal exercise performance in interstitial lung disease. Am J Respir Crit Care Med 1994;150(6 Pt 1):1616–22.

114. Harris-Eze AO, Sridhar G, Clemens RE, et al. Role of hypoxemia and pulmonary mechanics in exercise limitation in interstitial lung disease. Am J Respir Crit Care Med 1996;154(4 Pt 1): 994–1001.

115. Crockett AJ, Cranston JM, Antic N. Domiciliary oxygen for interstitial lung disease. Cochrane Database Syst Rev 2001;(3):CD002883.

116. Nishiyama O, Miyajima H, Fukai Y, et al. Effect of ambulatory oxygen on exertional dyspnea in IPF patients without resting hypoxemia. Respir Med 2013;107(8):1241–6.

117. Mermigkis C, Bouloukaki I, Antoniou KM, et al. CPAP therapy in patients with idiopathic pulmonary fibrosis and obstructive sleep apnea: does it offer a better quality of life and sleep? Sleep Breath 2013; 17(4):1137–43.

118. Patterson KC, Huang F, Oldham JM, et al. Excessive daytime sleepiness and obstructive sleep apnea in patients with sarcoidosis. Chest 2013; 143(6):1562–8.

119. De Vries J, Rothkrantz-Kos S, van Dieijen-Visser MP, et al. The relationship between fatigue and clinical parameters in pulmonary sarcoidosis. Sarcoidosis Vasc Diffuse Lung Dis 2004;21(2):127–36.

120. Drent M, Lower EE, De Vries J. Sarcoidosis-associated fatigue. Eur Respir J 2012;40(1):255–63.

121. Lower EE, Malhotra A, Surdulescu V, et al. Armodafinil for sarcoidosis-associated fatigue: a double-blind, placebo-controlled, crossover trial. J Pain Symptom Manage 2013;45(2):159–69.

122. Salles C, Ramos RT, Daltro C, et al. Prevalence of obstructive sleep apnea in children and adolescents with sickle cell anemia. J Bras Pneumol 2009;35(11):1075–83.

123. Kaleyias J, Mostofi N, Grant M, et al. Severity of obstructive sleep apnea in children with sickle cell disease. J Pediatr Hematol Oncol 2008;30(9): 659–65.

124. Samuels MP, Stebbens VA, Davies SC, et al. Sleep related upper airway obstruction and hypoxaemia in sickle cell disease. Arch Dis Child 1992;67(7):925–9.

125. Okoli K, Irani F, Horvath W. Pathophysiologic considerations for the interactions between obstructive sleep apnea and sickle hemoglobinopathies. Med Hypotheses 2009;72(5):578–80.

126. Spicuzza L, Sciuto C, Leonardi S, et al. Early occurrence of obstructive sleep apnea in infants and children with cystic fibrosis. Arch Pediatr Adolesc Med 2012;166(12):1165–9.

127. Perin C, Fagondes SC, Casarotto FC, et al. Sleep findings and predictors of sleep desaturation in adult cystic fibrosis patients. Sleep Breath 2012; 16(4):1041–8.

Ventilatory Support During Sleep in Patients with Chronic Obstructive Pulmonary Disease

Peter Jan Wijkstra, MD, PhD*,
Marieke Leontine Duiverman, MD, PhD

KEYWORDS

- Chronic obstructive pulmonary disease • Noninvasive ventilation • Chronic respiratory failure
- Monitoring • Adequate ventilation

KEY POINTS

- There is no conclusive evidence that chronic noninvasive ventilation (NIV) should be provided routinely to stable patients with chronic obstructive pulmonary disease.
- Level of baseline $Paco_2$, height of inspiratory pressures, and compliance seem to be important components in providing effective ventilatory support.
- The combination of rehabilitation and nocturnal ventilatory support seems to provide more benefits than rehabilitation alone.
- The option of providing chronic NIV after acute respiratory failure has to be investigated.

INTRODUCTION

Chronic ventilatory support is a well-accepted and effective therapy in patients with chronic respiratory failure due to thoracic cage abnormalities or in patients with neuromuscular disease. This is in contrast with patients with chronic obstructive pulmonary disease (COPD), where despite several positive uncontrolled trials, the evidence to start it routinely is lacking. This article will first discuss the different rationales why chronic nocturnal noninvasive ventilation (NIV) might be effective in these patients. It will then discuss the benefits of chronic NIV in stable disease, in combination with rehabilitation, and after acute respiratory failure. Thereafter the authors will elaborate on different issues that might be important in making NIV more effective in patients with COPD.

RATIONALE FOR VENTILATORY SUPPORT DURING SLEEP IN STABLE COPD

During sleep, ventilation is decreased due to several factors such as increased upper airway resistance, a decrease in the reticular activating system and metabolic rate, and a decreased chemosensitivity. During rapid eye movement (REM) sleep, breathing becomes more variable; upper airway resistance increases even further, and a generalized muscle hypotonia of the respiratory muscles leads to a decreased contribution of the intercostal muscles relative to the diaphragm.[1]

In COPD, respiratory failure during sleep occurs frequently, and various mechanisms are thought to contribute. First, it seems apparent that in patients with daytime respiratory failure, physiologic changes during sleep exacerbate this problem.

Conflict of Interest: P.J. Wijkstra reports grants and fees from Philips/Respironics, RESMED, VIVISOL, Medicq TEFA, Emdamed, Air Liquide and Goedegebeure.
Department of Pulmonary Diseases/Home Mechanical Ventilation, University Medical Centre Groningen, Post-Box 30.001, Groningen 9700 RB, The Netherlands
* Corresponding author.
E-mail address: p.j.wijkstra@int.azg.nl

1556-407X/14/$ – see front matter © 2014 Elsevier Inc. All rights reserved.

Second, as during the daytime reliance on inter-costal and accessory respiratory muscles is greater in COPD compared with healthy subjects, the generalized muscle atonia occurring in REM sleep leads to loss of this contribution and more reliance on a diaphragm that is in a mechanically disadvantageous position that it simply cannot deliver enough power to keep ventilation at a sufficient level. Third, a blunted chemoresponsiveness during sleep might lead to less frequent arousals, during which ventilation has the opportunity to increase. Fourth, functional residual capacity decreases during sleep, leading to increased ventilation–perfusion mismatching, with more pronounced effects in COPD, especially on oxygen levels.[2]

It seems logical to counterbalance these detrimental effects during sleep in COPD with noninvasive positive pressure ventilation. It has been shown that nocturnal hypoventilation is reversed by nocturnal NIV.[3] However, it is intriguing to find that a therapy applied during the night remains effective during the day. In addition to its effect on reversing nocturnal hypoventilation, three other possible mechanisms for improvement have been proposed.[4] NIV provides rest to (fatigued) respiratory muscles; NIV increases ventilatory sensitivity to carbon dioxide during spontaneous breathing, and NIV improves pulmonary mechanics.

Reversal of Nocturnal Hypoventilation

Reversal of nocturnal hypoventilation leads to improvements in arterial blood gases during sleep, and ideally this improvement can (at least partially) be sustained during the day.

It has been suggested that improved blood gases improve muscle function by improving the internal milieu; however, studies on the effects of hypercapnia/acidemia on peripheral and respiratory muscle contractility, strength, and endurance are controversial.[5–7]

Second, despite decreased chemosensitivity during sleep (especially REM sleep) in COPD, profound hypercapnia may provoke arousals. By reversing hypoventilation, arousals may occur less frequently, leading to improvement in sleep quality. However, sleep quality is affected by several other factors.

Interestingly, it has been shown that after cessation of NIV at awakening, arterial carbon dioxide level (Pa_{CO_2}) decreases even further during the first hours of subsequent spontaneous breathing, an effect more pronounced after patients have been using NIV for a longer period.[8] This suggests that there are additional mechanisms on top of just relying on improvements attained during the night.

Improving Respiratory Muscle Function

In patients with severe COPD, the respiratory muscles have an unfavorable position due to hyperinflation, and therefore the diaphragm is thought to be susceptible to fatigue. This hypothesis is derived from findings in several studies. On the 1 hand, studies have consistently shown that both central neural drive and respiratory muscle work/energy expenditure are increased in severe COPD.[9,10] On the other hand, NIV might reduce respiratory muscle drive[11] and respiratory muscle work load,[12] while capacity is increased, making the respiratory muscles less susceptible to fatigue.

There are also some arguments against the effects of NIV on fatigued muscles. First, it has been shown that the respiratory muscles of hypercapnic COPD patients work hard but are not fatigued; they seem to act as wise fighters, thereby deliberately keeping respiratory muscle work below the fatigue threshold at the expense of decreased tidal volumes and thus alveolar hypoventilation.[13] Second, most studies on NIV in COPD have not shown any effects on maximal respiratory muscle pressures independent from changes in lung volumes,[14] arguing against the hypothesis that if the muscles are rested, they should gain (reserve) capacity. As a consequence, instead of resting fatigued respiratory muscles, NIV might, among other things, lead to a decrease in respiratory muscle work through the induction of a more favorable breathing pattern, a pattern that can be maintained during the day.

Improving Central Drive

Prolonged hypercapnia might lead to a progressive resetting to a higher sensitivity threshold of the central chemoreceptors. After NIV treatment, the threshold might be reset downwards again, although this process has been suggested to occur progressively over several years.[15] In hypercapnic COPD patients, there is a lack of strong evidence that resetting of the CO_2 sensitivity plays a role.[9] However, from the wise fighter concept, it does not seem to be beneficial to increase CO_2 sensitivity, as increased ventilation means an increased load on the already heavily loaded system. Only when a simultaneous reduction in load (eg, by improved pulmonary mechanics) occurs, increased chemosensitivity during sleep and awake states leads to improved ventilation without the occurrence of respiratory muscle fatigue or failure.

Reducing the Load Against Which the Respiratory Muscle Pump Has to Function

Improvement in breathing patterns and pulmonary mechanics seems to be an important part of the improvement in gas exchange, as it was found consistently in most recent studies, especially those using higher pressures.[11,16–18] The mechanical load in severe COPD is high mainly due to a high airway resistance, leading to hyperinflation. Several studies have shown that NIV can reduce hyperinflation, and this reduction is associated with improvements in gas exchange.

A reduction in hyperinflation occurs when a reduction in airway resistance is achieved. A reduction in hypercapnia, causing less retention of salt and water, might lead to a decrease in airway resistance because of less airway edema and/or less airway inflammation.[19] Second, less airway inflammation might be important. Improved sputum expectoration, improved ventilation of peripheral regions, but also less airway edema probably exhibits a positive effect on airway inflammation. Less airway edema might lead to less airway wall remodeling by reducing inflammation when muscle fibers become less overstretched. Third, a reduction in hyperinflation is hypothesized to be a consequence of a slower and deeper breathing pattern, which is facilitated by improved respiratory muscle function that can be preserved from NIV to spontaneous breathing. Furthermore, when patients on NIV have fewer exacerbations, this might prevent any further increase in hyperinflation over time.

Finally, NIV might lead to (small) airway recruitment, probably to less small airway closure, In this respect, by improving ventilation in peripheral lung regions, NIV reduces ventilation–perfusion mismatching, thereby also improving arterial oxygen pressure.[20]

In conclusion, although several theories exist, there are currently no studies on NIV or nasal intermittent positive pressure ventilation (NIPPV) that have provided definitive evidence that the benefits found in gas exchange are related to improvements in respiratory muscle function or altered chemosensitivity. Reversal of nocturnal hypoventilation seems apparent; however, this mechanism does not explain the entire picture, and, furthermore, the effects on sleep efficiency are incompletely explained. The relationship between improved gas exchange and less hyperinflation needs further investigation.

VENTILATORY SUPPORT DURING SLEEP IN STABLE PATIENTS WITH COPD

In the last couple of decades, several trials have investigated the benefits of nocturnal NIV in stable patients with COPD. While in 2000 the opinion was that NIV was not effective in these patients,[21,22] due to new clinical trials there seems to be a shift in this opinion as recently discussed by Schönhofer.[23] This section, will discuss short- and long-term studies investigating the benefits of nocturnal NIV separately and will finish by referring to a recent published meta-analysis.

Uncontrolled Trials

In the past, several uncontrolled trials investigating the effects of NIV showed some encouraging results. A French study showed that 6 months of nocturnal NIV in 14 patients with a mean baseline $Paco_2$ of 7.8 kPa (58.5 mm Hg) significantly improved quality of life.[24] In addition to an improved quality of life, a significant improvement in arterial blood gases was found. In the study by Sivasothy,[25] 26 patients with severe COPD and hypercapnia ($Paco_2$ 8.6 kPa or 64.5 mm Hg) were also ventilated by a volume ventilator during the night. After 18 months, both gas exchange and quality of life improved significantly. A long-term study by Jones showed that after 24 months of pressure ventilation there were significant improvements in arterial blood gases and a reduction in hospital admissions and general practitioner visits.[26] In the last decade, several German studies were published investigating the benefits of high-intensity NIV. Windisch studied the benefits of controlled NIV with mean breathing frequency of 21 breaths per minute and mean inspiratory positive airway pressures of 28 cm H_2O in 73 COPD patients (mean forced expiratory volume in 1 second [FEV_1] 30% predicted). They found significant improvements in blood gas tensions, lung function, and hematocrit after 2 months. In this study, the 2- and 5-year survival rates of all patients were 82% and 58%, respectively.[17] In a randomized controlled crossover trial, the same group compared 6 weeks of high-intensity NIV (using controlled ventilation with mean inspiratory pressures of around 29 cm H_2O) with low-intensity NIV (using assisted ventilation with mean inspiratory pressures of 15 cm H_2O) in 17 patients with severe stable hypercapnic COPD.[17,27] They found a significant reduction in nocturnal $Paco_2$ in favor of high-intensity NIV, which was not unexpected, as high-intensity NIV was targeted in reducing nocturnal $Paco_2$. An important finding was that daily use of NIV was increased in high-intensity NIV compared with low-intensity NIV, meaning that patients tolerated high pressures better than low pressures. In addition, only high-intensity

NIV resulted in significant improvements in exercise-related dyspnea, FEV_1, vital capacity, and health-related quality of life. Despite these positive outcomes, the overall opinion is that there is a need for randomized controlled trials (RCTs) evaluating the role of high-intensity NIV in stable hypercapnic COPD patients.

Short-Term RCTs of NIV in COPD

There have been 6 RCTs of NIPPV up to a duration of 3 months that have been published.[3,28–32] Strumpf and colleagues[28] did not find significant changes in any of the measured variables apart from neuropsychological function. Important in this respect is that only 7 of the 19 patients completed the study, and most patients were not hypercapnic. Gay and colleagues[29] investigated the effects of NIPPV in hypercapnic patients and showed that NIPPV did not lead to an improvement in clinical parameters compared with sham ventilation. Still, only a small number of patients completed the study. The study of Meecham Jones and colleagues[3] was the only one to show clear benefits of nocturnal NIPPV in patients with COPD. Three months of NIPPV combined with oxygen were better than oxygen alone for gas exchange, sleep efficiency, and health status. They also showed that patients with an increased level of hypoventilation during the night showed the most benefit in reducing daytime $Paco_2$. Lin and colleagues[30] investigated the effects of only 2 weeks of NIPPV and showed only a positive effect of NIPPV and oxygen on the nighttime oxygenation. The fact that the patients had only 2 weeks of acclimatization on NIPPV might be the reason for this negative study. Renston and colleagues[12] investigated the effects of daytime NIPPV (ie, 2 hours per day) for 5 consecutive days. Although they did not find significant changes in gas exchange, the NIPPV group showed a significant decrease in the level of dyspnea and an improved exercise capacity. A study from Diaz and colleagues[16] investigated the effects of NIPPV during the daytime for 3 hours, 5 days a week for 3 weeks. Although this was a very short-term application of NIV, they found significant improvements in gas exchange, dyspnea, and walking distance. As conflicting results still exist in this field, recently an update of a meta-analysis of individual data from RCTs was published comparing NIV with conventional management of patients with COPD and stable respiratory failure.[31,32] Only studies investigating nocturnal NIPPV applied via a nasal or facemask for at least 4 hours each day for 3 weeks were included. Six RCTs were found that fulfilled the previously mentioned criteria (**Table 1**),[3,28,29,33–35] including the 3-month data of the study of Casanova and colleagues[33] as well. This meta-analysis showed that 3 months of NIPPV in patients with stable COPD did not improve lung function, gas exchange, sleep efficiency, or 6-minute walking distance.

Long-Term RCTs of NIV in COPD

Casanova and colleagues[33] were the first to investigate the effects of long-term NIPPV. This study had a duration of 12 months and randomized 52 patients to either NIPPV plus standard care or to standard care alone. Important issues were that the level of bilevel positive airway preparation (PAP) was only modest (inspiratory positive airway pressure [IPAP] 12–14 cm H_2O), and its effect was not monitored during the night. Therefore, it is not certain that effective ventilation was provided. Notwithstanding these limitations, the study did show some positive effects. The number of hospital admissions was lower after 3 months (5% vs 15%). However, this was not the case after 6 months. Although modest improvements were found in dyspnea and neuropsychological function, no significant changes in arterial blood gases and respiratory muscle strength were found after 12 months. Another long-term study compared the combination of NIPPV and long-term oxygen therapy (LTOT) with LTOT alone for a period of 2 years.[34] Patients with a $Paco_2$ greater than 6.6 kPa (49.5 mm Hg) were included. In this study, 90 patients were randomized, and 47 patients completed the study. The level of NIV was again modest (IPAP of 14 ± 3 cm H_2O). Patients did use the ventilator a considerable number of hours (9 ± 2 h). Compared with the 1-year period before the study, total hospital admissions increased by 27% in the LTOT group, while it decreased by 45% in the NIV group. Intensive care unit ICU admissions decreased in the NIV group by 75%, while in the LTOT group they increased by 20%. However, the outcomes were not statistically significantly different between both groups. After 2 years, dyspnea decreased, and health-related quality of life improved in the NIV group compared with the LTOT group. In an Australian study, 144 patients were randomized to either NIPPV with LTOT (n = 72) or to LTOT alone (n = 72).[36] Although the applied inspiratory pressures in this study were low (mean of 13 cm H_2O), NIPPV did improve sleep quality and sleep-related hypercapnia. In addition, the NIV patients showed good compliance with NIV therapy, with a mean nightly use 4.5 hours. Compared with

Table 1
Characteristics of studies included in meta-analysis

Trial	Study Design (Compared to Treatment)	IPAP/Expiratory Positive Airway Pressure	Study Population	Outcomes
Short term				
Casanova et al,[33] 2000	Parallel group (LTOT)	12/4	52 randomized patients, 36 completers $Paco_2$ 51 mm Hg, FEV_1 0.84 L	Blood gasses, lung function, PImax/PEmax, dyspnea after 3 mo Exacerbation rate, hospital admissions, intubations, and mortality after 12 mo
Clini et al,[34] 2002	Parallel group (LTOT)	14.4/3.8	90 randomized patients, 78 completers $Paco_2$ 56 mm Hg, FEV_1 0.75 L	Blood gasses and hospitalizations after 3 mo
Gay et al,[29] 1996	Parallel group (sham)	10/2	13 randomized patients, 10 completers $Paco_2$ 52 mm Hg, FEV_1 0.68 L	Blood gasses, 6 MWD, lung function, PImax/PEmax and sleep study
Meecham Jones et al,[3] 1995	Cross-over (LTOT)	18/2	18 randomized patients, 14 completers. $Paco_2$ 56 mm Hg, FEV_1 0.84 L	Blood gasses, 6 MWD, health-related quality of life, lung function, and sleep study
Sin et al,[35] 2007	Parallel group (sham)	20/4	23 randomized patients, 17 completers $Paco_2$ 43 mm Hg, FEV_1 0.88 L	Blood gasses, 6 MWD, lung function, HRV + natriuretic peptide measurements
Strumpf et al,[28] 1991	Cross-over (standard care)	15/2	19 randomized patients, 7 completers $Paco_2$ 46 mm Hg, FEV_1 0.54 L	Blood gasses, walking test, lung function, PImax/PEmax, sleep study, dyspnea
Long term				
Clini et al,[34] 2002	Parallelgroup (LTOT)	14.6/3.9	90 randomized patients, 57 completers. $Paco_2$ 56 mm Hg, FEV_1 0.75 L	Blood gasses, 6MWD, HRQL, lung function, PImax, sleep study, dyspnea, hospitalizations, mortality
McEvoy et al,[36] 2009	Parallelgroup (LTOT)	12.8/5.1	144 randomized patients, 81 completers. $Paco_2$ 54 mm Hg, FEV_1 0.65 L	Blood gasses, HRQL, lung function, sleep study (only in NIPPV group), hospitalization rates, survival

Abbreviations: HRV, heart rate variability; PEmax, maximal expiratory pressure; PImax, maximal inspiratory pressure; 6 MWD, 6-minute walking distance.

From Struik FM, Lacasse Y, Goldstein RS, et al. Nocturnal noninvasive positive pressure ventilation in stable COPD: a systematic review and individual patient data meta-analysis. Respir Med 2014;108:332; with permission.

LTOT alone, NIV showed an improvement in survival, however, at the cost of a worsened quality of life. The previously mentioned meta-analysis also investigated the long-term benefits from the RCTs.[31,32] Despite the previously mentioned positive results, the overall meta-analysis did not find any significant benefits of NIPPV compared with controls.

VENTILATORY SUPPORT DURING SLEEP COMBINED WITH REHABILITATION

Pulmonary rehabilitation has emerged as a recommended standard of care for patients with lung diseases, as it has been shown to improve exercise tolerance, improve quality of life, reduce respiratory symptoms, and reduce the number of hospitalizations.[37] In patients with severe COPD and respiratory failure, NIV can improve gas exchange,[8,11,16–18] lung function,[16,17,38] functional capacity,[18,38] and sleep quality.[3,36] NIV as an adjunct to pulmonary rehabilitation has been used in 2 different settings: (1) NIV during the exercise training, a topic that will not be discussed further here, and (2) NIV during the night while exercise training is performed during the daytime.

The first study investigating the effect of nocturnal NIV used negative pressure ventilation with a pulmowrap ventilator and showed no additional effects of this combination on lung function, inspiratory muscle pressure, exercise tolerance, and clinical improvement. However, the program lasted only for 3 weeks.[39] The first study using nocturnal domiciliary NIPPV in conjunction with a pulmonary rehabilitation program showed promising results despite low ventilator compliance (median use of 2.08 h/d) and the inclusion of only mildly hypercapnic patients (mean $Paco_2$ 45.6 mm Hg).[40] This study showed a significantly improved exercise tolerance and quality of life after 3 months of NIPPV with rehabilitation compared with the rehabilitation alone. The positive effects became especially apparent after 4 weeks, indicating that a certain duration of this combination therapy is necessary to achieve benefits. However, effects on gas exchange were minimal, with no change in $Paco_2$, indicating that no true improvement in ventilation was achieved. Therefore, the authors suggested that other mechanisms should have caused the improvement, and as they found a small increase in maximal inspiratory pressure only in the NIPPV with rehabilitation group, they speculated that relief of respiratory muscle fatigue caused the improvements.

Positive findings were also found in a longer-term study, showing that NIPPV with rehabilitation as compared to rehabilitation alone had a significant beneficial effect on quality of life, daytime arterial blood gases, exercise tolerance, functional activity, and lung function.[38] Although effects on quality of life, blood gases, and daily activity level were already apparent after 3 months of the combined therapy, the positive effects in terms of increased exercise tolerance and lung function continued to increase over time, possibly because the deterioration occurring in the rehabilitation alone group could have been prevented in the NIPPV with rehabilitation group. Importantly, in this study there was proof that NIPPV actually reversed nocturnal hypoventilation measured by nocturnal arterial blood gases, as well as daytime gas. This might be a consequence of better compliance (median use of NIPPV 6.9 h/d) and higher settings (mean IPAP 23 cm H_2O). It is possible that improved gas exchange played an important role in improving quality of life and exercise tolerance, as better blood gases probably give patients a more favorable condition to train.

Thus, to achieve beneficial effects of the addition of nocturnal NIPPV to rehabilitation, a good compliance, higher inspiratory pressures leading to changes in gas exchange, and a certain length of the treatment period seem to be important predictive factors. Although it seems that the longer the treatment period the more benefit, it is obvious that careful implementation of the NIPPV with close initial observation of patients leads to a better starting point and probably earlier and better results. In the study of Köhnlein and colleagues,[41] careful implementation led to improvements in as little as 3 to 5 weeks, although no strict conclusion can be drawn from this study, as it was only observational using a historical control group. In contrast, when NIV is instituted without extra attention to details, it will not lead to physiologic changes or objective benefits.

NIPPV on top of rehabilitation compared with rehabilitation alone has been shown to be able to increase FEV_1[38] and decrease hyperinflation.[41] Possible mechanisms for this lung function improvement are reduced airway obstruction due to improved hypercapnia-induced airway edema, reduced inflammation, and increased small airway recruitment. Lung function improvement has been shown in conjunction with blood gas improvements, but also without obvious changes in gas exchange, indicating that different mechanisms might be important.

To conclude, although evidence is not extensive yet, RCTs have shown that NIPPV on top of rehabilitation is of benefit in severe COPD patients. Important aspects to achieve benefits are careful implementation with sufficient high pressures, assuring that true improvements of gas exchange are achieved by careful monitoring, good compliance, and a sufficiently long period of treatment.

VENTILATORY SUPPORT DURING SLEEP AFTER ACUTE RESPIRATORY FAILURE

It is known that 80% of the patients who receive NIV during acute respiratory failure will be rehospitalized within 12 months after discharge and that

50% of these patients will die in this period.[42] Therefore, the application of chronic NIV might be effective in this situation. In an uncontrolled study, Tuggey and colleagues[43] investigated the benefits of chronic NIV in a group of patients who were admitted frequently because of acute respiratory failure and needed NIV in this situation. They showed that in the year after they started chronic NIV, there was a significant reduction in the number of admissions and total days in hospital. It has to be mentioned, however, that this was in a highly selective group of patients who were compliant with the ventilator and were motivated to use it at home. A randomized pilot trial was carried out by Cheung and colleagues[44] comparing chronic home NIV to placebo NIV (continuous positive airway pressure [CPAP] of 5 cm H_2O). Primary outcome was recurrent severe COPD exacerbation with acute hypercapnic respiratory failure (AHRF) resulting in need for NIV, intubation, or death within the following year. At 1 year, the proportion of patients developing this composite outcome was 38.5% in the NIPPV group versus 60.2% in the placebo CPAP group ($P = .04$). Although the mean IPAP in the NIPPV group was low (15 cm H_2O), the adherence to both types of therapy was high. However, dropout rates were also high, especially in the NIPPV group (35%). At present, there are 2 international RCTs underway investigating the benefits of chronic NIV after acute respiratory failure. The results of these trials have to be awaited to know whether chronic NIV has a place in this specific situation.

IMPORTANT ISSUES IN PROVIDING ADEQUATE VENTILATORY SUPPORT DURING SLEEP

Although the evidence for providing routine chronic NIV to COPD patients is still lacking, much has been learned from the studies that have been published. This section will elaborate on the different aspects that seem important to provide effective chronic ventilatory support.

Selection of Patients

Both Meecham Jones[3] and Clini[34] reported significant benefits of NIV by including patients with a $Paco_2$ of more than 6.6 kPa (49.5 mm Hg) in contrast to other studies. In addition, Meecham Jones and colleagues showed that patients who had an increase in $Paco_2$ during the night before they were on NIPPV experienced the most benefit in terms of decreasing daytime $Paco_2$ after starting NIV. In a recent meta-analysis based on individual data, it was also shown that patients who were more hypercapnic at baseline ($Paco_2$ >55 mm Hg) showed more reduction in their daytime $Paco_2$ compared with patients who were less hypercapnic.[31]

Adequacy of Ventilation

Monitoring seems to be more important to confirm whether ventilation was effective or not than the type of ventilation. While Strumpf and colleagues[28] monitored CO_2 using end tidal CO_2, which is an unreliable measure in patients with COPD, Meecham Jones and colleagues[3] monitored the effectiveness of ventilation by transcutaneous CO_2. The authors' group[18] monitored the effectiveness of ventilation by nocturnal arterial blood gases. In the last-mentioned controlled studies in which the effectiveness of NIPPV during sleep was confirmed reliably with either transcutaneous CO_2 or arterial blood gases, higher mean inspiratory pressures were used, and probably not surprisingly, these studies showed positive effects in most outcomes.[3,18] It is highly likely that appropriate CO_2 monitoring leads to higher pressures needed to achieve effective ventilation; this effect was also shown in a recent retrospective trial using mean inspiratory pressures of 28 cm H_2O.[17] This was also shown in the recent update of a meta-analysis showing that higher levels of IPAP (higher than 18 cm H_2O) lead to a larger reduction in daytime $Paco_2$. Nevertheless, it is not known whether more effective reduction in daytime Pa CO_2 leads to clinically important benefits (**Fig. 1**).[31]

Number of Hours on NIV

Because the optimal duration of ventilatory support is not known, different approaches have been used. Two randomized controlled studies treating patients with COPD explored shorter duration of time daytime ventilatory support.[12,16] In 1 study, the patients received bilevel PAP for 2 hours daily for 5 days a week, while in the other study, bilevel PAP was given for 3 hours daily, 5 days a week for 3 consecutive weeks. Despite these short periods of bilevel PAP support, significant benefits in clinical parameters and changes in Pao_2 and $Paco_2$ were found. This finding may be due to the fact that patients adjust to the NIV device during daytime more easily, and mask leakage is less. Other studies found positive outcomes by applying considerably more hours of bilevel PAP. Clini and colleagues[34] showed positive results with a mean number of hours on bilevel PAP of 9 hours, while Meecham Jones and colleagues[3] and the authors' group[38] showed positive outcomes by a median number of hours of bilevel PAP use of 6.9 hours.[3] A recent update of a meta-analysis of chronic NIPPV showed that the largest decrease in $Paco_2$ was found in

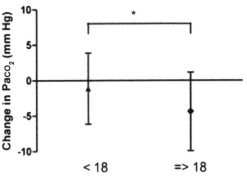

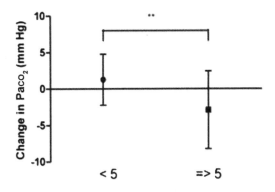

Compliance (ventilation hours/night)

Fig. 1. Change in $Paco_2$ after 3 months of NIPPV ($Paco_2$ baseline - $Paco_2$ after 3 months) for high and low inspiratory positive airway pressure (< 18 and => 18 IPAP) and high and low compliance (< 5 and => 5 ventilation hours per night). Figures display mean change scores and 95% confidence intervals. Significant difference: *: $p<0.05$, **$p<0.01$. (*From* Struik FM, Lacasse Y, Goldstein RS, et al. Nocturnal noninvasive positive pressure ventilation in stable COPD: a systematic review and individual patient data meta-analysis. Respir Med 2014;108:334; with permission.)

patients who used the ventilator for more than 5 hours per night (see **Fig. 1**).[31]

SUMMARY

In conclusion, currently there is no conclusive evidence that NIV should be provided routinely to stable patients with COPD. Nevertheless, patients who are clearly hypercapnic, who receive confirmed effective ventilation by applying higher inspiratory pressures, and have a better compliance might show clinical benefits. The combination of rehabilitation and nocturnal ventilatory support seems to provide more benefits than rehabilitation alone, so this might be a situation in which chronic NIV is effective.

ACKNOWLEDGMENTS

The authors kindly thank Elsevier for using the table and figure as were in Respiratory Medicine in 2014.[33]

REFERENCES

1. Collop N. Sleep and sleep disorders in chronic obstructive pulmonary disease. Respiration 2010; 80:78–86.
2. McNicholas WT, Verbraecken J, Marin JM. Sleep disorders in COPD: the forgotten dimension. Eur Respir Rev 2013;22:365–75.
3. Meecham Jones DJ, Paul EA, Jones PW, et al. Nasal pressure support ventilation plus oxygen compared with oxygen therapy alone in hypercapnic COPD. Am J Respir Crit Care Med 1995;152:538–44.
4. Hill NS. Noninvasive ventilation. Does it work, for whom, and how? Am Rev Respir Dis 1993;147: 1050–5.
5. Creese R. Bicarbonate ion and striated muscle. J Physiol 1949;110:450–7.
6. Rafferty GF, Lou Harris M, Polkey MI, et al. Effect of hypercapnia on maximal voluntary ventilation and diaphragm fatigue in normal humans. Am J Respir Crit Care Med 1999;160:1567–71.
7. Nizet TA, Heijdra YF, van den Elshout FJ, et al. Respiratory muscle strength and muscle endurance are not affected by acute metabolic acidemia. Clin Physiol Funct Imaging 2009;29:392–9.
8. Windisch W, Dreher M, Storre JH, et al. Nocturnal non-invasive positive pressure ventilation: physiological effects on spontaneous breathing. Respir Physiol Neurobiol 2006;150:251–60.
9. Elliott MW. Noninvasive ventilation in chronic ventilatory failure due to chronic obstructive pulmonary disease. Eur Respir J 2002;20:511–4.
10. Duiverman ML, van Eykern LA, Vennik PW, et al. Reproducibility and responsiveness of a noninvasive EMG technique of the respiratory muscles in COPD patients and in healthy subjects. J Appl Physiol 2004;96:1723–9.
11. Lukácsovits J, Carlucci A, Hill N, et al. Physiological changes during low- and high-intensity noninvasive ventilation. Eur Respir J 2012;39:869–75.
12. Renston JP, DiMarco AF, Supinski GS. Respiratory muscle rest using nasal BiPAP ventilation in patients with stable severe COPD. Chest 1994;105: 1053–60.
13. Bégin P, Grassino A. Chronic alveolar hypoventilation helps to maintain the inspiratory muscle effort of COPD patients within sustainable limits. Chest 2000;117:271S–3S.
14. Schönhofer B, Polkey MI, Suchi S, et al. Effect of home mechanical ventilation on inspiratory muscle strength in COPD. Chest 2006;130:1834–8.

15. Guilleminault C, Cummiskey J. Progressive improvement of apnea index and ventilatory response to CO2 after tracheostomy in obstructive sleep apnea syndrome. Am Rev Respir Dis 1982;126:14–20.

16. Díaz O, Bégin P, Andresen M, et al. Physiological and clinical effects of diurnal noninvasive ventilation in hypercapnic COPD. Eur Respir J 2005;26: 1016–23.

17. Windisch W, Kostić S, Dreher M, et al. Outcome of patients with stable COPD receiving controlled noninvasive positive pressure ventilation aimed at a maximal reduction of Pa(CO2). Chest 2005;128: 657–62.

18. Duiverman ML, Wempe JB, Bladder G, et al. Nocturnal non-invasive ventilation in addition to rehabilitation in hypercapnic patients with COPD. Thorax 2008;63:1052–7.

19. Burns GP, Gibson GJ. A novel hypothesis to explain the bronchoconstrictor effect of deep inspiration in asthma. Thorax 2002;57:116–9.

20. De Backer LA, Vos WG, Salgado R, et al. Functional imaging using computer methods to compare the effect of salbutamol and ipratropium bromide in patient-specific airway models of COPD. Int J Chron Obstruct Pulmon Dis 2011;6:637–46.

21. Rossi A. Noninvasive ventilation has not been shown to be ineffective in stable COPD. Am J Respir Crit Care Med 2000;161:688–9.

22. Hill NS. Noninvasive ventilation has been shown to be ineffective in stable COPD. Am J Respir Crit Care Med 2000;161:689–90.

23. Schonhofer B. Non-invasive positive pressure ventilation in patients with stable hypercapnic COPD: light at the end of the tunnel? Thorax 2010;65:765–7.

24. Perrin C, El Far Y, Vandenbos F, et al. Domiciliary nasal intermittent positive pressure ventilation in severe COPD: effects on lung function and quality of life. Eur Respir J 1997;10:2835–9.

25. Sivasothy P, Smith IE, Shneerson JM. Mask intermittent positive pressure ventilation in chronic hypercapnic respiratory failure due to chronic obstructive pulmonary disease. Eur Respir J 1998;1:34–40.

26. Jones SE, Packham S, Hebden M, et al. Domiciliary nocturnal intermittent positive pressure ventilation in patients with respiratory failure due to severe COPD: long-term follow up and effect on survival. Thorax 1998;53:495–8.

27. Dreher M, Storre JH, Schmoor C, et al. High–intensity versus low intensity non invasive ventilation in patients with stable hypercapnic COPD: a randomsied cross-over trial. Thorax 2010;65:303–8.

28. Strumpf DA, Millman RP, Carlisle CC, et al. Nocturnal positive-pressure ventilation via nasal mask in patients with severe chronic obstructive pulmonary disease. Am Rev Respir Dis 1991;144(6):1234–9.

29. Gay PC, Hubmayr RD, Stroetz RW. Efficacy of nocturnal nasal ventilation in stable, severe chronic obstructive pulmonary disease during a 3-month controlled trial. Mayo Clin Proc 1996;71(6):533–42.

30. Lin CC. Comparison between nocturnal nasal positive pressure ventilation combined with oxygen therapy and oxygen monotherapy in patients with severe COPD. Am J Respir Crit Care Med 1996; 154(2 Pt 1):353–8.

31. Struik FM, Lacasse Y, Goldstein RS, et al. Nocturnal noninvasive positive pressure ventilation in stable COPD: a systematic review and individual patient data meta-analysis. Respir Med 2014;108: 329–37.

32. Struik FM, Lacasse Y, Goldstein R, et al. Nocturnal noninvasive positive pressure ventilation for stable COPD. Cochrane Database Syst Rev 2013;(6): CD002878.

33. Casanova C, Celli BR, Tost L, et al. Long-term controlled trial of nocturnal nasal positive pressure ventilation in patients with severe COPD. Chest 2000;118:1582–90.

34. Clini E, Sturani C, Rossi A, et al. The Italian multi-centre study on noninvasive ventilation in chronic obstructive pulmonary disease patients. Eur Respir J 2002;20:529–38.

35. Sin DD, Wong E, Mayers I, et al. Effects of nocturnal noninvasive mechanical ventilation on heart rate variability of patients with advanced COPD. Chest 2007;131:156–63.

36. McEvoy RD, Pierce RJ, Hillman D, et al. Nocturnal non-invasive nasal ventilation in stable hypercapnic COPD: a randomised controlled trial. Thorax 2009; 64:561–6.

37. Ries AL, Bauldoff GS, Carlin BW, et al. Pulmonary rehabilitation: joint ACCP/AACVPR evidence-based clinical practice guidelines. Chest 2007;131: 4S–42S.

38. Duiverman ML, Wempe JB, Bladder G, et al. Two year home based nocturnal non invasive ventilation added to rehabilitation in COPD patients: a randomized controlled trial. Respir Res 2011;12: 112–22.

39. Celli B, Lee H, Criner G, et al. Controlled trial of external negative pressure ventilation in patients with severe chronic airflow obstruction. Am Rev Respir Dis 1989;140:1251–6.

40. Garrod R, Mikelsons C, Paul EA, et al. Randomized controlled trial of domiciliary noninvasive positive pressure ventilation and physical training in severe chronic obstructive pulmonary disease. Am J Respir Crit Care Med 2000;162:1335–41.

41. Köhnlein T, Schönheit-Kenn U, Winterkamp S, et al. Non invasive ventilation in pulmonary rehabilitation in COPD patients. Respir Med 2009;103:1329–36.

42. Chu CM, Chan VL, Lin AW, et al. Readmission rates and life threatening events in COPD survivors treated with non-invasive ventilation for acute hypercapnic respiratory failure. Thorax 2004;59:1020–5.

43. Tuggey JM, Plant PK, Elliott MW. Domiciliary non-invasive ventilation for recurrent acidotic exacerbations of COPD: an economic analysis. Thorax 2003;58(10):867–71.

44. Cheung AP, Chan VL, Liong JT, et al. A pilot trial of non-invasive ventilation after acute respiratory failure in COPD. Int J Tuberc Lung Dis 2010;14(5): 642–9.

Opioids, Sedatives, and Sleep Hypoventilation

Nevin Arora, MD[a], Michelle Cao, MD[a], Shahrokh Javaheri, MD[b],*

KEYWORDS

- Opioids • Hypoventilation • Sedatives • Sleep-disordered breathing • Sleep apnea
- Benzodiazepines • Ventilatory response

KEY POINTS

- The emphasis on effectively treating chronic pain syndromes has led to a large increase in the number of patients on opioid medications chronically.
- An increasingly recognized adverse effect of long-term opioid usage is sleep-related respiratory disorders, including sleep hypoventilation and sleep apnea.
- Sleep-related hypoventilation secondary to opioid use is associated with hypercapnia caused by a blunted hypercapnic ventilatory response, decreased respiratory drive, and possibly reduction in upper airway muscle tone.
- The combination of opioids and sedatives, individually working on different receptors, could synergistically cause severe respiratory depression during sleep.
- Treatment of opioid-induced sleep hypoventilation includes taper of dosage or withdrawal of the medication if possible, or use of noninvasive positive pressure ventilation devices to support breathing during sleep.

INTRODUCTION

The treatment of pain, both acute and chronic, is justifiably becoming more important. The presence of chronic pain is associated with decreased quality of life, and effective therapy with improvement.[1] Pain adversely effects both physical and mental health and has become a public health concern. Pain is considered a vital sign in medical clinics across the country. Beginning in 1997, the American Academy of Pain Medicine in conjunction with the American Pain Society issued a consensus supporting the use of opioids for the treatment of chronic pain.[2] Even before this statement was released, opioid usage was increasing, with a further increase in methadone and oxycodone usage by 824% and 660% from 1997 to 2003, respectively.[3] The escalation in opioid prescriptions is a result of increased awareness by health care providers to treat chronic pain and awareness by patients to seek treatment.

Opioids are effective and widely prescribed analgesics, but their use is limited by several problematic side effects. One of the more concerning and recognized adverse effects, to which tolerance does not develop with long-term treatment, is respiratory depression during sleep. This depression can manifest in a variety of ways, being in the category of sleep-related breathing disorders. There is a paucity of data on treatment options and the effectiveness of these options for patients with sleep-related breathing disorders including sleep hypoventilation associated with chronic opioid use. Furthermore, there is no clear consensus on how best to manage opioid-induced sleep-related breathing disorders, apart from using the lowest effective opioid dose. The adverse effects of chronic opioid use on respiration during sleep, specifically hypoventilation,

a Stanford Sleep Medicine, Stanford University, Redwood City, CA 94063-5704, USA; b Division of Pulmonary, Critical Care & Sleep Medicine, University of Cincinnati, Cincinnati, OH 45267-0564, USA
* Corresponding author.
E-mail address: shahrokhjavaheri@icloud.com

Sleep Med Clin 9 (2014) 391–398
http://dx.doi.org/10.1016/j.jsmc.2014.05.004
1556-407X/14/$ – see front matter © 2014 Elsevier Inc. All rights reserved.

and potential additive consequences when combined with sedatives, are reviewed here along with potential treatment options.

MECHANISMS OF OPIOID-INDUCED SLEEP HYPOVENTILATION
Opioid Receptors

Opioid receptors are a family of G-protein–coupled receptors (GPCRs). Ligand binding of opioid receptors activates inhibitory intracellular pathways leading to a reduction in neuronal excitability. Opioid receptors are widespread throughout the body and mediate multiple physiologic responses including pain, respiratory control, stress, appetite, and thermoregulation. There are 4 types of opioid receptors: delta (DOP) receptor, mu (MOP) receptor, kappa (KOP) receptor, and nociceptin/orphanin FQ peptide (NOP) receptor. Each receptor is associated with one or more endogenous ligands, including endorphins, enkephalins, dynorphins, and nociceptin/orphanin. Opioids induce respiratory depression chiefly through their actions on mu and kappa receptors, both of which are located centrally and peripherally. Opioids treat pain through these receptors as well.

Respiratory Rhythm Generation

Experimental studies in neonatal rats have improved understanding of how respiration is controlled. Respiratory rhythm generation occurs in the ventrolateral medullary portion of the rat brainstem in 2 distinct complexes: the pre-Bötzinger complex (pre-BotC) and the retrotrapezoid nucleus/parafacial respiratory group (RTN/pFRG), which are coupled and generate normal respiration rhythm.[4–6] The pre-BotC and RTN/pFRG together control respiration with the hypothesis that intrinsic pacemaker cells within these structures modulate respiratory rhythm. Respiratory rhythm in these complexes persists en bloc and in slices even after attenuation of postsynaptic inhibition, supporting the hypothesis that intrinsic rhythmical pacemaker neurons located in these complexes are driving the respiratory rhythm.[5] These findings have not been replicated in human studies.

Opioid Receptors and Respiratory Rhythm Control

Opioid receptors are found preferentially in the inspiratory generating pre-BotC.[5] A study by Mellen and colleagues[7] showed that when the potent mu-opioid agonist D-Ala2-MePhe4-Glycol5 Enkephalin (DAMGO) was added to the rat brainstem containing only pre-BotC, respiratory rhythm slowed. When DAMGO was added to the rat brainstem containing both pre-BotC and RTN/pFRG, the respiratory pattern became irregular with subthreshold action potentials still occurring regularly from the pre-BotC, but the action potentials were not transmitted. This effect is likened to the pathophysiology of Mobitz type II second-degree heart block occurring in control of respiration and supports the hypothesis that the RTN/pFRG also has inspiratory controlling capabilities in the absence of pre-BotC function.[7]

In animal studies, the pre-BotC seems to be the dominant site for inspiration and contains the neurokinin-1 receptor (NK1R) and mu-opioid receptor.[8] The anatomic region corresponding with the pre-BotC is identified by NK1R expression and in vitro electrophysiology. In rhythmically active brainstem section in vitro, NK1R expressing pre-BotC neurons are selectively inhibited by opioids.[9] Continuous local unilateral application of a mu-opioid receptor agonist DAMGO or fentanyl into the pre-BotC in adult rats caused sustained slowing of respiratory rate and increased respiratory rate variability (ataxic breathing). At sufficient concentrations of mu-opioid agonist, complete cessation of breathing was seen, as manifested by complete cessation of diaphragmatic muscle activity. Infusion of a mu-opioid agonist caused a state-dependent respiratory rate depression that is most profound in non–rapid eye movement sleep and during anesthesia.[10] These changes were fully reversed by the mu-opioid receptor antagonist naloxone.

HYPERCAPNIC AND HYPOXIC VENTILATORY RESPONSE

Metabolic control of breathing is largely determined by interactions between central and peripheral chemoreceptors. Central chemoreceptors are located in the brainstem; specifically the nucleus tractus solitaries, dorsal respiratory group, medullary raphe, and the aforementioned pre-BotC and RTN/pFRC group. Central chemoreceptors are stimulated by $Paco_2$/hydrogen ion concentration [H^+] in their environment.[11] The degree of ventilatory stimulation for a given level of $Paco_2$ greater than eupnea is known as the hypercapnic ventilatory response (HCVR). HCVR greater than eupnea is most commonly measured by rebreathing techniques while awake. The slope of the hypercapnic ventilatory response is determined by the change in ventilation for an increase in $Paco_2$ of 1 mm Hg. The slope of this response is mediated by the interactions of both central and peripheral chemoreceptors.[12]

Peripheral chemoreceptors are located in the carotid bodies at the bifurcation of the internal and external carotid body. Peripheral chemoreceptors detect changes in Pao_2 with synergistic responses to carbon dioxide $[H^+]$.[13] The degree of ventilatory stimulation for a given level of Pao_2 is known as the hypoxic ventilatory response (HVR). The HVR is usually measured under isocapnic conditions while monitoring oxyhemoglobin saturation. The degree of ventilatory stimulation for a 1% reduction in oxyhemoglobin saturation is linear and determines the slope of the HVR. Peripheral chemoreceptors via carotid sinus and glossopharyngeal nerves have inputs to central respiratory centers, which communicate with motor neurons that innervate respiratory muscles. Recent experiments indicate a major interaction between peripheral and central chemoreceptors that was previously not recognized.[12]

Opioids and Effects on Ventilation and Ventilatory Responses

Opioid receptors are located throughout the central and peripheral nervous system. All aspects of respiration including respiratory rate, tidal volume, and minute ventilation are suppressed in the presence of opioids,[13–16] although suppression of breathing rate is the predominant effect. In this regard, expiratory time is increased with a delay in inspiratory time, which allows $Paco_2$ to increase and Pao_2 to decrease. The suppression is underestimated, because the increase in $Paco_2$ stimulates ventilation. This suppression is dose dependent.

Opioids depress ventilatory responses to hypoxia (HVR) and hypercapnia (HCVR).[13–16] The depression is observed with both systemic[15] and intrathecal[14] administration of opioids. Suppression is mediated primarily via mu receptor. Opioids do not suppress ventilatory response to $Paco_2$ in knockout mice deficient in mu receptor.

Suppression of HCVR and HVR is thought to be caused by opioid binding to chemoreceptors, as discussed earlier.[14–16] However, suppression of ventilatory responses is observed when morphine, a hydrophilic opioid that does not cross the blood-brain barrier, is injected intrathecally. As expected, morphine was not detected in blood with this route of administration, which means that central processing is critical to opioid-mediated ventilatory responses, both HVR and HCVR.

With chronic opioid usage the trend seems to change. Teichtahl and colleagues[17] showed in a cohort of 50 patients on methadone maintenance treatment (MMT), compared with a cohort of matched controls, that HCVR was reduced but HVR was increased. It is hypothesized that the augmented HVR is related to long-term apnea-related intermittent hypoxia. This finding of increased HVR needs to be confirmed. In Teichtahl and colleagues'[17] study there was a further reduction in HCVR in the patients receiving MMT who were taking antidepressants (n = 7). Five of the 7 patients were taking a selective serotonin reuptake inhibitor, 1 taking a selective norepinephrine reuptake inhibitor, and 1 taking a monoamine oxidase inhibitor. Exclusion of this subgroup from the MMT group created a reduction in HCVR that did not reach statistical significance compared with the control group.[17] The effects of antidepressants on HCVR and opioid interaction need to be further investigated.

OPIOIDS AND SEDATIVES

The combination of opioids and sedatives highlights the dilemma of polypharmacy for treatment of comorbid medical and psychiatric conditions. Benzodiazepines are commonly used in the clinical setting for a variety of disorders. Benzodiazepines and related drugs bind to gamma receptors with multiple subtypes and have been used extensively as hypnotics and anxiolytics. However, their effects on breathing and interaction with opioids specifically during sleep need to be systematically investigated, given the potential adverse consequences of polypharmacy of opioids and benzodiazepine receptor agonists. Cohn[18] conducted a review on benzodiazepines and their effects on HCVR in normal controls, citing some studies reporting a decrease, some no change, and some an increase in the slope of HCVR. Other studies in pediatric patients reported that benzodiazepines and opioids reduced pharyngeal muscle tone and depressed ventilation, thereby diminishing the ventilatory response to carbon dioxide.[19,20] Although the studies were conducted in children, these findings are likely applicable to adults. The effect of long-term use of sedatives or a combination of sedatives and opioids on HVR has not been studied.

We remain concerned that the combination of opioids and sedatives, individually working on different receptors, could synergistically cause severe respiratory depression, particularly during sleep, and also during the postoperative period. There have been reports of postoperative mortality caused by one or a combination of these two classes of drugs.[21,22]

OPIOIDS AND SLEEP HYPOVENTILATION

Sleep hypoventilation secondary to chronic opioid use is associated with nocturnal hypercapnia ($Paco_2 \geq 45$ mm Hg) and results from decreased respiratory drive; presumably from the collective effects of opioids on the pre-BotC and the hypoglossal nerve pool. The hypoglossal nerve pool is thought to be associated with worsening of upper airway obstruction or obstructive sleep apnea (OSA)[23] and decreased chemoreceptor responsiveness. Hajiha and colleagues[24] showed that opioids applied to the genioglossus nucleus pool caused a dose-related suppression of tonic brainstem stimulatory input to the genioglossus muscle in rats, a primary muscle involved in upper airway patency.[24] Montandon and colleagues[10] identified a distinct site on the rat medulla that is associated with opioid-induced suppression of hypoglossal activity. This site is innervated by pre-BotC neurons, corresponding with the site of hypoglossal premotor neurons identified in neonatal rats in vivo and the parahypoglossal nucleus in adults, which is highly associated with opioid-induced suppression of hypoglossal muscle activity.

While awake, severe diurnal hypoventilation is unusual in patients who use opioids chronically.[25,26] In 50 patients on chronic methadone, only 10 patients had a $Paco_2$ between 45 and 50 mm Hg, with the remainder having normal arterial blood gas values (42.3 ± 3.8 mm Hg).[26] However, during sleep, potentially dangerous respiratory depressant effects of opioids are unmasked because sleep has profound destabilizing effects on breathing, some of which are shared with effects of opioids on breathing, therefore these adverse effects could be additive or synergistic. These shared destabilizing effects include a reduction in both HCVR and upper airway muscle activity. Sleep decreases the tonic activity to upper airway muscles. The physiologic effect of sleep added to a decreased hypoglossal nerve activity induced by opioids results in increasing upper airway resistance and hypoventilation. As noted earlier, both opioids and sleep are associated with decreased HCVR. The combination of increased upper airway resistance and reduced HCVR is conducive to sustained hypoventilation unless wakefulness returns.

Other destabilizing effects of sleep on breathing include reduction in lung volume that further increases upper airway collapsibility, and unmasking the CO_2-induced apneic threshold promoting apneas, as opioids do by their actions on other receptors.

In spite of adverse additive/synergistic effects of sleep and opioids on breathing, creating the perfect conditions for hypoventilation and potential for demise, no systematic studies are available to show the magnitude and the severity of hypoventilation in patients on chronic opioids. To demonstrate this, studies are needed to measure $Paco_2$ and ventilation while awake and during sleep.

Because measuring $Paco_2$ during sleep is invasive, transcutaneous Pco_2 (although not ideal) is acceptable if appropriate calibration in the sleep laboratory is performed. Another alternative is monitoring end-tidal Pco_2. In either case, with transcutaneous and end-tidal monitoring of Pco_2, extreme care, appropriate calibration, and attention to the setup are needed in order to minimize leak (for end-tidal monitoring).

In the absence of these measurements, investigators have used sustained hypoxemia as a surrogate for hypoventilation. Mogri and colleagues[27] evaluated this finding in a study of 98 patients on stable doses of opioids. In addition to a high prevalence of sleep-disordered breathing in this population (only 15% of patients did not have sleep apnea), 31% of patients showed hypoxemia independent of respiratory events. This number increased to approximately 75% when including hypoxemia associated with apneic events.[27] As emphasized, hypoventilation was not diagnosed via carbon dioxide monitoring during this study, but rather using hypoxemia (defined as 5 minutes of oxyhemoglobin saturation $\leq 90\%$ with nadir of 85%, or >30% of total sleep time spent <90%) as a surrogate marker for hypoventilation. The increase in hypoxemia as noted in Mogri and colleagues'[27] study can be explained by a combination of comorbid sleep-disordered breathing and blunted respiratory responses, allowing for an increase in $Paco_2$ and subsequent reduction in Pao_2.

With regard to chronic opioid usage and the development of sleep-disordered breathing, the dose of opioids may be important, although studies show sleep apnea even with small doses. A study by Walker and colleagues[28] showed the development of ataxic breathing in 92% of individuals with morphine-equivalent milligrams per day greater than 200 mg; this number reduced to 61% in those taking less than 200 mg/d and 5% in controls.[28] The study by Mogri and colleagues[27] had participants with a mean morphine dosage of 180 mg/d.[27] Another study showed that central sleep apnea severity was significantly increased with morphine dosing equivalents of 200 mg/d.[29]

It is thought that usage of a partial mu-opioid agonist buprenorphine/naloxone, commonly used for opioid dependency with limited respiratory toxicity, has a lower incidence of sleep-disordered breathing and respiratory depression; buprenorphine/naloxone is associated with fewer deaths than methadone.[30] Buprenorphine/naloxone has recently been studied with regard to its effects on respiratory patterns during sleep, with 70 patients placed on buprenorphine after acute opioid withdrawal.[31] Farney and colleagues[31] found that 63% of patients had mild sleep-disordered breathing, with most of these patients having central apnea events.[31] Nocturnal hypoxemia was present in 44 of 70 patients on buprenorphine/naloxone.[31] It is reasonable to assume that buprenorphine/naloxone is not free of respiratory depression.

TREATMENT OPTIONS FOR OPIOID-INDUCED SLEEP HYPOVENTILATION

Despite the serious clinical dilemma that comes with chronic use of opioids for the management of chronic pain, there are some recommendations in place and future directions with promise in treating the sleep-related breathing disorders that accompany opioid usage. Although a difficult task, tapering to the lowest dose as tolerated by the patient or discontinuation of the offending agent is the best approach. Evaluation of polypharmacy with multiple drugs of differing mechanisms for respiratory depression with potential for additive/synergistic effects should be evaluated and medications curtailed if possible.

Noninvasive Positive Pressure Ventilation

Positive airway pressure (PAP) devices including continuous positive airway pressure (CPAP), bilevel positive airway pressure with or without back-up respiratory rate (noninvasive positive pressure ventilation [NIPPV]), and the advanced devices targeting minute ventilation by way of pressure support have been used to treat hypoventilation of various causes. CPAP delivers continuous positive pressure to the airway. Bilevel airway pressure delivers a higher inspiratory pressure and a lower expiratory pressure, augmenting tidal volume with each breath and therefore improving alveolar ventilation. More sophisticated NIPPV modes (eg, average volume-assured pressure support [AVAPS] and intelligent volume-assured pressure support [iVAPS]) use an algorithm to vary and adjust pressure support in order to deliver a set tidal volume, therefore guaranteeing minute ventilation and treating hypoventilation during sleep.

Although alternative pain management strategies are being considered and implemented, NIPPV remains the mainstay in management of hypoventilation during sleep. As noted, NIPPV has been used for the treatment of sleep hypoventilation caused by various medical conditions such as obesity hypoventilation syndrome (OHS), congenital central alveolar hypoventilation syndrome, neuromuscular disorders, chest wall diseases, and obstructive lung disease.[32]

Studies have also investigated PAP therapies including NIPPV for sleep-disordered breathing associated with chronic opioid use (ie, obstructive and central sleep apnea syndromes), but there are no specific studies focusing on PAP therapy or NIPPV for sleep hypoventilation induced by chronic opioid use. For OHS, several studies showed that both CPAP and bilevel therapy improved blood gases (decreased hypercapnia and improved hypoxemia) as well as sleep architecture.[33,34] AVAPS therapy has also been shown to improve nocturnal hypoventilation; however, sleep quality was better on bilevel therapy.[35,36]

Treatment of hypoventilation requires adequate delivery of tidal volume and maintaining minute ventilation in order to effectively eliminate carbon dioxide, thereby showing the limitations of CPAP in treating hypoventilation. However, when diurnal hypoventilation is caused by obstructive sleep apnea, several studies (for review see Ref.[22]) have shown that use of CPAP improves awake $Paco_2$. However, CPAP is ineffective for treatment of sleep-disordered breathing (ie, obstructive and central sleep apnea syndromes) induced by chronic use of opioids.[37–40] For this purpose, bilevel devices with backup respiratory rate and adaptive servoventilation devices have proved to be effective.[37,38,40–42]

Advanced NIPPV devices are available specifically for treatment of hypoventilation and during sleep by targeting tidal volume and/or minute ventilation (AVAPS, iVAPS). Because the AVAPS or iVAPS modes adjust pressure support based on the patient's respiratory cycle breath by breath, they adapt to changes in severity of disease and therefore are ideal for sleep hypoventilation secondary to opioids, because patients often adjust medication dosages corresponding with pain level. Although studies have not documented the efficacy of NIPPV in sleep hypoventilation secondary to chronic use of opioids, it is logical that NIPPV may also be used for the treatment of opioid-induced hypoventilation during sleep.

Ampakines

Regarding pharmacologic approaches, a compound that reverses opioid-induced respiratory depression without altering pain control would be the ideal agent. There is promise for pharmacologic interventions based on neurotransmitter responses in pre-BotC, specifically serotonin receptors such as $5HT_{1A,4A}$.[43] Ampakines are a family of compounds that modulate the action of the excitatory neurotransmitter glutamate at the alpha-amino-3-hydroxy-5-methylisoxazole-4-proprionic acid (AMPA) receptors by altering channel kinetics. Recent work using rat models has shown that ampakines alleviate opiate-induced respiratory depression of central respiratory rhythmogenesis, which is hypothesized to originate from the pre-BotC.[44–46] Studies using adult rats showed that CX717, a synthetic ampakine compound, alleviates fentanyl-induced respiratory depression without inhibiting analgesia or sedation.[47,48] In a study on 16 healthy human subjects, CX717 counteracted alfentanil-induced respiratory depression without affecting opiate-mediated analgesia.[49] Lorier and colleagues[50] showed that opiates induced upper airway obstruction by acting on the presynaptic inhibition of hypoglossal XII motor neuron, an important tongue muscle involved in maintaining upper airway patency. The investigators also showed that ampakines (CX614 and CX717) successfully counteracted mu-opioid receptor–mediated depression of hypoglossal XII motor neuron inspiratory activity. Preliminary findings suggest that ampakines may be beneficial in counteracting opiate-induced respiratory depression, maintaining upper airway patency, while preserving opioids' analgesic effect.

Minocycline, a tetracycline antibiotic, working through inhibition of microglial activation, has been shown potentially to augment pain control as well as attenuate respiratory depression.[43] More research is needed before conclusively recommending any pharmacologic treatment of reversal of opioid-induced respiratory depression.

SUMMARY

The emphasis on improved pain control and the focus on treating chronic pain syndromes have led to a large increase in the number of patients on opioid medications chronically. With sleep, the use of opioids chronically is associated with a variety of breathing disorders, including central sleep apnea, obstructive sleep apnea, and hypoventilation. Many patients on opioids are found dead in bed and no cause is found at autopsy except opioids, benzodiazepines, and other drugs in the blood. We think that terminal apnea is the sine qua non of death by opioids. It remains to be seen whether effective treatment of these sleep-related breathing disorders decreases the associated mortality of opioids. Meanwhile, understanding the mechanisms underlying control of respiration and opioid-mediated respiratory depression is essential in treatment options and providing new directions for management.

REFERENCES

1. Katz N. The impact of pain management on quality of life. J Pain Symptom Manage 2002;24(Suppl 1):S38–47.
2. The use of opioids for the treatment of chronic pain. A consensus statement from the American Academy of Pain Medicine and the American Pain Society. Clin J Pain 1997;13:6–8.
3. Joranson DE, Ryan KM, Gilson AM, et al. Trends in the medical use and abuse of opioid analgesics. J Am Med Assoc 2000;283(13):1710–4.
4. Smith JC, Ellenberger HH, Ballanyi K, et al. Pre-Bötzinger complex: a brainstem region that may generate respiratory rhythm in mammals. Science 2001;25(5032):726–9.
5. Feldman JL, Del Negro CA. Looking for inspiration: new perspectives on respiratory rhythm. Nat Rev Neurosci 2006;7:232–42.
6. Janczewski WA, Feldman JL. Novel data supporting the two respiratory rhythm oscillator hypothesis. Focus on respiration-related rhythmic activity in the rostral medulla of newborn rats. J Neurophysiol 2006;96(1):1–2.
7. Mellen NM, Janczwski WA, Bocchiaro CM, et al. Opioid-induced quantal slowing reveals dual networks for respiratory rhythm generation. Neuron 2003;37(5):821–6.
8. Gray PA, Janczewski WA, Mellen N, et al. Normal breathing requires preBötzinger complex neurokinin-1 receptor-expressing neurons. Nat Neurosci 2001;4(9):927–30.
9. Gray PA, Rekling JC, Bocchiaro CM, et al. Modulation of respiratory frequency by peptidergic input to rhythmogenic neurons in the preBotzinger complex. Science 1999;286(5444):1566–8.
10. Montandon G, Qin W, Liu H, et al. PreBotzinger complex neurokinin-1 receptor-expressing neurons mediate opioid-induced respiratory depression. J Neurosci 2011;31(4):1292–301.
11. Bruce EN, Cherniack NS. Central chemoreceptors. J Appl Phys 1987;62(2):389–402.
12. Blain GM, Smith CA, Henderson KS, et al. Contribution of the carotid body chemoreceptors to eupneic ventilation in the intact, unanesthetized dog. J Appl Phys 2009;106(5):1564–73.
13. Pattison KT. Opioids and the control of respiration. Br J Anaesth 2008;100(6):747–58.
14. Bailey PL, Lu JK, Pace NL, et al. Effects of intrathecal morphine on the ventilatory response to hypoxia. N Engl J Med 2000;343(17):1228–34.
15. Weil JV, McCullough RE, Kline JS, et al. Diminished ventilatory response to hypoxia and hypercapnia after morphine in normal man. N Engl J Med 1975;292(13):1103–6.
16. Bailey PL, Thakur R. Pain management and regional anesthesia. In: Deham SW, Dahan A, Teppema LJ, editors. Pharmacology and pathophysiology of the control of breathing. Lung Biol in Health and Diseases, vol. 202. Boca Raton (FL): Taylor and Francis; 2005. p. 424–512.

17. Teichtahl H, Wang D, Cunnington D, et al. Ventilatory responses to hypoxia and hypercapnia in stable methadone maintenance treatment patients. Chest 2005;128(3):1339–47.
18. Cohn MA. Hypnotics and the control of breathing: a review. Br J Clin Pharmacol 1983;16:245S–50S.
19. Waters KA, McBrien F, Stewart P, et al. Effects of OSA, inhalational anesthesia, and fentanyl on the airway and ventilation in children. J Appl Phys 2002;92(5):1987–94.
20. Strauss SG, Lynn AM, Bratton SL, et al. Ventilatory response to CO_2 in children with obstructive sleep apnea from adeno-tonsillar hypertrophy. Anesth Analg 1999;89(2):328–32.
21. Subramanyam R, Chidambaran V, Ding L, et al. Anesthesia and opioids-related malpractice claims following tonsillectomy in USA: LexisNexis claims database 1984–2012. Paediatr Anaesth 2014; 24(4):412–20.
22. Almoosa KF, Javaheri S. Obesity and the control of breathing. In: Ward DS, Dahan A, Teppema LJ, editors. Pharmacology and pathophysiology of the control of breathing. Lung Biology in Health and Disease, vol. 202. Boca Raton (FL): Taylor and Francis; 2005. p. 383–412.
23. Yue H, Guilleminault C. Opioid medication and sleep-disordered breathing. Med Clin North Am 2010;94:435–46.
24. Hajiha M, Dubord MA, Liu H, et al. Opioid receptor mechanisms at the hypoglossal motor pool and effects on tongue muscle activity in vivo. J Physiol 2009;587:2677–92.
25. Santiago TV, Pugliese AC, Edelman NH. Control of breathing during methadone addiction. Am J Med 1977;62:347–54.
26. Teichtahl H, Wang D, Cunnington D, et al. Cardiorespiratory function in stable methadone maintenance treatment (MMT) patients. Addict Biol 2004;9:247–53.
27. Mogri M, Desai H, Webster L, et al. Hypoxemia in patients on chronic opiate therapy with and without sleep apnea. Sleep Breath 2009;13:49–57.
28. Walker JM, Farney RJ, Rhondeau SM, et al. Chronic opioid use is a risk factor for the development of central sleep apnea and ataxic breathing. J Clin Sleep Med 2007;3(5):455–61.
29. Jungquist CR, Flannery M, Perlis ML, et al. Relationship of chronic pain and opioid use with respiratory disturbance during sleep. Pain Manag Nurs 2012;13(2):70–9.
30. Auriacombe M, Franeques P, Tignol J. Deaths attributable to methadone versus buprenorphine in France. J Am Med Assoc 2001;285:45.
31. Farney RJ, McDonald AM, Boyle KM, et al. Sleep disordered breathing in patients receiving therapy with buprenorphine/naloxone. Eur Respir J 2012; 42(2):394–403.
32. Selim B, Junna M, Morgenthaler T. Therapy for sleep hypoventilation and central apnea syndromes. Curr Treat Options Neurol 2012;14(5):427–37.
33. Borel J, Tamisier R, Gonzalez-Bermejo L, et al. Noninvasive ventilation in mild obesity hypoventilation syndrome: a randomized controlled trial. Chest 2012;141(3):692–702.
34. Priou P, Hamel J, Person C, et al. Long-term outcome of noninvasive positive pressure ventilation for obesity hypoventilation syndrome. Chest 2010;138(1):84–90.
35. Janssens J, Metzger M, Sforza E. Impact of volume targeting on efficacy of bi-level non-invasive ventilation and sleep in obesity-hypoventilation. Respir Med 2009;103(2):165–72.
36. Storre JH, Seuthe B, Fiechter R, et al. Average volume-assured pressure support in obesity hypoventilation: a randomized crossover trial. Chest 2006;130(3):815–21.
37. Allam JS, Olson EJ, Gay PC, et al. Efficacy of adaptive servoventilation in treatment of complex and central sleep apnea syndromes. Chest 2007;132(6):1839–46.
38. Guilleminault C, Cao M, Yue HJ, et al. Obstructive sleep apnea and chronic opioid use. Lung 2010; 188(6):459–68.
39. Farney RJ, Walker JM, Boyle KM, et al. Adaptive servoventilation (ASV) in patients with sleep disordered breathing associated with chronic opioid medications for non-malignant pain. J Clin Sleep Med 2008;4(4):311–9.
40. Javaheri S, Malik A, Smith J, et al. Adaptive pressure support servoventilation: a novel treatment for sleep apnea associated with use of opioids. J Clin Sleep Med 2008;4(4):305–10.
41. Javaheri S, Harris N, Howard J, et al. Adaptive servo-ventilation for treatment of opioids-associated central sleep apnea. J Clin Sleep Med 2014;10(6):637–43.
42. Cao M, Cardell CY, Willes L, et al. A Novel adaptive servoventilation (ASVAuto) for the treatment of central sleep apnea associated with chronic use of opioid. J Clin Sleep Med 2014; in press.
43. Dahan A, Aarts L, Smith TW. Incidence, reversal, and prevention of opioid-induced respiratory depression. Anesthesiology 2009;112(1):226–38.
44. Ren J, Poon BY, Tang Y, et al. Ampakines alleviate respiratory depression in rats. Am J Respir Crit Care Med 2006;174:1384–91.
45. Ren J, Greer J. Modulation of respiratory rhythmogenesis by chloride-mediated conductances during the perinatal period. J Neurosci 2006;26(14):3721–30.
46. Ren J, Greer J. Modulation of perinatal respiratory rhythm by gaba- and glycine receptor-mediated chloride conductances. Adv Exp Med Biol 2008; 605(14):149–53.
47. Greer J, Ren J. Ampakine therapy to counter fentanyl-induced respiratory depression. Respir Physiolo Neurobiol 2009;168(1–2):153–7.

48. Ren J, Ding X, Funk GD, et al. Ampakine CX717 protects against fentanyl-induced respiratory depression and lethal apnea in rats. Anesthesiology 2009;110(6):1364–70.

49. Oertel BJ, Felden L, Tran PV, et al. Selective antagonism of opioid-induced ventilatory depression by an ampakine molecule in humans without loss of opioid analgesia. Clin Pharmacol Ther 2010;87(2):204–11.

50. Lorier AR, Funk GD, Greer JJ. Opiate-induced suppression of rat hypoglossal motoneuron activity and its reversal by ampakine therapy. PLoS One 2010;5(1):e8766.

Obesity Hypoventilation Syndrome and Anesthesia Considerations

 CrossMark

Roop Kaw, MD[a],*, Maged Argalious, MD, MBA[b],
Loutfi S. Aboussouan, MD[b], Frances Chung, MBBS[c]

KEYWORDS

- Obesity hypoventilation syndrome • Perioperative • Anesthesia • Surgery
- Positive airway pressure

KEY POINTS

- Obesity hypoventilation is often undiagnosed before surgery, hence appropriate suspicion and preparedness are required.
- Preoperative identification of undiagnosed compensated respiratory acidosis and obstructive sleep apnea are key.
- Primary treatment is positive airway pressure therapy, and appropriate sleep referral may be mandated before major surgery.

INTRODUCTION

Small cohort studies have reported the prevalence of obesity hypoventilation syndrome (OHS) in the general population to be around 0.3% to 0.4%.[1] Among the only surgical series to report prevalence of OHS is a recent report from premenopausal women presenting for bariatric surgery with 8% prevalence of OHS.[2] Among patients with known obstructive sleep apnea (OSA) the reported prevalence of OHS is between 10% and 20% and is known to increase with obesity to as high as 50% as the body mass index (BMI) exceeds 50 kg/m^2.[3] OHS is often undiagnosed or undertreated before elective noncardiac surgery and is usually associated with many medical comorbidities. This article describes and examines many important steps and strategies that can improve perioperative outcomes in this high-risk population.

IMPORTANT PATHOPHYSIOLOGIC CONSIDERATIONS

Effect of Obesity, Supine Posture, and Anesthesia on Lung Function

Functional residual capacity (FRC) can be exponentially reduced in the supine position and Trendelenburg positions as a function of increasing BMI. Reductions as low as 51% have been described in morbidly obese patients undergoing jejunoileal bypass surgery.[4] With a decreased FRC, the closing volume, at which dependent alveoli start collapsing, may start encroaching on the normal tidal volume excursions, resulting in increased airway closure such that well-perfused basal areas may be closed at normal tidal breaths, thereby creating hypoxemia caused by a mismatch between ventilation and perfusion (**Fig. 1**).[5] The FRC reduction may last up to 7 days after surgery and recovery of spirometric

Disclosure: None.
[a] Cleveland Clinic Lerner College of Medicine, Departments of Hospital Medicine and Outcomes Research Anesthesia, Cleveland Clinic, 9500 Euclid Avenue, Cleveland, OH 44195, USA; [b] Cleveland Clinic, 9500 Euclid Avenue, Cleveland, OH 44195, USA; [c] Department of Anesthesia, University Health Network, University of Toronto, Toronto Western Hospital, 399 Bathurst Street, Toronto, ON, Canada
* Corresponding author.
E-mail address: kawr@ccf.org

Sleep Med Clin 9 (2014) 399–407
http://dx.doi.org/10.1016/j.jsmc.2014.05.005
1556-407X/14/$ – see front matter © 2014 Elsevier Inc. All rights reserved.

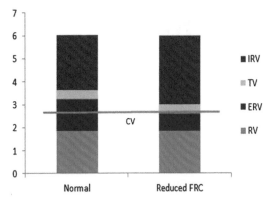

Fig. 1. Closing volume (CV; represented by the blue horizontal line) is within the normal tidal volume (TV) range when the FRC is low, resulting in airway closure and hypoxemia with tidal breaths. ERV, expiratory reserve volume; IRV, inspiratory reserve volume; RV, residual volume.

values may be significantly faster in patients receiving postoperative epidural analgesia compared with those receiving opioid analgesia.[6] More importantly, in addition to hypoxemia, the low FRC reduces the total available oxygen reservoir, such that any intervening events such as apneas are associated with more rapid desaturation and a lower oxygen nadir.[7] In a simulated model, oxyhemoglobin desaturation occurred and persisted in obese adults for several seconds before recovery from intravenous succinylcholine administration.[8] Compared with patients with eucapnic obesity, the chest wall compliance is reduced 2.5-fold in patients with OHS and the pulmonary resistance is increased because of decreased FRC, thereby increasing the work of breathing (**Table 1**).[9]

Blunted Ventilatory Drive

Obese patients have increased work of breathing and higher basal oxygen consumption, and they produce more carbon dioxide compared with nonobese subjects. To accommodate all these differences, obese patients in general have a higher central respiratory drive. In contrast, patients with OHS have blunted central respiratory drive to both hypoxia and hypercapnia.[10]

Table 1
Clinical and demographic differences between obese (eucapnic) patients and patients with OHS

Parameters	OHS (Mean ± SD)	Eucapnic Obesity (Mean ± SD)	P Value
N	741	2972	—
Age (y)	50.1 ± 9.3	51.3 ± 8.5	<.0001
Male (%)	70.5	78.6	N/A
Female (%)	29.5	21.4	N/A
BMI (kg/m^2)	39.6 ± 7.7	33.4 ± 5.9	<.0001
Neck circumference (cm)	47 ± 6	44 ± 5	.01
Waist/hip ratio	1.0 ± 0.06	0.9 ± 0.1	<.0001
Gas Exchange			
Pao_2 (mm Hg)	66.8 ± 8.7	78.7 ± 8.0	<.0001
$Paco_2$ (mm Hg)	49.8 ± 6.4	39.7 ± 2.7	<.0001
HCO_3^- (mM)	30.9 ± 3.8	25.9 ± 3.4	<.0001
Pulmonary Function			
FEV_1 (% predicted)	71.0 ± 13.1	87.8 ± 13.2	<.0001
FVC (% predicted)	80.3 ± 12.4	92.8 ± 10.4	<.0001
FEV_1/FVC	79.4 ± 7.2	80.7 ± 5.3	<.0001
FRC (% predicted)	80.8 ± 7.3	83.5 ± 3.6	.0156
TLC (% predicted)	77 ± 14.7	95 ± 11.5	<.0001
Sleep-disordered Breathing			
AHI (events/h)	66.4 ± 21.6	47.5 ± 18.2	<.0001
TST Spo_2 <90% (%)	49.2 ± 31.8	17.1 ± 21.1	<.0001
Minimum nocturnal Spo_2 (%)	65.1 ± 10.4	74.5 ± 7.7	<.0001
Central Respiratory Drive to CO_2			
CO_2 sensitivity (L/min/mm Hg)	1.2 ± 0.8	2.4 ± 1.5	<.0001

Abbreviations: AHI, Apnea-Hypopnea Index; FEV_1, forced expiratory volume in 1 second; FVC, forced vital capacity; N/A, not applicable; SD, standard deviation; TLC, total lung capacity; TST, total sleep time.

Severity of OSA and Postoperative Complications

Although literature abounds with mentions of suboptimal postoperative outcomes among patients with OSA, thus far the severity of OSA as measured by the Apnea-Hypopnea Index (AHI) has not been proved to correlate with the severity of poor outcomes.[11] In addition, even though in patients with OSA the incidence of OHS seems to increase with higher BMI, neither BMI nor AHI have been shown to significantly correlate with integrated overnight $Paco_2$ among patients with OSA.[12] Nocturnal end-tidal CO_2 can reflect physiologic characteristics of OSA not addressed by the AHI or BMI.[12]

PREOPERATIVE ASSESSMENT
Obese Patients with Known OSA

Obese patients (mean BMI, 39) known to have severe OSA (mean AHI, 64) and restrictive chest mechanics (forced expiratory volume in 1 second [FEV_1] <71% and forced vital capacity [FVC] <85% of predicted) are more likely to have OHS.[1] In a cohort of obese patients referred to the sleep laboratory for suspected OSA, a serum bicarbonate threshold of 27 mEq/L was 92% sensitive in predicting hypercapnia on arterial blood gases (ABG).[3] Because BMI in that range is invariably associated with restrictive lung mechanics, diurnal oxygen desaturations less than 90% (corresponding Pao_2 <60 mm Hg) and serum bicarbonate greater than 27 mEq/mL (in the absence of any other explanation) help increase the suspicion for diurnal hypercapnia, which then should be confirmed by obtaining an ABG before the patient goes for surgery (**Fig. 2**).

Obese Patients with Suspected OSA

Higher AHI has been reported among patients with OHS compared with those with eucapnic OSA (mean difference, 12.51; 95% confidence interval [CI], 6.59–18.44; $P<.0001$).[1] The STOP-Bang questionnaire has been validated as a screening tool in surgical patients, although at scores greater than 3 it loses the specificity for moderate (43%) and severe (37%) OSA. The addition of serum bicarbonate greater than 28 mmol/L increases the specificity for diagnosing any OSA to 85.2% and

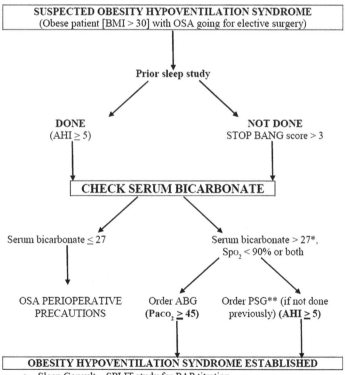

Fig. 2. Preoperative decision tree in patients with suspected OHS. PAP, positive airway pressure; PH, pulmonary hypertension; PSG, polysomnography; Spo_2, oxygen saturation via pulse oximetry.

that of severe OSA to 79.4%.[13] In obese patients suspected to have OSA from clinical signs and symptoms and a STOP-Bang score, serum bicarbonate greater than 27 mEq/L should prompt a preoperative evaluation with polysomnography before elective noncardiac surgery, when possible (see **Fig. 2**).

POSTOPERATIVE COMPLICATIONS IN PATIENTS WITH OHS

OHS is characterized by a triad of chronic daytime hypercapnia ($Paco_2 \geq 45$ mm Hg), sleep-disordered breathing, and obesity with a BMI greater than 30 kg/m^2.[3] ABG measurements are important for confirming chronic daytime diurnal hypercapnia; however, these measurements often cannot be obtained in routine outpatient preoperative settings. Moreover, the diagnosis of OHS can only be established after excluding other possible causes of hypercapnia like severe obstructive airway disease, severe kyphoscoliosis, or interstitial lung disease and neuromuscular disorders. Given these practical difficulties in establishing the diagnosis there are no studies to date evaluating postoperative outcomes among patients with OHS.

Compared with the eucapnic obese subjects, patients with OHS have been reported to have higher odds of heart failure, angina pectoris, and cor pulmonale (odds ratio [OR], 9; 95% CI, 1.4–57.1); pulmonary hypertension (PH; 30% to 88%); and higher mortality (23% vs 8%).[14,15] The only surgical series to report postoperative outcomes among patients with high likelihood of OHS is bariatric surgery. Obesity surgery mortality risk score (OS-MRS) assigns 1 point to each of 5 preoperative variables among patients undergoing bariatric surgery: male gender, BMI greater than 50, PH, OHS, prior thromboembolism/presence of inferior vena cava filter.[16] Mortality ranged from 0.2% (in low-risk class, 0–1 morbidity) to 2.4% (among high-risk class, 4–5 comorbidities). Emerging data link OHS with higher likelihood of postoperative complications, especially respiratory failure (44% vs 2.6%) compared with eucapnic OSA.[17] OHS is mostly unrecognized at the time of surgery and wherever postoperative respiratory failure occurs in an obese patient without other predispositions, the possibility of sleep-related hypoventilation should be considered.

INTRAOPERATIVE CONSIDERATIONS
Airway Management

The 2013 Practice Guidelines for Management of the Difficult Airway from the American Society of Anesthesiologists (ASA) defines a difficult airway as difficulty with facemask ventilation or tracheal intubation, or both.[18] A recent multicenter retrospective study identified several factors that predict difficult mask ventilation combined with difficult laryngoscopy: age greater than or equal to 46 years, male sex, BMI greater than or equal to 30 kg/m^2, limited thyromental distance, Mallampati oropharyngeal class III to IV, presence of beard, limited neck extension and jaw protrusion, OSA, thick neck, and neck radiation changes or neck mass. Patients with OHS typically have 3 (obesity, sleep apnea, thick neck) or more of these predictors.[19]

Airway management in patients with OHS can be accomplished by awake fiberoptic intubation under local anesthesia if difficult mask ventilation is suspected or by the use of various video and optical laryngoscopic equipment after induction of general anesthesia if preoperative assessment does not point to the possibility of difficult ventilation. Supraglottic airway devices can act as a conduit for intubation if difficult laryngoscopy is encountered or if unexpected difficulty in mask ventilation occurs after induction of general anesthesia. Most importantly, supraglottic airway devices should be used as part of the ASA difficult airway algorithm in cases of cannot-intubate-cannot-ventilate scenarios before proceeding with a surgical airway.

Preoxygenation
Patients with OHS are at risk of rapid oxygen desaturation after induction of general anesthesia because of a higher incidence of obstructed airway, a reduction in FRC, as well as higher oxygen consumption.[20] Preoxygenation with 100% oxygen with a tight-fitting mask in chest-elevated position can prolong the time to desaturation.[21] During periods of apnea the volume of oxygen absorbed from the lungs is more than the amount of carbon dioxide produced, thus creating a negative pressure that assists in ventilation during the apnea period. Additional use of continuous positive airway pressure (CPAP) up to 10 cm H_2O for 3 minutes targeted to an end-tidal oxygen concentration of greater than 90% can improve the efficiency of preoxygenation and minimize the risk of absorption atelectasis from high-flow oxygen.[22]

Positioning for laryngoscopy
Although the sniffing position improves pharyngeal patency in anesthetized patients with OSA,[23] the head elevation laryngoscopy position (HELP; also called the ramped position), achieving horizontal alignment between the auditory meatus and the sternal notch, results in a significant improvement

in laryngeal view compared with the sniffing position in morbidly obese patients.[24] Proper positioning of the patient in the sitting position can decrease the passive closing pressure (PCLOSE) by 6 cm H_2O; whereas the sniffing or the ramp position decreases the PCLOSE by 4 cm H_2O, also allowing both tracheal intubation and ventilation.[23]

Choice of Anesthesia Technique

Although central neuraxial anesthesia techniques (spinal and epidural anesthesia) using local anesthetics have the benefit of avoiding airway instrumentation and limiting the use of anesthetic agents that can contribute to an already blunted respiratory drive in patients with OHS,[25] these techniques are technically more difficult, require the presence of specialized equipment (eg, longer 12.7-cm [5-inch] epidural needles) and may be better tolerated if performed under fluoroscopic and/or ultrasonography guidance.[26] The use of central neuraxial catheters is recommended for lengthy surgical procedures, especially in cases performed in positions other than the supine position, to avoid the scenario of a resolving block in a patient positioned in the lateral or prone position, in which general anesthesia cannot readily be induced. If PH is suspected, general anesthesia is preferred overall; epidural anesthesia is preferred rather than spinal anesthesia because of the rapid onset of the latter with associated profound sympatholytic effect.

Drug dosing of general anesthesia agents should take into consideration lipophilicity and volume of distribution (**Table 2**). Factors that affect the volume of distribution in patients with OHS include an increase in total body fat, an increase in lean body mass (more than 98% of metabolic activity occurs within lean body mass), increased blood volume, increased cardiac output, and reduced total body water. Drugs that are mainly distributed to lean tissues should have the loading dose calculated based on lean body weight (LBW), whereas the dosing should be calculated based on total body weight (TBW) if the drug is equally distributed in adipose and lean tissues (eg, lipophilic drugs with increased volume of distribution). Neuromuscular blockers are hydrophilic compounds and should be dosed on LBW. One exception is succinylcholine, which is dosed based on TBW because of increased metabolism from increase in total plasma cholinesterase levels associated with greater total body weight.[27] Rocuronium (dosed by LBW) is a good alternative for rapid induction if succinylcholine is contraindicated or unavailable.[28] For maintenance, a drug with similar clearance in both obese and nonobese patients should be based on LBW, whereas drugs whose clearance increases with obesity should have the maintenance dose calculated according to TBW.[29,30]

A high incidence of left ventricular systolic and diastolic dysfunction as well as concomitant PH in patients with OHS requires careful titration of induction agents to avoid unnecessary hemodynamic fluctuations. In patients with known or suspected PH, avoidance of systemic hypotension is key because it can further precipitate right

Table 2
Dosing guidelines for commonly used intravenous anesthetics

Drug	Dosing
Induction Agents	
Thiopental	LBW
Etomidate	LBW
Propofol	LBW (TBW used for maintenance dose because of high affinity for fat tissue and high hepatic extraction)
Muscle Relaxants	
Depolarizing: succinylcholine	TBW: plasma cholinesterase activity increases in proportion to body weight
Nondepolarizing: rocuronium, vecuronium, pancuronium, atracurium, cisatracurium	LBW
Narcotics	
Fentanyl, sufentanil, alfentanil, remifentanil	LBW
Reversible Choline Esterase Inhibitor	
Neostigmine	TBW

Abbreviations: LBW, lean body weight; TBW, total body weight.

ventricular ischemia. In this regard, etomidate with its minimal impact on myocardial contractility and systemic vascular resistance, can be preferred for induction rather than propofol and sodium thiopental.[31] Nitrous oxide may increase pulmonary vascular resistance, result in an obligatory reduction in the fraction of inspired oxygen (Fio_2), and contribute to right ventricular ischemia.[32]

Patient Positioning

The HELP/ramp-up position uses a 25° elevation to raise the upper part of the body above the chest. As well as improving the laryngoscopic view, this position compensates for the exaggerated flexion of the neck caused by the cervical pad of fat and adds advantage to respiratory mechanics.[24] Repositioning patients into this position after failed intubation can be tedious. Operating room tables with greater capacities (allowing a greater maximum patient weight) are available that are capable of mechanically flexing to raise the trunk.

Although prone positioning potentially improves lung compliance, oxygenation, and ventilation, it may have a deleterious effect if incorrect positioning does not allow free diaphragmatic excursion. Resulting increased intra-abdominal and intrathoracic pressure can worsen inferior vena caval and aortic compression, resulting in a worsening cycle of reduced venous return, reduced cardiac output, hypoperfusion, hypoxemia, and hypercapnia that can only be reversed by a change in patient position.

At the conclusion of surgery, placing the patient into the reverse Trendelenburg position improves respiratory compliance, reduces alveolar-arterial oxygen tension difference, and improves oxygenation through an improvement in FRC. However, care must be taken to avoid unrecognized migration of the endotracheal tube (ET) into the right main stem, especially with change of patient position into a Trendelenburg or lithotomy position, because breath sounds may not be easily auscultated in this patient population. ET position can be confirmed by fiberoptic bronchoscopy. Extreme changes to patient position, such as the use maximal flexion of the so-called kidney rest on the operating table, can result in rhabdomyolysis, especially with prolonged surgeries.

Intraoperative Ventilation Strategies

The use of TBW instead of ideal body weight may overestimate the tidal volumes by 20% to 50%,[33] which can increase postoperative pulmonary complications.[34] Pressure control ventilation has been shown to improve intraoperative oxygenation compared with volume controlled ventilation, although these results were only shown in patients undergoing laparoscopic surgery.[35] Positive end-expiratory pressure (PEEP) of up to 10 cm H_2O is known to reduce atelectasis in obese patients undergoing laparoscopic bariatric surgery but careful titration is required to avoid marked reductions in venous return, cardiac output, and systemic blood pressure, with resultant ventilation perfusion mismatch.[34] In a recent multicenter, double-blind trial, the use of an intraoperative protective mechanical ventilation strategy (tidal volumes of 6 to 8 mL/kg of predicted body weight, PEEP of 6–8 cm H_2O, and lung recruitment in the form of 30 seconds of CPAP at 30 cm H_2O) for patients undergoing laparoscopic or open abdominal surgery with a baseline intermediate to high risk of developing pulmonary complications resulted in a clinically and statistically significant reduction in the incidence of major pulmonary and extrapulmonary complications.[36] **Table 3** shows the optimum intraoperative ventilation strategies in patients with OHS.

Postanesthesia Extubation and Positive Airway Pressure Therapy

Because tracheal extubation is preferred only after the patient is fully conscious, inhalational anesthetics with a rapid recovery profile, including sevoflurane and desflurane, can be used for maintenance of anesthesia, keeping in mind that even subanesthetic concentrations of inhalational anesthetics impair the already blunted hypoxic (and hypercapnic) drive and may contribute to hypoxemia in the postoperative period.[37] Short-acting adjuvants like remifentanil or combined general-regional anesthetics can help decrease the volatile anesthetic requirement and minimize the washout time from fat/muscle.[38] The use of total intravenous anesthesia avoids the use of inhalational

Table 3 Intraoperative ventilation strategies	
Mode of Ventilation	**Pressure Control**
Tidal volume	6–8 mL/kg according to ideal body weight
Respiratory rate	10–14/min
Inspiratory/ expiratory ratio	1/2; can change to 1/1.5 to increase inspiratory time
PEEP	4–10 cm H_2O
Intermittent lung recruitment (vital capacity maneuver)	CPAP at 30 cm H_2O for 30 s every 30 min

anesthetics but is typically associated with a slower recovery profile.

Following extubation criteria meticulously with an emphasis on complete reversal of muscle relaxant effect is essential in ensuring that low tidal volumes do not accentuate the preexisting hypercapnia, resulting in a vicious cycle of increasing respiratory acidosis, blunted central respiratory drive, and CO_2 narcosis that can ultimately result in hypoxemia when supplemental oxygen is given. In addition, acute respiratory acidosis augments neuromuscular blocking agent activity and interferes with its reversal. Even mild reductions in train of four fade ratio (TOF) ratio (<0.9) may accentuate the hypercapnia in patients with OHS.

Extubation is preferred in the semisitting or sitting position, thereby compensating for the reduced FRC; the operating table can also rapidly be repositioned for reintubation if needed. Any signs of airway obstruction should prompt the use of CPAP or noninvasive/bilevel positive airway pressure (PAP) ventilation, which helps to avoid high postoperative Fio_2 and postoperative atelectasis.

Patients with any signs of airway obstruction and those previously known to use PAP devices should be resumed on PAP therapy after surgery. Use of PAP reduced postextubation respiratory failure in obese patients in the intensive care unit.[39] Patients with known OHS typically require an inspiratory PAP of 16 to 18 cm H_2O and an expiratory PAP of 9 to 10 cm H_2O, and these settings can be empirically tried in patients with suspected OHS.

Monitoring and Opioid-induced Ventilatory Impairment

Invasive arterial monitoring is recommended in the event of difficulty in obtaining noninvasive blood pressure. Invasive arterial monitoring is also indicated in OHS with right and/or left ventricular dysfunction, those with moderate to severe PH, as well as in patients undergoing surgeries with large fluid shifts, and is also helpful in the perioperative management of oxygenation and ventilation through ABG analyses. The use of noninvasive and minimally invasive monitors of fluid responsiveness that rely on respiratory variation in pulse pressure and plethysmographic waveforms has limited applications in patients with OHS, especially in light of the high prevalence of concomitant PH (17%–53%)[40] and left and right ventricular dysfunction in this patient population. In addition, laparoscopic surgery, with the associated increase in intra-abdominal pressure, further reduces the reliability of these monitors.[41]

Opioid-induced ventilatory impairment (OIVI) is a frequent cause of postoperative hypoventilation. Opioids not only shift the carbon dioxide response curve to the right (ie, increase the apneic threshold) but can also decrease the slope of the CO_2 response curve (ie, reduce the minute volume response to a high $Paco_2$). This effect is particularly important, because patients with OHS have an already compromised central respiratory drive. Approaches to reduce the incidence of postoperative OIVI are:

1. Use of multimodal analgesic regimens to decrease the reliance on narcotic use (peripheral and central neuraxial blocks, local anesthetic infiltration, acetaminophen, low dose ketamine, and others).[18]
2. Early detection of postoperative OIVI through implementation of centralized monitoring units on regular surgical nursing floors. These monitoring units include centralized pulse oximetry and/or end-tidal or transcutaneous capnography monitors.[42] The Anesthesia Patient Safety Foundation recommends that continuous digital monitoring (eg, continuous pulse oximetry) be used for inpatients receiving postoperative opioids.
3. Implement use of sedation scoring systems in postoperative patients using opioids because respiratory rate alone may not be a reliable sign of OIVI.[43]

Postoperative Supplemental Oxygen

Patients with known OHS should ideally be resumed on their PAP devices after surgery. However, 40% patients with OHS may need additional oxygen in the nonsurgical setting despite being on adequate settings of PAP.[44] The need for supplemental oxygen can only increase after surgery in these patients, especially if OHS was unrecognized at the time of surgery. Recent data suggest that extreme caution is needed in administration of high concentrations of supplemental oxygen to this group of patients because significant decrease in minute ventilation and consequent worsening of hypercapnia has been reported.[45] In patients receiving supplemental oxygen (most postoperative patients, especially those who are receiving intravenous patient-controlled analgesia), monitors of ventilation (eg, capnography) were thought to be necessary to detect hypoventilation.[46]

REFERENCES

1. Kaw R, Hernandez A, Walker E, et al. Determinants of hypercapnia in obese patients with obstructive

sleep apnea: a systematic review and meta-analysis of cohort studies. Chest 2009;136(3):787–96.

2. Lecube A, Sampol G, Lloberes P, et al. Asymptomatic sleep disordered breathing in pre-menopausal women awaiting bariatric surgery. Obes Surg 2010;20:454–61.

3. Mokhlesi B, Tulaimat A, Faibussowitsch I, et al. Obesity hypoventilation syndrome: prevalence and predictors in patients with obstructive sleep apnea. Sleep Breath 2007;11:117–24.

4. Damia G, Mascheroni D, Croci M, et al. Perioperative changes in functional residual capacity in morbidly obese patients. Br J Anaesth 1988;60(5): 574–8.

5. Holley HS, Milic-Emili J, Becklake MR, et al. Regional distribution of pulmonary ventilation and perfusion in obesity. J Clin Invest 1967;46(4): 475–81.

6. Ungern-Sternberg BS, Regli A, Reber A, et al. Effect of obesity and thoracic epidural analgesia on perioperative spirometry. Br J Anaesth 2005;94(1): 121–7.

7. Shepard JW Jr. Gas exchange and hemodynamics during sleep. Med Clin North Am 1985;69(6):1243–64.

8. Benumof JL, Dagg R, Benumof R. Critical hemoglobin desaturation will occur before return to an unparalyzed state following 1 mg/kg intravenous succinylcholine. Anesthesiology 1997;87(4):979–82.

9. Sharp JT, Henry JP, Sweany SK, et al. The total work of breathing in normal and obese men. J Clin Invest 1964;43:728–39.

10. Zwilich CW, Sutton FD, Pierson DJ, et al. Decreased hypoxic ventilator drive in the obesity hypoventilation syndrome. Am J Med 1975;59:343–8.

11. Kaw R, Pasupuleti V, Walker E, et al. Postoperative complications in patients with obstructive sleep apnea. Chest 2012;141(2):436–41.

12. Jaimchariyatam N, Dweik R, Kaw R, et al. Polysomnographic determinants of nocturnal hypercapnia in patients with sleep apnea. J Clin Sleep Med 2013; 9(3):209–15.

13. Chung F, Chau E, Yang Y, et al. Serum bicarbonate level improves specificity of STOP-Bang screening for obstructive sleep apnea. Chest 2013;143(5): 1284–93.

14. Berg G, Delaive K, Manfreda J, et al. The use of health-care resources in obesity hypoventilation syndrome. Chest 2001;120:377–83.

15. Nowbar S, Burkart KM, Gonzales R, et al. Obesity associated hypoventilation in hospitalized patients: prevalence, effects and outcome. Am J Med 2004; 116:1–7.

16. DeMaria EJ, Murr M, Byrne TK, et al. Validation of the obesity surgery mortality risk score in a multicenter study proves it stratifies mortality risk in patients undergoing gastric bypass for morbid obesity. Ann Surg 2007;246:578–82.

17. Kaw R, Pasupuleti V, Walker E, et al. Obesity hypoventilation syndrome: an emerging and unrecognized risk factor among surgical patients. Am J Respir Crit Care Med 2011;183:A3147.

18. Apfelbaum JL, Hagberg CA, Caplan RA, American Society of Anesthesiologists Task Force on Management of the Difficult Airway. Practice guidelines for management of the difficult airway: an updated report by the American Society of Anesthesiologists Task Force on Management of the Difficult Airway. Anesthesiology 2013;118:251–70.

19. Kheterpal S, Han R, Tremper KK, et al. Incidence and predictors of difficult and impossible mask ventilation. Anesthesiology 2006;105:885–91.

20. De Divitiis O, Fazio S, Pettito M, et al. Oesity and cardiac function. Circulation 1981;64:477–82.

21. Dixon BJ, Dixon JB, Carden JR, et al. Preoxygenation is more effective in the 25 degrees head-up position than in the supine position in severely obese patients: a randomized controlled study. Anesthesiology 2005;102(6):1110–5 [discussion: 5A].

22. Gander S, Frascaralo P, Suter M, et al. Positive end-expiratory pressure during induction of general anesthesia increases duration of non-hypoxic apnea in morbidly obese patients. Anesth Analg 2005;100: 580–4.

23. Isono S. Optimal combination of head, mandible and body positions for pharyngeal airway maintenance during perioperative period: lesson from pharyngeal closing pressures. Semin Anesth 2007; 26:83–93.

24. Collins JS, Lemmens HJ, Brodsky JB, et al. Laryngoscopy and morbid obesity: a comparison of the "sniff" and "ramped" positions. Obes Surg 2004; 14(9):1171–5.

25. Shimura R, Tatsumi K, Nakamura A, et al. Fat accumulation, leptin, and hypercapnia in obstructive sleep apnea-hypopnea syndrome. Chest 2005;127: 543–9.

26. Chin KJ, Perlas A, Chan V, et al. Ultrasound imaging facilitates spinal anesthesia in adults with difficult surface anatomic landmarks. Anesthesiology 2011; 115:94–101.

27. Lemmens HJ, Brodsky JB. The dose of succinylcholine in morbid obesity. Anesth Analg 2006;102: 438–42.

28. Poso T, Kesek D, Winso O, et al. Volatile rapid sequence induction in morbidly obese patients. Eur J Anaesthesiol 2011;28:781–7.

29. Ingrande J, Lemmens HJ. Dose adjustment of anaesthetics in the morbidly obese. Br J Anaesth 2010;105(Suppl 1):i16–23.

30. Leykin Y, Miotto L, Pellis T. Pharmacokinetic considerations in the obese. Best Pract Res Clin Anaesthesiol 2011;25:27–36.

31. Ebert TJ, Muzi M, Berrens R, et al. Sympathetic responses to induction of anesthesia in humans with

propofol or etomidate. Anesthesiology 1992;76(5): 725–33.

32. Schulte-Sasse U, Hess W, Tarnow J. Pulmonary vascular responses to nitrous oxide in patients with normal and high pulmonary vascular resistance. Anesthesiology 1982;57(1):9–13.

33. Jaber S, Coisel Y, Chanques G, et al. A multicentre observational study of intraoperative ventilatory management during general anaesthesia: tidal volumes and relation to body weight. Anaesthesia 2012;67:999–1008.

34. Talab HF, Zabani IA, Abdelrahman HS, et al. Intraoperative ventilatory strategies for prevention of pulmonary atelectasis in obese patients undergoing laparoscopic bariatric surgery. Anesth Analg 2009; 109:1511–6.

35. Cadi P, Guenoun T, Journois D, et al. Pressure-controlled ventilation improves oxygenation during laparoscopic obesity surgery compared with volume controlled ventilation. Br J Anaesth 2008;100: 709–16.

36. Futier E, Constantin JM, Paugam-Burtz C, et al. A trial of intraoperative low-tidal-volume ventilation in abdominal surgery. N Engl J Med 2013;1369(5): 428–37.

37. Gupta A, Stierer T, Zuckerman R, et al. Comparison of recovery profile after ambulatory anesthesia with propofol, isoflurane, sevoflurane and desflurane: a systematic review. Anesth Analg 2004;98:632–41.

38. Seet E, Chung F. Management of sleep apnea in adults – functional algorithms for the perioperative period: continuing professional development. Can J Anaesth 2010;57:849–64.

39. El-Solh AA, Equilina A, Pineda L, et al. Non-invasive ventilation for prevention of post-extubation respiratory failure in obese patients. Eur Respir J 2006;28: 588–95.

40. Atwood CW, McCrory D, Garcia JG, et al. Pulmonary artery hypertension and sleep disordered breathing: ACCP evidence-based clinical practice guidelines. Chest 2004;126:72S–7S.

41. Maguire S, Rinehart J, Vakharia S, et al. Technical communication: respiratory variation in pulse pressure and plethysmographic waveforms: intraoperative applicability in a North American academic center. Anesth Analg 2011;112(1):94–6.

42. Taenzer AH, Pyke JB, McGrath SP, et al. Impact of pulse oximetry surveillance on rescue events and intensive care unit transfers: a before-and-after concurrence study. Anesthesiology 2010; 112:282–7.

43. Macintyre P, Loadsman JA, Scott DA. Opioids, ventilation and acute pain management. Anaesth Intensive Care 2011;39:545–58.

44. Banerjee D, Yee BJ, Piper AJ. Obesity hypoventilation syndrome: hypoxemia during continuous positive airway pressure. Chest 2007;131:1678–84.

45. Wijesinghe M, Williams M, Perrin K, et al. The effect of supplemental oxygen on hypercapnia in subjects with obesity associated hypoventilation: a randomized, crossover, clinical study. Chest 2011;139: 1018–24.

46. No patient shall be harmed by opioid induced respiratory depression. Anesthesia Patient Safety Foundation Newsletter 2011;26:21–40. Available at: http://www.apsf.org/newsletters/pdf/fall_2011.pdf.

Sleep Hypoventilation in Neuromuscular and Chest Wall Disorders

Lisa F. Wolfe, MD[a],*, Pallavi P. Patwari, MD[b], Gökhan M. Mutlu, MD[c]

KEYWORDS

- Sleep hypoventilation • Neuromuscular disorders • Chest wall disorders • Ventilation

KEY POINTS

- Hypoventilation due to neuromuscular and chest wall disorders includes a large number of conditions, and although these are frequently thought of as a homogeneous group, there are unique factors that separate these conditions.
- The diagnostic evaluations and therapeutic interventions for each condition are highly variable.
- Close consideration and individualization of therapy should be considered.

INTRODUCTION

Hypoventilation during sleep is common in the setting of neuromuscular and chest wall abnormalities. Often referred as restrictive thoracic disorders (RTDs), these conditions combine muscle weakness and/or nervous system failure with the possible addition of a stiff and misshapen chest wall. There are a large number of conditions that fall under RTDs, with unique features that impact control of breathing and strategies needed to optimally intervene and support the patient. The RTDs augment the reduced output from the respiratory center and central chemosensitivity and exaggerate the increase in upper airway resistance that occurs during sleep. Identification of patients with RTDs at risk for sleep-disordered breathing (SDB) and sleep-related hypoventilation can be challenging. These patients need early screening for nocturnal hypoventilation, but the typical testing used for screening in the setting of SDB is rarely helpful. Interventions with noninvasive

ventilation (NIV) are most common, but the role of polysomnography in the decision-making process for the initiation of therapy is less clear in the setting of RTDs as compared with other forms of SDB. Once initiated, ongoing management of these NIV devices is important and the new options of electronic monitoring have provided an objective window to guide management. Last, there are non-NIV options that are alternatives to treat sleep-related hypoventilation in the setting of RTDs. In this overview, we review the effects of sleep on ventilation in neuromuscular and chest wall disorders.

NEUROMUSCULAR DISORDERS

There is a very large and diverse number of RTDs and although each disorder has unique features they loosely fall into 1 of 10 categories, based on the anatomy of the nervous system and the corresponding area of pathology. Areas are outlined in **Fig. 1** and include motor neuron diseases

[a] Pulmonary and Critical Care Medicine, Northwestern University Feinberg School of Medicine, 240 East Huron Street, McGaw M300, Chicago, IL 60611, USA; [b] Sleep Medicine Center, Department of Pediatrics, Ann & Robert H. Lurie Children's Hospital of Chicago, 225 East Chicago Avenue, Box #43, Chicago, IL 60611-2605, USA; [c] Section of Pulmonary and Critical Care Medicine, University of Chicago, 5841 South Maryland Avenue, MC6026, Chicago, IL 60637, USA
* Corresponding author.
E-mail address: lwolfe@northwestern.edu

Sleep Med Clin 9 (2014) 409–423
http://dx.doi.org/10.1016/j.jsmc.2014.05.010
1556-407X/14/$ – see front matter © 2014 Elsevier Inc. All rights reserved.

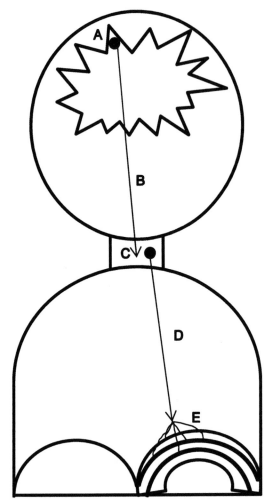

Fig. 1. Schematic of the anatomy of the nervous system and the corresponding area of pathology. Point A is the body of the motor nerve cell. B is the upper motor neuron connecting the motor cortex to the spinal cord cell bodies at point C. At point D, the peripheral lower motor neuron continues, dividing to delivering signal to neuromuscular junctions of individual skeletal muscle fibers at point E.

(MNDs), peripheral neuron disease, neuromuscular junction disease, inflammatory myopathies, muscular dystrophies, metabolic diseases of muscle, infectious myopathy, spinal cord injury (SCI), diaphragm injury, and scoliosis (**Box 1**). This section reviews of the most common conditions in each of these categories highlighting the important features related to the aspects of sleep and related hypoventilation.

Motor Neuron Disease

The most common MNDs are amyotrophic lateral sclerosis (ALS) in adults and spinal muscular atrophy (SMA) in children.

Box 1
Criteria to initiate noninvasive ventilation (1 criterion is sufficient)

1. Forced vital capacity less than 50% (predicted).

2. Maximal inspiratory pressure greater than −60 cm H_2O.

3. $Paco_2 \geq 45$ mm Hg

4. Sleep oximetry demonstrates oxygen saturation $\leq 88\%$ for at least 5 minutes

---

Amyotrophic lateral sclerosis

ALS occurs in approximately 2 of 100,000 adults per year, usually starting in the fifth to sixth decades of life. Patients present with a combination of upper and lower motor neuron symptoms. Most patients present with limb weakness, but approximately 20% present with bulbar disease in the form of difficulties with speech and dysphagia. Approximately 15% of patients have additional frontotemporal dementia. Approximately 10% to 20% of cases have been associated with genetic causes, and more than 20 genes have been described.[1] The average patient with ALS has a life expectancy of 3 to 5 years after diagnosis and the most common cause of death is respiratory compromise. Initially, respiratory failure presents with nocturnal hypoventilation, but daytime evaluations to predict the development of this impairment have been a challenge.[2] Screening questionnaires have been developed, and the most reliable finding is a complaint of orthopnea.[3] Questionnaires have not been as reliable as lung function testing for predicting the development of nocturnal or daytime hypoventilation. Forced vital capacity (FVC) is the most commonly used test, but assessment in the supine position, with slow rather than fast measurements has been shown to improve the test's ability to predict nocturnal hypoventilation.[4,5] Additional lung function assessments, such as maximal inspiratory pressure (MIP) assessment or sniff nasal inspiratory pressure (SNIP) testing, can add additional early insight for predicting the development of nocturnal hypoventilation.[6] Ultimately, using multiple testing techniques has been most effective. Initiation of therapy for nocturnal hypoventilation when any lung function test is abnormal, such as upright or supine FVC/MIP, is associated with an improvement in overall outcome of those with ALS.[7] Given this finding, information that will be obtained from a diagnostic polysomnography to characterize hypoventilation has had unclear value. The benefit of polysomnography to initiate and optimize therapy never has been demonstrated. Because current protocols do not adequately guide goals of therapy, ongoing dyssynchrony does not resolve with polysomnographic guidance.[8] Early initiation of NIV therapy is still important, as it has been shown to extend life and improve quality of life.[9]

Spinal muscular atrophy

SMA is a neuromuscular disease characterized by progressive muscular weakness due to degeneration of motor neurons, and is caused by mutations in the *survival motor neuron (SMN)*. Inherited in an autosomal recessive pattern, most affected patients carry homozygous *SMN1* deletions or loss-of-function mutations and carry varying copy numbers of the alternatively spliced *SMN2* gene. The low levels of SMN protein produced from spliced *SMN2* result in the characteristic motor neuron degeneration and progressive skeletal muscle atrophy.[10]

The SMA phenotype is variable and classified based on age of presentation and severity of weakness as type 1 (severe), 2 (intermediate), 3 (mild), or 4 (adult). SMA type 1 presents in infancy before 6 months of age and is characterized by inability to sit without support and early demise (<2 years of age). Children with SMA type 2 present with weakness at a slightly later age (6–18 months), have the ability to sit independently but not stand, and have normal neurocognitive ability. The third childhood type, which presents after 18 months of age, is SMA type 3. These children can sit and stand independently, but have difficulty with walking due to proximal limb weakness that has greater effect on the legs than arms. SMA type 4 describes individuals with onset of weakness in early adulthood with an anticipated normal life span.

Multidisciplinary care is needed for the affected children and should involve attention to optimization of nutrition, management of orthopedic problems such as scoliosis, and screening for SDB and hypoventilation. Morbidity and mortality in childhood SMA is often due to pulmonary complications. Therefore, concerted attention to evaluation of the respiratory phenotype is essential.

The respiratory phenotype in SMA is characterized by diaphragmatic breathing with weak intercostal and bulbar muscles that results in a "bell-shaped" chest wall deformity and difficulty with cough and airway clearance. Respiratory-specific evaluation and monitoring should be completed every 3 to 6 months and should include physical examination, pulmonary function testing (peak cough flow, maximal inspiratory pressure, maximal expiratory pressure), chest radiograph, pulse oximetry, carbon dioxide monitoring, and full attended polysomnography with carbon dioxide monitoring.[11]

Although an accurate assessment of lung function can be difficult in pediatric patients who are too young or too weak to complete standard testing, the physical examination should include demonstration of the effectiveness of cough and checking for subtle signs of increased work of breathing and risk for hypoventilation, such as increase in baseline respiratory rate (RR) and thoracoabdominal paradoxic breathing pattern. For those with SMA who are able to walk (indicating greater baseline strength), complete pulmonary function testing is indicated. Gas exchange abnormalities can be identified with a low oxygen saturation and an increase in end-tidal carbon dioxide or transcutaneous carbon dioxide monitoring, but also can be subtle. While continuous overnight pulse oximetry is not routinely recommended as an alternative to full in laboratory attended polysomnography, it is useful for periodic "spot checks" that can guide day-to-day management. Carbon dioxide monitoring should be limited to end-tidal or transcutaneous monitoring, as serum bicarbonate values can be falsely reassuring. Hyperventilation in response to having a blood draw will artificially drop resting carbon dioxide if measured by arterial blood gas (ABG). Development of hypoventilation and SDB can be subtle and must be actively sought through nocturnal polysomnography before progression to daytime respiratory failure.

Mainstay of chronic and acute respiratory care involves maneuvers to optimize airway clearance and provide positive airway pressure support via mask or tracheostomy. Nocturnal NIV should be initiated when there are signs of gas exchange abnormalities or SDB develops. The goals of NIV are to improve gas exchange, decrease work of breathing, and improve sleep quality and daytime functioning. NIV also can be prescribed during an acute respiratory decompensation as may occur with an acute infection. Polysomnography with carbon dioxide monitoring can be helpful for titration of respiratory support. Discussions regarding patient and family choices related to tracheostomy and palliative care should be initiated before the development of acute events (**Fig. 2**).[12]

Peripheral Nerve Disease

Both acute and chronic inflammatory demyelinating polyneuropathy (AIDP and CIDP) affect respiratory function and lead to sleep-related or chronic hypoventilation.

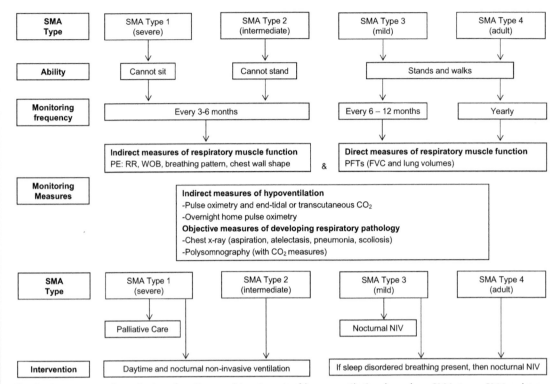

Fig. 2. Assessment of respiratory function and treatment of hypoventilation based on SMA type. SMA subtypes are defined by physical ability. These differences drive the frequency of respiratory monitoring. Once hypoventilation has been defined, therapy options should be considered. PE, physical exam; PFT, pulmonary function test; RR, respiratory rate; WOB, work of breathing.

Guillain–Barré syndrome

Guillain–Barré Syndrome (GBS) is frequently referred to as AIDP and is defined as an acute polyradiculoneuropathy with flaccid ascending paresis. The annual incidence of GBS is estimated to be between 0.34 and 1.34 per 100,000 persons. There are many subtypes that may include sensory or autonomic involvement. In 10% to 15% of patients, respiratory involvement occurs, leading to ventilatory failure.[13] Severe involvement of the upper extremities and tongue are the factors that are most predictive of respiratory insufficiency.[14] On physical examination, signs of impending respiratory failure include a weak nasal voice with an inability to count from 1 to 20 in one breath. Abnormalities seen in pulmonary function testing include a vital capacity (VC) less than 20 mL/kg, and/or a reduction in VC of more than 30% from baseline, an MIP less than 30 cm H_2O or a maximum expiratory pressure (MEP) of less than 40 cm H_2O.[15] Given the bulbar findings in many of these patients, and the rapid progression of disease, the initial use of NIV is not recommended.[16] Many of these patients may need prolonged mechanical ventilation. A calculation of the pulmonary function score (PF = VC + MIP + MEP) on days 1 and 12 of

intubation helps to predict the need for prolonged ventilatory support. If the Pao_2/Fio_2 ratio of day 1:12 is less than 1, at least another 3 weeks of mechanical ventilation would be expected.[17] NIV can be considered to speed the transition off mechanical ventilation. A return of bulbar function and good level of alertness suggests that a trial of NIV should be considered.[18] The recovery of patients with GBS may take weeks to months. At 6 months, some patients will still have persistent weakness and may never completely recover their muscle function. In some of these patients, respiratory muscle weakness may require ongoing NIV nocturnally for sleep-related hypoventilation. Many patients whose disease course shows no significant recovery will continue to have a deficit in muscle function even after 6 months.

Chronic inflammatory demyelinating polyneuropathology

In contrast to the natural course of disease in GBS, which is characterized by a relatively quick onset and a slow recovery period, CIDP includes a group of acquired polyneuropathies that are characterized clinically by a progressive symmetric weakness that evolves over a period of at least 2 months. Weakness typically involves proximal and distal limb muscles, whereas ocular or bulbar involvement is uncommon. This slow progression is in stark contrast to AIDP; however, the conditions are often grouped together, as many of the symptoms are similar. CIDP is much less common then AIDP. The incidence is estimated to be between 1.5 and 3.6 cases in a million people. Although most patients will respond well to therapy, approximately a quarter of adults will not respond to currently available treatments.[19]

Ventilatory involvement is rare in CIDP, with a reported prevalence varying from 1.7% to 9.0%, but prospective studies have shown abnormal phrenic nerve conductions in up to 80% to 92% of patients. Although chronic involvement of respiratory muscles leading to ventilatory failure is thought to be a rare complication of CIDP, patients may require ventilatory support during acute exacerbations of disease. Although most patients recover, long-term use of nocturnal ventilatory support has been reported in some patients. NIV is a more realistic initial ventilatory support option, as bulbar involvement is much less common in patients with CIDP as compared with AIDP.[20,21]

Collectively, there is need for nocturnal NIV in a group of patients with AIDP and CIDP. The long-term phase of disease should be the focus, but given the lack of data, there are no clear guidelines. A close look at the reported data can help to construct a reasonable plan for an individual patient (**Fig. 3**). The use of pulmonary function testing and/or polysomnography should be used to direct the NIV support in these patients.

Neuromuscular Junction Disease

Myasthenia gravis (MG) is a neuromuscular condition associated with autoantibody production, which impairs the neuromuscular junction. It affects both children and adults. The prevalence of MG is estimated to be between 25 and 142 (average ~30) in 1 million per year. The most common antibodies are nicotinic skeletal muscle acetylcholine receptor and muscle-specific receptor tyrosine kinase (MuSK). The most common presenting symptoms are weakness in the ocular and bulbar muscles. Patients complain of dysphagia, dysphonia, dysarthria, and chewing/swallowing difficulty, as well as generalized weakness.[22] Respiratory failure can be associated with all forms of the disease; however, those with the MuSK antibody are at higher risk.[23] The drive to breathe remains intact and central nervous system–related control of breathing appears to be unaffected; however, muscle weakness and easy fatigability are associated with a rapid shallow breathing pattern. As $Paco_2$ rises during hypoventilation, the muscle becomes taxed further, even less able to meet the ventilatory needs.[24,25] Initial investigations used VC as a single test to screen for hypoventilation, but this was found to be not helpful, as bulbar dysfunction may limit the patient's ability to accurately perform the test.[26] The use of multiple tests is more useful and accurate in screening for hypoventilation. When VC is greater than 20 mL/kg, a maximal expiratory pressure is greater than 40 cm H_2O, or a maximal inspiratory pressure is more negative than −40 cm H_2O, patients are unlikely to require ventilatory support. A decline of 30% or greater in maximal inspiratory pressure is

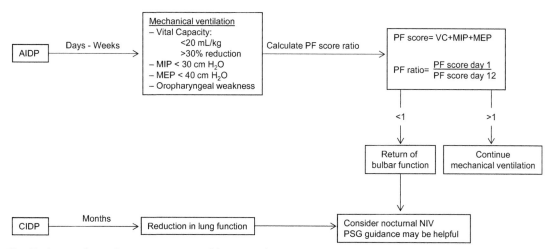

Fig. 3. Approach to the management of hypoventilation in AIDP and CIDP. Although AIDP and CIDP have different presentations, patients with both conditions may eventually benefit from NIV. PSG, polysomnography.

associated with a higher risk of requiring ventilatory support.[27] In those with hypoventilation, the presence of bulbar disease may limit the ability to use NIV, as it raises aspiration risk and reduces the ability of the patient to tolerate a mask. NIV has been shown to be tolerated as an effective therapy for acute exacerbation, post-thymectomy exacerbation, and extubation failure.[28–30] In the setting of chronic stable MG, sleep is disrupted and patients complain of chronic fatigue and sleepiness, but no excess hypoventilation or central or obstructive sleep apnea (OSA) is usually seen.[31,32]

Muscular Dystrophies

There are a large number of conditions that are associated with the clinical findings of progressive limb and core body muscle weakness. These disorders are unified by the finding of dystrophic features on muscle biopsy. They have a variable impact on cardiac and respiratory muscle function and may involve organs other than the musculoskeletal system. The conditions are heritable and the genetics have become better understood over the past 2 decades. The most common childhood and adult conditions in this group are Duchenne muscular dystrophy (DMD) and myotonic, respectively.[33]

DMD is an X-linked disease that affects 1 in 3600 to 6000 live male births, and occurs as a result of mutations in the dystrophin gene (*DMD*; locus Xp21.2). Mutations lead to an absence of or defect in the protein dystrophin. Affected individuals will display symptoms of proximal muscle weakness by age 5. A milder variant, Becker muscular dystrophy, may present at an older age, usually in the late teens. The disorder is associated with heart failure and kyphoscoliosis, but the predominant driver of early mortality is respiratory failure.[34] Respiratory weakness begins at early school age and by the second to third decades this can progress to full respiratory failure.[35] Many factors contribute to this pathology. As a skeletal muscle, eventually the diaphragm fails despite intact central drive and neural output.[36] Other factors, such as heart failure and scoliosis, progress at the same time. Ultimately, these all contribute to the development of nocturnal hypoventilation. Lung function testing has been shown to have variable prognostic value for predicting sleep-related hypoventilation. Some data suggest that a resting RR of more than 23 breaths per minute and resting rapid shallow breathing index (RSBI) (the ratio of RR to tidal volume (Vt) [RBSI in breaths/min/mL) greater than 0.07 accurately predict the development of nocturnal hypoventilation, but these tests

are rarely performed outside research settings. The most common clinically used value is the VC. Some studies indicate that a VC less than 1.82 L is predictive of nocturnal hypoventilation, whereas other studies show no relationship between VC and nocturnal hypercapnia.[37,38] Because of this variability, consensus statements suggest that full polysomnography should be performed for boys with DMD if they are considering surgical repair of scoliosis or yearly after they have disease progression requiring the use of a wheelchair.[39] Therapy with nocturnal NIV is beneficial, reducing work of breathing, and improving dyspnea, and quality and length of life.[40] The impact of early and aggressive therapy with NIV for those with DMD has the greatest impact when coadministered with broader therapeutic approaches, such as an aggressive support of heart failure. The addition of airway-clearance techniques with lung volume recruitment, aggressive therapy for heart failure, appropriate surgical intervention for scoliosis, and use of steroid therapy after early diagnosis have combined to significantly improve outcomes over the years, delaying the onset of respiratory failure and all-cause mortality by 10 to 20 years.[41]

Infectious Motor Neuropathy

Paralytic poliomyelitis is caused by a small RNA virus with a complete genome of only approximately 7500 nucleotides. It was known to occur sporadically from 1600 to 1300 BC. Epidemic poliomyelitis was a more modern disease related to improvement of sanitary conditions of the western world. Given the advancements in vaccination, acute paralytic polio (APP) was eradicated from the United States in 1979.[42] But eradication of APP did not eliminate the ongoing medical needs of APP survivors. It is estimated that there are 1.63 million people in the United States and 12 to 20 million people worldwide suffering from disabilities related to poliomyelitis. Taken together, these symptoms are referred to as the post-polio syndrome (PPS), which is defined as the onset of new and progressive fatigue, pain, muscle weakness, and atrophy that starts decades after recovery from paralytic polio.[43] Many of the patients with PPS have ventilatory failure. Some, but not all, of these patients required ventilatory support during their course with APP.

Although the past need for ventilatory support is a risk factor, it does not predict the development of chronic hypoventilation as well as pulmonary function tests do. Those with FVC and MIP less than 50% of predicted have been shown to have inadequate ventilation.[44] Many factors contribute to the development of respiratory muscle weakness, such a motor neuron stress, cranial nerve dysfunction, decreased central respiratory drive, and scoliosis.[45] In these patients, the use of nocturnal NIV has been shown to improve daytime ventilation and quality of life.[46,47]

During full polysomnography, hypoventilation is often noted in those patients with FVC values that are less than 50% of predicted. Patients with PPS and better FVC values may have SDB in the form of OSA alone or in combination with hypoventilation. Those with OSA alone have normal FVC values and wakefulness $Paco_2$ levels.[48] In addition, there are no daytime symptoms or signs that would suggest the presence of sleep-related hypoventilation.[48] Among the manifestations of SDB and hypoventilation in PPS, the most prevalent symptom is fatigue, which is considered the hallmark of the disorder. SDB explains only approximately 65% of the cases of extreme fatigue in PPS.[49] Other causes of fatigue, such as depression, menopause, and physical weakness, have been suggested as alternative explanations.[50] Insomnia and unrefreshing sleep are common complaints associated with daytime fatigue, and excessive limb movements are frequently documented in polysomnography.[51] Persistent, severe fatigue has occasionally been treated with stimulants, but the response has been variable.[52] This suggests that aggressive and complete evaluation is needed to appropriately address complaints of fatigue in PPS (**Fig. 4**).

Spinal Cord Injury

It is estimated that there were approximately 273,000 people with SCI in the United States in 2013. There are 12,000 new cases of SCI in the United States every year. Approximately 40% of these patients have high-level injury and quadriparesis. Respiratory impairment in this group is associated with a high cost of care and risk of mortality due to pneumonia and sepsis.[53] This is true for those with either acute SCIs or long-standing disease. Associated hypoventilation drives this process with the development of atelectasis and secondary pneumonia.[54]

Sleep itself is disrupted in those with chronic SCI and this appears to be due to many factors, such as aging, weight gain, smoking, alcohol misuse, and chronic conditions (chronic obstructive pulmonary disease, asthma), but there are unique factors as well.[55] In those with high SCI, the superior cervical ganglion, which originates from C8–T2, is impaired and often disrupted to the point that autonomic dysfunction becomes prominent. This ganglion plays a role in sleep regulation, as it is a stop on the pathway to melatonin production, passing the light signal from the suprachiasmatic nucleus to the pineal gland (**Fig. 5**). The impairment in melatonin production has been described as one of the factors contributing to sleep disruption in SCI.[56]

Sleep also is impaired by disordered breathing. There are many factors that drive this abnormal control of breathing, such as medications and

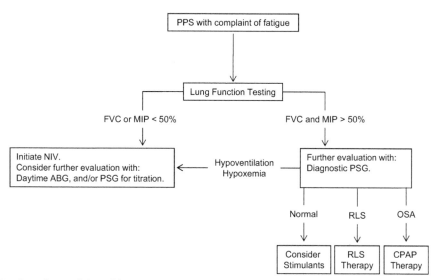

Fig. 4. Evaluation of complaint of fatigue in PPS. Fatigue is prominent in PPS and history based evaluations are not useful. Evaluations must begin with assessment of lung function. CPAP, continuous positive airway pressure; RLS, restless leg syndrome.

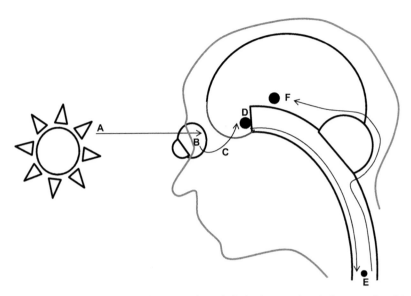

Fig. 5. Regulation of sleep by melatonin. Blue wave length light from point A, is transmitted to the retina at point B. The signal is then transmitted through the retinohypothalamic tract at C, to the hypothalamic, suprachiasmatic nucleus at point D. The signal is then transmitted through the periventricular nucleus to the superior cervical ganglion at point E. Last, postsynaptic sympathetic neurons innervate the pineal gland, in the epithalamus at point F, the site of melatonin production and regulation.

spasticity, but primary abnormalities of control of breathing include obstructive and central apnea, as well as hypoventilation. In high SCI, the use of autotitrating positive airway pressure devices is controversial because of the presence of central respiratory events in some patients.[57,58] In addition, medications, such as narcotics and baclofen, that are commonly used in the setting of SCI, are associated with the development of central apnea.[59] Other studies suggested that the findings of discrete events, such as apnea/hypopnea, are not as important as the larger issue of chronic hypoventilation with the accompanying risk of hypercapnia, higher 24-hour work of breathing, atelectasis, and potential higher risk of chest infection.[60] This remains an unresolved quandary, and intricate investigation is needed before a management scheme is developed. A suggested approach is reviewed in **Fig. 6**, and emphasizes that given the lack of agreement, all management plans should be individualized, and careful assessment of lung function assessment, including cough strength, carbon dioxide level, and nocturnal oximetry, should be considered.

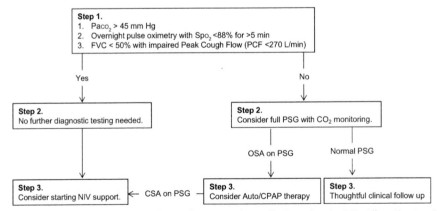

Fig. 6. Protocol for developing a patient-focused nocturnal ventilation plan in SCI. All patients with high SCI should have screening for respiratory impairment (Step 1) that could include pulmonary function testing, cough strength assessment, carbon dioxide screening, and overnight oximetry. Formal sleep testing may be helpful (Step 2). This testing should be integrated to develop a nocturnal ventilation support strategy (Step 3). CPAP, continuous positive airway pressure; CSA, central sleep apnea; PSG, polysomnography.

Diaphragm/Phrenic Injury

In 1948, Parsonage and Turner[61] suggested that neuralgic amyotrophy (NA) was a form of "mononeuritis multiplex." The incidence is approximately 2 to 4 in 100,000. NA is a clinical syndrome that is characterized by acute severe pain, and patchy paresis in the upper extremity (shoulder and arms). The paresis may be associated with atrophy resulting in winging of the scapula. The disorder is most often sporadic, but in rare cases it can be genetic (SEPT9 gene [17q25]) with an autosomal dominant pattern. In many situations, the disorder has atypical presentations. Other nerves, such as lower cranial nerves or the lumbosacral plexus, may be involved, and occasionally attacks may be painless. In approximately 15% of cases, the phrenic nerve is involved.[62] Phrenic nerve involvement can lead to dyspnea, hypoventilation, and weak phonation. Additional involvement of the vocal cords may exacerbate these complaints.[63] The phrenic involvement may be bilateral, causing more prominent symptoms.[64] Because of atypical presentation, the condition is often misdiagnosed, as the symptoms may mimic an acute coronary syndrome or diaphragmatic rupture.[65] The formal evaluation of these patients will demonstrate abnormalities in diaphragmatic function suggested by abnormalities in pulmonary function tests, chest radiography, and fluoroscopy; however, definitive diagnosis of NA may require the confirmation of electrophysiological abnormalities suggestive of axonal damage rather than demyelination of the phrenic nerve.[66] Therapy is mostly supportive. Although corticosteroids may be administered to reduce pain, they do not improve other symptoms. There have been reports of success with plasma exchange and intravenous immunoglobulin, impacting weakness, dyspnea, and pain.[67] Although patients may acutely require NIV, lung function may significantly improve over time, resolving dyspnea and hypercapnia. This can be a long-term process with measurable improvements noted after 2 to 3 years from the time of the acute presentation. The degree of recovery is variable, from complete resolution of diaphragmatic dysfunction to disabling dyspnea and persistent hypoventilation.[68] Unique to phrenic nerve issues such as NA, one available treatment option is diaphragmatic plication, which is a surgical procedure that involves the use of U-stitches to oversew the redundant folds of the weak diaphragm, placing it in a more stable position, facilitating lung expansion, and improved ventilation. The benefit of this surgery has been demonstrated to continue for more than 5 years. Many investigators suggest that in the setting of NA, plication should be delayed for 2 to 3 years to assess the possibility of spontaneous return of phrenic function.[69] Overall, NA is an excellent model for understanding the physiology of primary disorders of the phrenic nerve, because hypoventilation has a unique presentation and therapeutic approach (**Fig. 7**).

CHEST WALL DISORDERS
Scoliosis

Scoliosis is a condition that is usually associated with underlying disorders, such as neuromuscular disease or connective tissue disorders. Regardless of cause, if left untreated, scoliosis is associated with a high mortality rate, mostly attributed to cardiac and/or respiratory failure.[70] The development of respiratory failure occurs due to many factors. Scoliosis limits the formation of alveoli, and chest wall abnormalities limit lung function with reduction in total lung capacity (TLC), residual volume (RV), and VC. Secondary impairment in lung and chest wall compliance drives an ineffective breathing pattern with elevated dead space and hypoventilation. As with all restrictive thoracic disorders, patients are initially affected during sleep, but untreated will develop hypoxia-related cor pulmonale.[71] The SDB noted in scoliosis has been termed "Quasimodo Syndrome,"[72] and is notable for hypoventilation predominantly in rapid eye movement (REM) sleep with hypoxemia and hypercapnia.

Sleep is fragmented and patients complain of fatigue and unrefreshing sleep.[73,74] Ventilatory abnormalities appear first during REM sleep before non-REM sleep or wakefulness and ventilatory failure is more likely to occur when the VC is less than

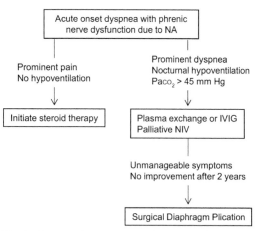

Fig. 7. Therapy for NA. An evaluation and treatment plan for the respiratory impairment due to diaphragm weakness in Parsonage–Turner syndrome. IVIG, intravenous immunoglobulin.

1.0 to 1.5 L or the MIP is less than −20 to 25 cm H_2O.[72] Noninvasive ventilation has been shown to normalize oxygen saturation and carbon dioxide levels both during sleep and during the daytime. Patients using NIV to resolve nocturnal hypoventilation have improved quality of life and exercise tolerance. They also have a reduction in cardiac disease, with both an improvement in right ventricular function and autonomic control.[75,76] Surgical correction of the scoliosis can help to reduce the long-term complications listed previously; however, the surgery itself carries risks. Up to 80% may report some type of complication and mortality has been reported to be as high as 7%. Patients are at risk for prolonged postoperative hospitalization due to respiratory failure, infections, gastrointestinal complications, cardiac failure, wound problems, pancreatitis, superior mesenteric artery syndrome, and excessive blood loss.[77] The risk of postoperative respiratory failure is significant because the average patient will experience a 12% drop in FVC postoperatively.[78] Those with underlying neuromuscular disease are at high risk, and complications can be estimated with preoperative testing. If the patient is older than 16 years and has an FVC of less than 40% predicted and the Cobb angle is greater than 69°, then the management team will face the greatest challenge.[79] Early initiation of nocturnal NIV before surgery will best help to mitigate the postoperative risk.[80]

POLYSOMNOGRAPHY

The role of polysomnography in the evaluation and treatment of those with RTD is unclear and controversial. It has been suggested that there is no role for polysomnography, and the care of those with neuromuscular disorders can appropriately address hypoventilation without the use of formal polysomnography.[81] In the United States, a national coverage determination by the Centers for Medicare and Medicaid Services has established a standard that those with RTDs qualify for the use of NIV as therapy for hypoventilation merely by the demonstration of impaired respiratory function. Patients need to demonstrate only one of many criteria for the initiation of NIV therapy on an empiric basis (see **Box 1**).[82] Although this standard has been in place in the United States since 1999, many communities continue to perform routine polysomnography. The best clinical practice document published by the American Academy of Sleep Medicine in 2010 recommended that standard overnight monitoring be expanded to include diaphragm electromyography to assess respiratory effort. The addition of carbon dioxide

measurements either by transcutaneous or end-tidal techniques is also recommended.[83] The newest scoring guidelines provide an option for using carbon dioxide data to score "hypoventilation events" although it is unclear how these events would impact diagnosis or management of those with RTDs. The hypoventilation is defined as an increase in the P_{CO_2} to a value greater than 55 mm Hg for equal or longer than 10 minutes, or there is a 10 mm Hg or greater increase in P_{CO_2} during sleep (in comparison with an awake supine value) to a value exceeding 50 mm Hg for at least 10 minutes.[84] When titration of NIV is performed, the goals are unique and are different from those of typical titrations done for the treatment of OSA. The study is successful when the RR is not too low, with a backup rate sufficient to eliminate central apnea events, a Vt that is adequate so that oxygen saturation is within in the normal range, and any tachypnea is resolved. The ultimate goal is to provide sufficient respiratory support that both oxygen saturation and carbon dioxide levels are within normal range. If titration is successful, the use of supplemental oxygen should not be necessary.[83] In fact, supplemental oxygen administration should be considered as a last resort. In the end, it may be that the biggest factor limiting quality care for patients with RTDs in the sleep laboratories is physical access. Most laboratories lack wheelchair accessibility, lifts or other transfer apparatus, adaptive call lights, space for caregivers, and suction pumps to name a few. Despite all of these issues, the care of those with RTDs has a potential future with formal polysomnography, as many care providers will continue to need assistance in providing optimized NIV.

HOME MANAGEMENT OF NIV

The home management of NIV for those with neuromuscular and chest wall disorders is not standardized. It is unclear how often the NIV device should be monitored or adjusted. The widely available access to device reports, which include ventilation characteristics, as well as compliance data, has opened a new area of potential monitoring of these patients. Some have argued that the many differences in the technology between manufacturers may make the report interpretation challenging, limiting widespread use.[85] Others have highlighted the fact that by its nature, monitoring of NIV for RTDs focuses on factors unique to neuromuscular disorders. Those accustomed to evaluating download data from devices for patients with OSA may need to adjust their interpretation strategies (**Table 1**).[86] The most convincing data for long-term follow-up stems from overnight pulse oximetry,

Table 1
Download interpretation strategies of obstructive sleep apnea versus restrictive thoracic disorders

Device Download Parameter	Obstructive Sleep Apnea	Restrictive Thoracic Disorders
Leak	Mask issues	If there is daytime use, consider that the patient may be talking with NIV on.
AHI	Upper airway obstruction	Consider: 1. Central apnea and a need to increase back-up rate 2. Central apnea due to glottic closures from elevated pressure support 3. Central hypopnea due to insufficient pressure support 4. Asynchrony due to inappropriate trigger
High Run Time	Hypersomnia Long total sleep	Increasing disability. Consider daytime ventilation.
Low % of patient-triggered breaths	N/A	Increasing disability. Consider increasing back up rate.
Dropping tidal volume	N/A	Increasing disability. Consider increasing pressure support.
Shorter inspiratory time	N/A	Increasing disability. Consider increasing device delivered inspiratory time.

Abbreviations: AHI, apnea hypopnea index; N/A, not applicable; NIV, noninvasive ventilation.

rather than device download data. In one study that monitored patients with ALS with overnight oximetry every 3 months, investigators found that those patients with normal pulse oximetry values had improved outcomes.[87] Normal was defined as less than 5% of nocturnal monitoring period with an SpO_2 less than 90%. Survival at 1 year in those with normal pulse oximetry was 75% as compared with 57% for those who did not maintain adequate saturation. Optimizing ventilation settings to normalize saturation did improve survival for patients who had abnormal overnight recordings.

ALTERNATIVE THERAPIES FOR HYPOVENTILATION

In the era before the widely available access to positive pressure–based NIV, therapy for hypoventilation related to RTDs included many devices that are not commonly available at this time. Negative-pressure ventilation was common, and whole body–type devices, such as iron lungs or pneumosuits, were used. These devices were problematic. They supported ventilation by expanding the chest wall, allowing air to passively fill the lungs, but as they had no mechanism to support the upper airway, obstructive apnea events could ensue. However, because there is no oral interface, these devices could more easily be adapted for those with facial deformities,

claustrophobia, or poor salivary control.[88] More-modern versions of these devices have been developed. For example, the Biphasic Cuirass Ventilation includes additional external pressure at the initiation of a breath to support the opening of the upper airway, and can provide high-frequency chest wall oscillation, doubling as a device for both NIV and airway clearance. Unfortunately, there have been no large trials to document the efficacy of these devices in specific RTDs **(Fig. 8)**.[89]

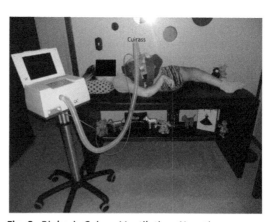

Fig. 8. Biphasic Cuirass Ventilation. Negative-pressure ventilator is located in the foreground and the patient is wearing a Chest Cuirass.

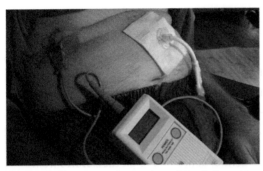

Fig. 9. Diaphragm pacing system. Stimulation wires are operatively affixed to the diaphragm and tunneled under the skin. At the skin site, the wire ends are tipped, allowing an external stimulation box to be connected. The stimulation box delivers the electrical charge, causing diaphragmatic contraction.

Diaphragm pacing systems is another therapy that is an alternative to NIV. The mechanistic basis has been described elsewhere in detail, but in brief, direct electrical stimulation of the phrenic nerve, as it inserts into the diaphragm, is used to stimulate contraction of the muscle. The stimulation electrodes are implanted surgically and an external generator provides the electrical pulses **(Fig. 9)**.[90] Currently, the device is being used as therapy in both SCI and ALS. In ALS, the device is used for therapeutic electrical stimulation; that is, the device provides electricity as a form of training, to support a muscle under stress due to the degeneration of its feeding motor neuron. This device also has been shown to improve sleep quality for those with ALS, but it is not a form of NIV.[91] Early testing suggests a possible benefit to patients by improving their survival.[92] In contrast, diaphragmatic pacing device is used as a form of NIV in the setting of SCI. In high-level SCI, direct stimulation of the diaphragm with a pacer can be used as functional electrical stimulation, which means that the device is not being used to enrich muscle function but rather to replace a failing system of spontaneous ventilation.[90]

SUMMARY

In summary, hypoventilation due to neuromuscular and chest wall disorders includes a large number of conditions. Although these conditions are frequently thought of as a homogeneous group, there are unique factors that separate these conditions. The diagnostic evaluations and therapeutic interventions for each condition are highly variable. Close consideration and individualization of therapy should be considered.

REFERENCES

1. Robberecht W, Philips T. The changing scene of amyotrophic lateral sclerosis. Nat Rev Neurosci 2013;14(4):248–64.
2. Sivak ED, Shefner JM, Mitsumoto H, et al. The use of non-invasive positive pressure ventilation (NIPPV) in ALS patients. A need for improved determination of intervention timing. Amyotroph Lateral Scler Other Motor Neuron Disord 2001;2(3):139–45.
3. Steier J, Jolley CJ, Seymour J, et al. Screening for sleep-disordered breathing in neuromuscular disease using a questionnaire for symptoms associated with diaphragm paralysis. Eur Respir J 2011;37(2):400–5.
4. Sanjak M, Salachas F, Frija-Orvoen E, et al. Quality control of vital capacity as a primary outcome measure during phase III therapeutic clinical trial in amyotrophic lateral sclerosis. Amyotroph Lateral Scler 2010;11(4):383–8.
5. Schmidt EP, Drachman DB, Wiener CM, et al. Pulmonary predictors of survival in amyotrophic lateral sclerosis: use in clinical trial design. Muscle Nerve 2006;33(1):127–32.
6. Mustfa N, Moxham J. Respiratory muscle assessment in motor neurone disease. QJM 2001;94(9): 497–502.
7. Lechtzin N, Scott Y, Busse AM, et al. Early use of non-invasive ventilation prolongs survival in subjects with ALS. Amyotroph Lateral Scler 2007; 8(3):185–8.
8. Atkeson AD, RoyChoudhury A, Harrington-Moroney G, et al. Patient-ventilator asynchrony with nocturnal noninvasive ventilation in ALS. Neurology 2011;77(6):549–55.
9. Miller RG, Jackson CE, Kasarskis EJ, et al. Practice parameter update: the care of the patient with amyotrophic lateral sclerosis: drug, nutritional, and respiratory therapies (an evidence-based review): report of the Quality Standards Subcommittee of the American Academy of Neurology. Neurology 2009;73(15):1218–26.
10. Wirth B. An update of the mutation spectrum of the survival motor neuron gene (SMN1) in autosomal recessive spinal muscular atrophy (SMA). Hum Mutat 2000;15(3):228–37.
11. Schroth MK. Special considerations in the respiratory management of spinal muscular atrophy. Pediatrics 2009;123(Suppl 4):S245–9.
12. Wang CH, Finkel RS, Bertini ES, et al. Consensus statement for standard of care in spinal muscular atrophy. J Child Neurol 2007;22(8):1027–49.
13. Korinthenberg R. Acute polyradiculoneuritis: Guillain-Barre syndrome. Handb Clin Neurol 2013; 112:1157–62.
14. Orlikowski D, Terzi N, Blumen M, et al. Tongue weakness is associated with respiratory failure in

patients with severe Guillain-Barre syndrome. Acta Neurol Scand 2009;119(6):364–70.

15. Rabinstein AA, Wijdicks EF. Warning signs of imminent respiratory failure in neurological patients. Semin Neurol 2003;23(1):97–104.

16. Wijdicks EF, Roy TK. BiPAP in early Guillain-Barre syndrome may fail. Can J Neurol Sci 2006;33(1): 105–6.

17. Lawn ND, Wijdicks EF. Post-intubation pulmonary function test in Guillain-Barre syndrome. Muscle Nerve 2000;23(4):613–6.

18. Reddy VG, Nair MP, Bataclan F. Role of noninvasive ventilation in difficult-to-wean children with acute neuromuscular disease. Singapore Med J 2004;45(5):232–4.

19. Vanasse M, Rossignol E, Hadad E. Chronic inflammatory demyelinating polyneuropathy. Handb Clin Neurol 2013;112:1163–9.

20. Henderson RD, Sandroni P, Wijdicks EF. Chronic inflammatory demyelinating polyneuropathy and respiratory failure. J Neurol 2005;252(10):1235–7.

21. Zivkovic SA, Peltier AC, Iacob T, et al. Chronic inflammatory demyelinating polyneuropathy and ventilatory failure: report of seven new cases and review of the literature. Acta Neurol Scand 2011; 124(1):59–63.

22. Silvestri NJ, Wolfe GI. Myasthenia gravis. Semin Neurol 2012;32(3):215–26.

23. Evoli A, Tonali PA, Padua L, et al. Clinical correlates with anti-MuSK antibodies in generalized seronegative myasthenia gravis. Brain 2003;126(Pt 10): 2304–11.

24. Borel CO, Teitelbaum JS, Hanley DF. Ventilatory drive and carbon dioxide response in ventilatory failure due to myasthenia gravis and Guillain-Barre syndrome. Crit Care Med 1993;21(11): 1717–26.

25. Garcia Rio F, Prados C, Diez Tejedor E, et al. Breathing pattern and central ventilatory drive in mild and moderate generalised myasthenia gravis. Thorax 1994;49(7):703–6.

26. Rieder P, Louis M, Jolliet P, et al. The repeated measurement of vital capacity is a poor predictor of the need for mechanical ventilation in myasthenia gravis. Intensive Care Med 1995;21(8): 663–8.

27. Thieben MJ, Blacker DJ, Liu PY, et al. Pulmonary function tests and blood gases in worsening myasthenia gravis. Muscle Nerve 2005;32(5):664–7.

28. Mishra SK, Krishnappa S, Bhat RR, et al. Role of intermittent noninvasive ventilation in anticholinesterase dose adjustment for myasthenic crisis. Acta Anaesthesiol Taiwan 2010;48(1):53–4.

29. Wu JY, Kuo PH, Fan PC, et al. The role of noninvasive ventilation and factors predicting extubation outcome in myasthenic crisis. Neurocrit Care 2009;10(1):35–42.

30. Rabinstein A, Wijdicks EF. BiPAP in acute respiratory failure due to myasthenic crisis may prevent intubation. Neurology 2002;59(10):1647–9.

31. Burns TM, Grouse CK, Wolfe GI, et al. The MG-QOL15 for following the health-related quality of life of patients with myasthenia gravis. Muscle Nerve 2011;43(1):14–8.

32. Prudlo J, Koenig J, Ermert S, et al. Sleep disordered breathing in medically stable patients with myasthenia gravis. Eur J Neurol 2007;14(3):321–6.

33. Mercuri E, Muntoni F. Muscular dystrophies. Lancet 2012;381(9869):845–60.

34. Bushby K, Finkel R, Birnkrant DJ, et al. Diagnosis and management of Duchenne muscular dystrophy, part 1: diagnosis, and pharmacological and psychosocial management. Lancet Neurol 2010; 9(1):77–93.

35. Hahn A, Duisberg B, Neubauer BA, et al. Noninvasive determination of the tension-time index in Duchenne muscular dystrophy. Am J Phys Med Rehabil 2009;88(4):322–7.

36. Beck J, Weinberg J, Hamnegard CH, et al. Diaphragmatic function in advanced Duchenne muscular dystrophy. Neuromuscul Disord 2006; 16(3):161–7.

37. Toussaint M, Steens M, Soudon P. Lung function accurately predicts hypercapnia in patients with Duchenne muscular dystrophy. Chest 2007; 131(2):368–75.

38. Katz SL, Gaboury I, Keilty K, et al. Nocturnal hypoventilation: predictors and outcomes in childhood progressive neuromuscular disease. Arch Dis Child 2010;95(12):998–1003.

39. Finder JD, Birnkrant D, Carl J, et al. Respiratory care of the patient with Duchenne muscular dystrophy: ATS consensus statement. Am J Respir Crit Care Med 2004;170(4):456–65.

40. Toussaint M, Chatwin M, Soudon P. Mechanical ventilation in Duchenne patients with chronic respiratory insufficiency: clinical implications of 20 years published experience. Chron Respir Dis 2007;4(3): 167–77.

41. Jeppesen J, Green A, Steffensen BF, et al. The Duchenne muscular dystrophy population in Denmark, 1977-2001: prevalence, incidence and survival in relation to the introduction of ventilator use. Neuromuscul Disord 2003;13(10):804–12.

42. Nathanson N, Kew OM. From emergence to eradication: the epidemiology of poliomyelitis deconstructed. Am J Epidemiol 2010;172(11):1213–29.

43. Shiri S, Wexler ID, Feintuch U, et al. Post-polio syndrome: impact of hope on quality of life. Disabil Rehabil 2012;34(10):824–30.

44. Soliman MG, Higgins SE, El-Kabir DR, et al. Noninvasive assessment of respiratory muscle strength in patients with previous poliomyelitis. Respir Med 2005;99(10):1217–22.

45. Chai T, Aseff JN, Halstead LS. Diaphragm dysfunction due to remote poliomyelitis in a patient with unexplained dyspnea. PM R 2011;3(2):179–82.

46. Olofson J, Dellborg C, Sullivan M, et al. Qualify of life and palliation predict survival in patients with chronic alveolar hypoventilation and nocturnal ventilatory support. Qual Life Res 2009;18(3):273–80.

47. Bach JR, Alba AS. Sleep and nocturnal mouthpiece IPPV efficiency in postpoliomyelitis ventilator users. Chest 1994;106(6):1705–10.

48. Hsu AA, Staats BA. "Postpolio" sequelae and sleep-related disordered breathing. Mayo Clin Proc 1998;73(3):216–24.

49. Dahan V, Kimoff RJ, Petrof BJ, et al. Sleep-disordered breathing in fatigued postpoliomyelitis clinic patients. Arch Phys Med Rehabil 2006;87(10): 1352–6.

50. Kalpakjian CZ, Quint EH, Toussaint LL. Menopause and post-polio symptoms as predictors of subjective sleep disturbance in poliomyelitis survivors. Climacteric 2007;10(1):51–62.

51. Araujo MA, Silva TM, Moreira GA, et al. Sleep disorders frequency in post-polio syndrome patients caused by periodic limb movements. Arq Neuropsiquiatr 2010;68(1):35–8.

52. Vasconcelos OM, Prokhorenko OA, Salajegheh MK, et al. Modafinil for treatment of fatigue in post-polio syndrome: a randomized controlled trial. Neurology 2007;68(20):1680–6.

53. DeVivo MJ, Go BK, Jackson AB. Overview of the national spinal cord injury statistical center database. J Spinal Cord Med 2002;25(4):335–8.

54. Berlly M, Shem K. Respiratory management during the first five days after spinal cord injury. J Spinal Cord Med 2007;30(4):309–18.

55. LaVela SL, Burns SP, Goldstein B, et al. Dysfunctional sleep in persons with spinal cord injuries and disorders. Spinal Cord 2012;50(9):682–5.

56. Verheggen RJ, Jones H, Nyakayiru J, et al. Complete absence of evening melatonin increase in tetraplegics. FASEB J 2012;26(7):3059–64.

57. Berlowitz DJ, Ayas N, Barnes M, et al. Auto-titrating continuous positive airway pressure treatment for obstructive sleep apnoea after acute quadriplegia (COSAQ): study protocol for a randomized controlled trial. Trials 2013;14:181.

58. Sankari A, Bascom AT, Chowdhuri S, et al. Tetraplegia is a risk factor for central sleep apnea. J Appl Physiol (1985) 2014;116(3):345–53.

59. Bensmail D, Marquer A, Roche N, et al. Pilot study assessing the impact of intrathecal baclofen administration mode on sleep-related respiratory parameters. Arch Phys Med Rehabil 2012;93(1): 96–9.

60. Bach JR. Noninvasive respiratory management of high level spinal cord injury. J Spinal Cord Med 2012;35(2):72–80.

61. Parsonage M, Turner J. Neuralgic amyotrophy: the shoulder girdle syndrome. Lancet 1948;254:973–8.

62. van Alfen N. The neuralgic amyotrophy consultation. J Neurol 2007;254(6):695–704.

63. Chen YM, Hu GC, Cheng SJ. Bilateral neuralgic amyotrophy presenting with left vocal cord and phrenic nerve paralysis. J Formos Med Assoc 2007;106(8):680–4.

64. Kumar N, Folger WN, Bolton CF. Dyspnea as the predominant manifestation of bilateral phrenic neuropathy. Mayo Clin Proc 2004;79(12):1563–5.

65. Beydoun SR, Rodriguez R. Neuralgic amyotrophy misdiagnosed as diaphragmatic rupture. Muscle Nerve 1996;19(9):1181–2.

66. Nardone R, Bernhart H, Pozzera A, et al. Respiratory weakness in neuralgic amyotrophy: report of two cases with phrenic nerve involvement. Neurol Sci 2000;21(3):177–81.

67. Kalluri M, Huggins JT, Strange C. A 56-year-old woman with arm pain, dyspnea, and an elevated diaphragm. Chest 2008;133(1):296–9.

68. Hughes PD, Polkey MI, Moxham J, et al. Long-term recovery of diaphragm strength in neuralgic amyotrophy. Eur Respir J 1999;13(2):379–84.

69. Stolk J, Versteegh MI. Long-term effect of bilateral plication of the diaphragm. Chest 2000;117(3): 786–9.

70. Nilsonne U, Lundgren KD. Long-term prognosis in idiopathic scoliosis. Acta Orthop Scand 1968; 39(4):456–65.

71. Martini A, Bonadeo D, Bottoni G, et al. Bioadhesives: rationale, state of the art and therapeutic potential. Boll Chim Farm 1995;134(11):595–603 [in Italian].

72. Shneerson JM. Respiration during sleep in neuromuscular and thoracic cage disorders. Monaldi Arch Chest Dis 2004;61(1):44–8.

73. Guilleminault C, Kurland G, Winkle R, et al. Severe kyphoscoliosis, breathing, and sleep: the "Quasimodo" syndrome during sleep. Chest 1981;79(6): 626–30.

74. Ellis ER, Grunstein RR, Chan S, et al. Noninvasive ventilatory support during sleep improves respiratory failure in kyphoscoliosis. Chest 1988;94(4):811–5.

75. Watson JP, Nolan J, Elliott MW. Autonomic dysfunction in patients with nocturnal hypoventilation in extrapulmonary restrictive disease. Eur Respir J 1999;13(5):1097–102.

76. Fuschillo S, De Felice A, Gaudiosi C, et al. Nocturnal mechanical ventilation improves exercise capacity in kyphoscoliotic patients with respiratory impairment. Monaldi Arch Chest Dis 2003; 59(4):281–6.

77. Master DL, Son-Hing JP, Poe-Kochert C, et al. Risk factors for major complications after surgery for neuromuscular scoliosis. Spine (Phila Pa 1976) 2012;36(7):564–71.

78. Roberto R, Fritz A, Hagar Y, et al. The natural history of cardiac and pulmonary function decline in patients with Duchenne muscular dystrophy. Spine (Phila Pa 1976) 2011;36(15):E1009–17.

79. Kang GR, Suh SW, Lee IO. Preoperative predictors of postoperative pulmonary complications in neuromuscular scoliosis. J Orthop Sci 2011;16(2): 139–47.

80. Ferris G, Servera-Pieras E, Vergara P, et al. Kyphoscoliosis ventilatory insufficiency: noninvasive management outcomes. Am J Phys Med Rehabil 2000; 79(1):24–9.

81. Bach JR, Chaudhry SS. Standards of care in MDA clinics. Muscular Dystrophy Association. Am J Phys Med Rehabil 2000;79(2):193–6.

82. Clinical indications for noninvasive positive pressure ventilation in chronic respiratory failure due to restrictive lung disease, COPD, and nocturnal hypoventilation—a consensus conference report. Chest 1999;116(2):521–34.

83. Berry RB, Chediak A, Brown LK, et al. Best clinical practices for the sleep center adjustment of noninvasive positive pressure ventilation (NPPV) in stable chronic alveolar hypoventilation syndromes. J Clin Sleep Med 2010;6(5):491–509.

84. Berry RB, Budhiraja R, Gottlieb DJ, et al. Rules for scoring respiratory events in sleep: update of the 2007 AASM manual for the scoring of sleep and associated events. Deliberations of the sleep apnea definitions task force of the American Academy of Sleep Medicine. J Clin Sleep Med 2012; 8(5):597–619.

85. Contal O, Vignaux L, Combescure C, et al. Monitoring of noninvasive ventilation by built-in software of home bilevel ventilators: a bench study. Chest 2012;141(2):469–76.

86. Janssens JP, Borel JC, Pepin JL. Nocturnal monitoring of home non-invasive ventilation: the contribution of simple tools such as pulse oximetry, capnography, built-in ventilator software and autonomic markers of sleep fragmentation. Thorax 2011;66(5):438–45.

87. Gonzalez-Bermejo J, Morelot-Panzini C, Arnol N, et al. Prognostic value of efficiently correcting nocturnal desaturations after one month of noninvasive ventilation in amyotrophic lateral sclerosis: a retrospective monocentre observational cohort study. Amyotroph Lateral Scler Frontotemporal Degener 2013;14(5–6):373–9.

88. Dettenmeier PA, Jackson NC. Chronic hypoventilation syndrome: treatment with non-invasive mechanical ventilation. AACN Clin Issues Crit Care Nurs 1991;2(3):415–31.

89. Chatburn RL. High-frequency assisted airway clearance. Respir Care 2007;52(9):1224–35 [discussion: 1235–7].

90. DiMarco AF. Phrenic nerve stimulation in patients with spinal cord injury. Respir Physiol Neurobiol 2009;169(2):200–9.

91. Gonzalez-Bermejo J, Morelot-Panzini C, Salachas F, et al. Diaphragm pacing improves sleep in patients with amyotrophic lateral sclerosis. Amyotroph Lateral Scler 2012;13(1):44–54.

92. Onders RP, Elmo M, Kaplan C, et al. Final analysis of the pilot trial of diaphragm pacing in amyotrophic lateral sclerosis with long-term follow-up: diaphragm pacing positively affects diaphragm respiration. Am J Surg 2014;207(3):393–7 [discussion: 397].

Hypoventilation Syndromes of Infancy, Childhood, and Adulthood

Congenital Central Hypoventilation Syndrome (CCHS), Later-Onset CCHS, and Rapid-Onset Obesity with Hypothalamic Dysfunction, Hypoventilation, and Autonomic Dysregulation

Rehan Saiyed, BS[a], Casey M. Rand, BS[a],
Michael S. Carroll, PhD[a,b], Debra E. Weese-Mayer, MD[a,b],*

KEYWORDS

- Autonomic dysregulation • Hypothalamic dysregulation • Hypoventilation • *PHOX2B*

KEY POINTS

- Congenital central hypoventilation syndrome (CCHS) (including later-onset CCHS) and rapid-onset obesity with hypothalamic dysfunction, hypoventilation, and autonomic dysregulation (ROHHAD) are rare neurocristopathies with shared features including alveolar hypoventilation, disordered respiratory control, variable autonomic nervous system dysregulation (ANSD), tumors of neural crest origin, and risk of sudden death.
- Mutations in the *PHOX2B* gene are causative in all known cases of CCHS. The *PHOX2B* genotype is predictive of many features of the CCHS phenotype, including severity of hypoventilation, risk of cardiac sinus pauses, Hirschsprung disease, neural crest tumors, and symptoms of ANSD.
- For ROHHAD, research is under way to determine the etiology of the disease.
- Early consideration of CCHS and stepwise *PHOX2B* testing in cases with unexplained alveolar hypoventilation or delayed recovery of spontaneous breathing after sedation, anesthesia, or a severe respiratory infection will enhance diagnosis of milder CCHS cases and LO-CCHS, decreasing morbidity and mortality in these instances.
- Heightened clinical suspicion in cases of rapid-onset obesity with hypoventilation, especially in the event of a tumor of neural crest origin, will allow for early identification of ROHHAD patients. Coupled with conservative management, this strategy will optimize the long-term outcome and neurocognitive development for children with ROHHAD.
- For CCHS, LO-CCHS, and ROHHAD, targets for treatment and drug intervention are being evaluated as progress is made in understanding the underlying mechanisms and phenotypic manifestations of these disorders.

[a] Center for Autonomic Medicine in Pediatrics (CAMP), Ann & Robert H. Lurie Children's Hospital of Chicago, 225 East Chicago Avenue, Chicago, IL 60611, USA; [b] Northwestern University Feinberg School of Medicine, 303 E. Chicago Avenue, Chicago, IL 60611, USA
* Corresponding author. Center for Autonomic Medicine in Pediatrics (CAMP), Ann & Robert H. Lurie Children's Hospital of Chicago, 225 East Chicago Avenue, Box 165, Chicago, IL 60611.
E-mail address: D-Weese-Mayer@Northwestern.edu

Sleep Med Clin 9 (2014) 425–439
http://dx.doi.org/10.1016/j.jsmc.2014.06.001
1556-407X/14/$ – see front matter © 2014 Elsevier Inc. All rights reserved.

INTRODUCTION: NATURE OF THE PROBLEM

Congenital central hypoventilation syndrome (CCHS) and rapid-onset obesity with hypothalamic dysfunction, hypoventilation, and autonomic dysregulation (ROHHAD) are rare disorders of hypoventilation. CCHS typically presents in the newborn period and ROHHAD in childhood, although later identification of CCHS is becoming increasingly more common, and these cases are now termed later-onset CCHS (LO-CCHS). Each of these syndromes causes apparent alveolar hypoventilation with disordered respiratory control during sleep and often during wakefulness, in addition to a varied and complex assortment of phenotypic manifestations (**Table 1**). Both disorders are included within the rubric of Respiratory and Autonomic Disorders of Infancy, Childhood and Adulthood (RADICA), and both are examples of neurocristopathies.

CCHS

Etiology

CCHS was first described by Mellins and colleagues[1] as a case report in 1970. Early study of CCHS was focused on the respiratory control deficit in these patients. Symptoms of diffuse autonomic nervous system (ANS) dysregulation (ANSD) became evident as larger patient populations were reviewed, leading to the introduction of the ANSD acronym and a focus on central hypoventilation in the context of ANSD.[2] In 2003, heterozygous mutations within the *PHOX2B* gene were discovered to be responsible for the CCHS phenotype.[3,4] The *PHOX2B* gene encodes a highly conserved transcription factor known to play an integral role in the embryologic expression of neural crest cells involved in development of the ANS.[5] *PHOX2B* variations in CCHS cases include polyalanine repeat expansion mutations (PARMs; ~90% of cases) in exon 3, as well as non-PARMs (NPARMs) with missense, frameshift, nonsense, and stop-codon mutations (8%–10% of cases) throughout the coding region, and whole or partial gene deletions (<1% of cases; **Fig. 1**).[6] The type and location of the mutation within the *PHOX2B* gene influences the magnitude of cellular disruption.[7,8] Accordingly, the type of *PHOX2B* mutation has been shown to be prognostic of phenotypic severity in CCHS, for both the hypoventilation and some features of ANSD (**Fig. 2**). However, a recent study of a 3-generation family with a CCHS-affected individual in each generation, all of whom were shown to have the same *PHOX2B* NPARM mutation, revealed distinct CCHS phenotypes in each case, indicating variable expressivity even within a single family sharing an identical NPARM.[9] Whole or partial gene deletions tend to produce a less severe phenotype, although the relative severity of these large-scale deletions cannot be statistically assessed because of the limited number of patients identified to date.[10]

An autosomal dominant pattern of inheritance has been ascertained for CCHS through observation of somatic mosaicism in parents in addition to direct inheritance from an affected CCHS parent to child.[4] Whereas up to 25% of CCHS cases are inherited from a parent with somatic mosaicism, de novo germline mutations are responsible for most cases of CCHS.[6] As of early 2014, approximately 1200 cases of CCHS have been diagnosed since the first case report in 1970, including patients from at least 50 countries. The true prevalence of CCHS remains unknown, and estimation proves difficult because of undiagnosed mild or later-onset cases.

Overview of major features

Central hypoventilation Alveolar hypoventilation, without a primary neuromuscular, respiratory, or cardiac basis or a brainstem lesion that can account for the full CCHS phenotype, remains the most prominent indication of the disorder. Patients with CCHS have diminished tidal volumes with limited respiratory rate variability. This feature is most evident during non–rapid eye movement (REM) sleep but also can be observed during REM sleep and wakefulness.[11–13] As a result, patients become hypoxemic and hypercarbic, and lack the physiologic and behavioral responsiveness to such challenges (absent adjustments of respiration and/or arousal during sleep). Tissue injury arising from intermittent hypoxia in central nervous system areas responsible for cardiac and respiratory control has been reported,[14] potentially exacerbating control of breathing deficits, among other ANS irregularities.

Neurocognitive function Impaired neurocognitive function has been reported in a subset of patients with CCHS.[13,15–18] Whether the noted neurocognitive deficits arise solely from intermittent hypoxia, a primary neurologic issue intrinsic to CCHS, or a combination of both remains unknown. Recent evidence has suggested altered cerebral autoregulation in CCHS,[19] which could contribute to the observed neurologic deficit in conjunction with experienced hypoxemia in the disorder.

Hirschsprung disease and gastrointestinal dysfunction A subset of CCHS patients are born with Hirschsprung disease (HSCR), defined as an absence of ganglion cells from variable lengths of distal bowel. These patients typically present shortly after birth with failure to pass meconium,

Table 1
Overview of common and differentiating features in congenital central hypoventilation syndrome (CCHS), later-onset CCHS (LO-CCHS), and rapid-onset obesity with hypothalamic dysfunction, hypoventilation, and autonomic dysregulation (ROHHAD)

	Phenotypic Features (%)						
	Alveolar Hypoventilation	ANSD[a]	Neural Crest Tumors	Hirschsprung Disease	Hypothalamic Dysregulation	Rapid-Onset Obesity	Etiology	Onset/Clinical Detection
CCHS	100	100	NPARM: ≥50 PARM: <1	NPARM: >80 PARM: ~20	<5	0	*PHOX2B* gene mutations	Newborn
LO-CCHS	100	100	0	≤5	0	0	*PHOX2B* gene mutations	Infancy–adulthood
ROHHAD	100	100	40	0	100	100	Unknown	1.5–11 y

Abbreviations: ANSD, autonomic nervous system dysregulation; NPARM, non–polyalanine repeat expansion mutation; PARM, polyalanine repeat expansion mutation.
[a] Features of ANSD vary greatly between CCHS/LO-CCHS and ROHHAD.

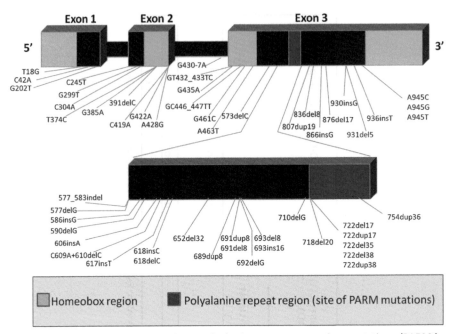

Fig. 1. CCHS-associated *PHOX2B* gene mutations. Polyalanine repeat expansion mutations (PARMs) are located within the second polyalanine expansion region of exon 3 (shown in *red*). Nearly all NPARMs identified thus far have been found at the extreme 3′ end of exon 2 or in exon 3. (*From* Weese-Mayer DE, Rand CM, Berry-Kravis EM, et al. Congenital central hypoventilation syndrome from past to future: model for translational and transitional autonomic medicine. Pediatr Pulmonol 2009;44:526; with permission.)

abdominal distention, and vomiting, although a subset will be diagnosed after the neonatal period presenting with severe constipation. New murine models indicate that *PHOX2B* dysfunction can lead to decreased bowel ganglion cell density,[20] a condition that would not be termed HSCR but would likely lead to variable gastrointestinal dysfunction. Indeed, a recent abstract reported

that non-HSCR CCHS patients are more likely than healthy controls to experience constipation, dysphagia, diarrhea, and bloating.[21]

Neural crest cell–derived tumors Solid extracranial tumors of neural crest origin have been described in CCHS. These tumors may occur anywhere along the sympathetic chain, including

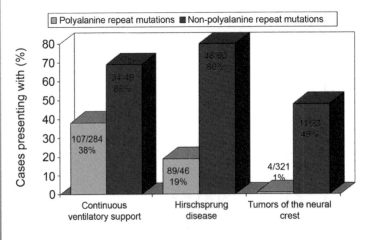

Fig. 2. Rate of phenotypic manifestations in CCHS cases with PARMs in *PHOX2B* compared with those cases with NPARMs in *PHOX2B*. CCHS cases included were compiled from cases reported in the literature through 2009 including reports from groups in the United States, Italy, France, Japan, Germany, China, Australia, and the Netherlands, in addition to data reported by the authors, where adequate clinical information was available. Neural crest tumor data were derived from cases whereby information was available and the child had survived at least the first year of life. All PARM cases with tumors had large (29–33 repeat; genotypes 20/29–20/33) expansion mutations. (*From* Weese-Mayer DE, Rand CM, Berry-Kravis EM, et al. Congenital central hypoventilation syndrome from past to future: model for translational and transitional autonomic medicine. Pediatr Pulmonol 2009;44:530; with permission.)

paraspinal masses of the chest and abdomen, and the adrenal gland. Tumors in NPARMs are typically neuroblastomas, whereas those in the PARMs are near exclusively ganglioneuromas and ganglioneuroblastomas.[22,23]

Cardiac rhythm abnormalities Reduced heart-rate variability, decreased respiratory sinus arrhythmia, and cardiac asystoles have been noted in CCHS. Gronli and colleagues[24] reported an association between the longest sinus pause on Holter monitoring and the most common PARM genotypes 20/25–20/27. Specifically, sinus pauses of 3 seconds or longer were least frequent in children with genotype 20/25 (0%), intermediate in children with the 20/26 genotype (19%), and longest in children with the 20/27 genotype (83%). Though not identified with the 20/25 genotype in childhood, instances of prolonged sinus pauses reported in cases of LO-CCHS with the 20/25 genotype may suggest an effect of long-standing intermittent hypoxia on this aspect of the CCHS phenotype.[25]

Autonomic nervous system dysregulation In addition to prolonged sinus pauses, additional symptoms of ANSD have been described in CCHS, including diminished gut motility in the absence of HSCR, attenuated temperature regulation including lowered body temperature and cool extremities, and eye irregularities including pupillary response to light and strabismus, among others.[24,26–28]

Diagnosis

CCHS is characteristically diagnosed in the newborn period with cyanosis and hypercarbia resulting from diminished tidal volumes and resultant hypoventilation, always in the absence of respiratory distress. Some patients demonstrate a shallow depth of breathing only during sleep, whereas others with more severe phenotypes will exhibit hypoventilation during both sleep and wakefulness. Individuals with CCHS will lack the physiologic and behavioral responsiveness to hypoxemia/hypercarbia[19] and will not automatically adjust spontaneous ventilation or awaken from sleep. Breathing in non-REM sleep will be synchronous with the mechanical ventilator, but spontaneous breaths will be increased in REM sleep.[11] Many patients presenting with LO-CCHS are identified only after exposure to an environmental trigger. LO-CCHS should be considered in patients who exhibit cyanosis, alveolar hypoventilation, or seizures after receiving sedation or anesthesia, or following a severe respiratory infection, or those who fail traditional sleep apnea therapy. Once CCHS or LO-CCHS is suspected, the stepwise genetic testing suggested herein should be followed to confirm a mutation within the *PHOX2B* gene (**Fig. 3**). While awaiting results of *PHOX2B* genetic testing, it is important for clinicians to rule out other causes of alveolar hypoventilation. Chest radiography, computed tomography (CT), magnetic resonance imaging (MRI), echocardiography,

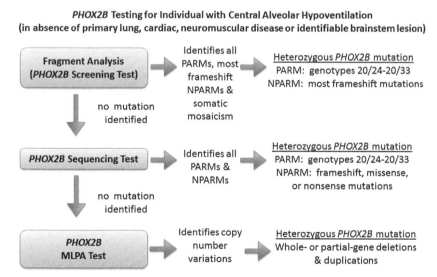

Fig. 3. Algorithm to determine when and what type of *PHOX2B* genetic testing should be performed in various clinical scenarios in which CCHS and LO-CCHS are suspected or confirmed. (*From* Weese-Mayer DE, Patwari PP, Rand CM, et al. Congenital central hypoventilation syndrome (CCHS) and *PHOX2B* mutations. In: Robertson D, Biaggioni I, Burnstock G, et al, editors. Primer on the autonomic nervous system. 3rd edition. Oxford: Elsevier; 2012:448; with permission.)

neurologic evaluation, and/or (potentially) muscle biopsy should be performed to rule out other disorders that might account for the hypoventilation and CCHS phenotype.

Following a *PHOX2B* mutation–confirmed diagnosis of CCHS, the American Thoracic Society (ATS) 2010 Statement on CCHS recommends parental genetic testing (**Fig. 4**).[6] Given the autosomal dominant inheritance pattern exhibited by the disorder, such *PHOX2B* genetic testing is invaluable for anticipating the risk of recurrence in subsequent offspring (by identifying somatic mosaicism in a parent of CCHS probands) and identifying any asymptomatic parents with LO-CCHS. Spontaneous miscarriages have been reported in the literature in both affected and unaffected parents.[9] In rare cases germline mutations may be carried by a parent and would not be detectable by current testing methods,[29] hence the recommendation for prenatal testing with each pregnancy.

ROHHAD

Etiology
The condition now referred to as ROHHAD was first described in 1965 by Fishman and colleagues.[30] In 2000, Katz and colleagues[31] described an additional new case and summarized 10 prior cases in the literature of what was then

termed "late-onset central hypoventilation with hypothalamic dysfunction." The acronym ROHHAD was introduced by Ize-Ludlow and colleagues[32] in 2007, with the aim of describing the phenotypic features in the order of typical timing of presentation and highlighting the rapid-onset weight gain (20–30 lb [9–13.6 kg] over a 3–6-month period) as a harbinger of the syndrome.

While significant advancements have been made in understanding the clinical presentation of the disorder, the etiology and pathogenesis of ROHHAD remain unknown. One current hypothesis that has been explored is an autoimmune or paraneoplastic basis for ROHHAD.[33–35] However, such investigation has been limited to a handful of patients at varied stages of an evolving phenotype, making it difficult to determine the specific effect of the intervention. Likewise, no long-term follow-up has been provided in these reports. Though an intriguing concept, the hypothesis does not account for continued evolution of the ROHHAD phenotype after surgical neural crest tumor resection or for ROHHAD manifestations in the multitude of patients who never develop tumors of neural crest origin.

In recognition of the consistency in features of the ROHHAD phenotype, studies have been undertaken in attempts to identify the underlying genetic etiology. Such studies, limited by extremely

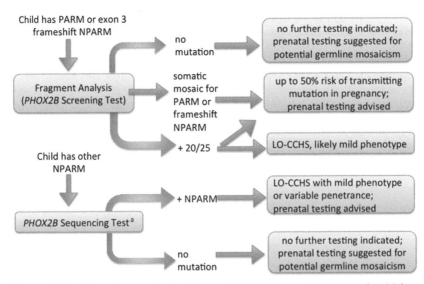

Genetic Testing for Both <u>Parents</u> of Individual with
***PHOX2B* Mutation-Confirmed Congenital Central Hypoventilation Syndrome**

Fig. 4. Algorithm to determine when and what type of *PHOX2B* genetic testing should be performed in parents of CCHS proband. [a] The *PHOX2B* Sequencing Test does not identify low-level mosaicism.[42] (*From* Weese-Mayer DE, Patwari PP, Rand CM, et al. Congenital central hypoventilation syndrome (CCHS) and *PHOX2B* mutations. In: Robertson D, Biaggioni I, Burnstock G, et al, editors. Primer on the autonomic nervous system. 3rd edition. Oxford: Elsevier; 2012:448; with permission.)

small sample sizes, have thus far failed to identify any genetic variants related to the disorder.[32,36,37] Identification of a case of monozygotic twins discordant for the ROHHAD phenotype raises the possibility of a more multifactorial or epigenetic basis for ROHHAD.[38] Further research is needed to examine these concepts and to determine the underlying cause of ROHHAD.

Overview of major features

Central hypoventilation Individuals with ROHHAD have an evolving phenotype, especially in terms of the hypoventilation (**Table 2**). Initially they may have mild obstructive sleep apnea. Then, after surgical intervention with adenotonsillectomy, the child's hypoventilation during sleep becomes more apparent. With advancing age, and often abruptly, the hypoventilation during sleep becomes severe enough to require artificial ventilation. In a subset of cases the children will advance to a need for continuous artificial ventilation as life support. Studies of formal control of breathing have not yet been published, although clinical care suggests attenuated physiologic response to hypercarbia/hypoxia and a lack of behavioral awareness of the compromise.

Hypothalamic dysfunction Rapid-onset obesity, with weight gain of 20 to 30 lb over a 3- to 6-month period, is the most prominent feature of the ROHHAD-related hypothalamic dysfunction. Subsequent hypothalamic defects can be encountered months or years after the initial symptom onset.

Neural crest cell–derived tumors Tumors of neural crest origin, typically ganglioneuromas or ganglioneuroblastomas in the chest or abdomen, can develop at any age in ROHHAD. However, most tumors are identified in the early stages of ROHHAD.

Autonomic nervous system dysregulation Individuals with ROHHAD experience symptoms of ANSD. These symptoms will be variably expressed and can develop throughout the clinical course.[32]

Diagnosis

Diagnosis of ROHHAD is ascertained through an evaluation of the clinical presentation and progression of symptoms in suspected cases. Criteria for diagnosis include:

1. Rapid-onset obesity and the development of alveolar hypoventilation after the age of 1.5 years
2. Evidence of hypothalamic dysfunction as defined by 1 or more of the following findings: rapid-onset obesity, hyperprolactinemia, central hypothyroidism, disordered water balance, failed growth hormone stimulation test, corticotropin deficiency, or altered onset of puberty

Table 2
Percentage of ROHHAD cases[a] with specific phenotypic manifestations

Hypothalamic Dysfunction (%)		Respiratory Manifestations (%)	
Rapid-onset obesity	100	Alveolar hypoventilation	100
Failed growth hormone stimulation test	60	Cardiorespiratory arrest	60
Hyperphagia	53	Reduced CO_2 ventilatory response	60
Hyperprolactinemia	47	Obstructive sleep apnea	53
Hypernatremia	47	Cyanotic episodes	27
Diabetes insipidus	33	**Autonomic Dysregulation (%)**	
Hypothyroidism	33		
Hypodipsia	27	Ophthalmologic manifestations	87
Adrenal insufficiency	27	Thermal dysregulation (hyper- or hypothermia)	73
Polyuria	27	Altered gastrointestinal dysmotility	67
Short stature	20	Altered perception of pain (often decreased)	53
Delayed puberty	13	Altered sweating	53
Hyponatremia	13	Cold hands and feet	40
Low IGF-1 and IGFBP-3	13	Bradycardia	33
Precocious puberty	13	Tumor of neural crest origin (ganglioneuroma and ganglioneuroblastoma)	33

Abbreviations: IGF, insulin-like growth factor; IGFBP, insulin-like growth factor binding protein.
[a] Percentages calculated from 15 cases with full phenotypic information available in Ize-Ludlow and colleagues.[32]
Data from Ize-Ludlow D, Gray J, Sperling MA, et al. Rapid onset obesity with hypothalamic dysfunction, hypoventilation, and autonomic dysregulation presenting in childhood. Pediatrics 2007;120:182.

3. Absence of a *PHOX2B* mutation confirmed through genetic testing

Onset of obesity in ROHHAD typically precedes the central hypoventilation. As a result, differentiating ROHHAD from obesity-related hypoventilation can prove challenging for those with limited experience with such patients. ROHHAD remains a distinct clinical phenomenon, as evidenced by the persistence of central hypoventilation despite decreases in body mass in children with ROHHAD.

Even with heightened clinical suspicion, the variable constellation of symptoms in ROHHAD makes a conclusive diagnosis difficult, and necessitates a comprehensive physiologic evaluation. At a minimum, serial overnight polysomnography and awake physiologic recording should be performed to monitor signs of obstructive sleep apnea or central hypoventilation. It is further recommended to provide additional cardiac, endocrine, and oncologic evaluation from the outset of consideration of a ROHHAD diagnosis, with the aim of ensuring optimal outcomes for the patient. ATS recommendations for clinical evaluation in CCHS provide the current framework for ROHHAD testing.

THERAPEUTIC OPTIONS

Treatment of individuals with CCHS and ROHHAD ideally requires comprehensive testing and an integrated and multidisciplinary team with coordination among regional, national, and international providers (**Tables 3** and **4**). The diversity in *PHOX2B* mutations and corresponding phenotypic diversity in CCHS, and the extreme rarity of ROHHAD, make it difficult to provide care that encompasses the many complex needs of individuals with CCHS or ROHHAD and, consequently, emphasizes the required involvement of centers with extensive experience with these disorders.

CCHS

Central hypoventilation
As the most prominent symptom, immediate recognition and provision of ventilatory support for the central hypoventilation in CCHS is imperative in optimizing the neurocognitive outcome for patients. All individuals with CCHS will require mechanical ventilation, but some children will only require support during sleep time (nap and night) whereas others will require round-the-clock artificial ventilation as life support. In infants and young children, ATS guidelines currently recommend positive pressure ventilation via tracheostomy. With the advent of *PHOX2B* genetic testing, CCHS can be promptly diagnosed and a

tracheostomy can be performed in the first weeks of life. The tracheostomy tube must be upsized with growth to ensure sufficient ventilation. Supportive ventilation with bilevel positive pressure via nasal or face mask and negative pressure ventilators can be considered in the older child. Diaphragm pacing is an excellent form of ventilatory support for the child requiring artificial ventilation awake and asleep, allowing for freedom from the mechanical ventilator when paced during wakefulness. In carefully selected patients, diaphragm pacing for sleep time may be a consideration, although removal of the tracheostomy tube is not guaranteed. Thoracoscopic implantation of the diaphragm pacer system minimizes morbidity and mortality for the child with CCHS.[39] Although more noninvasive means of ventilation such as mask ventilation have been described for use at all ages, current guidelines advise strongly against their use in children younger than 6 years because of the risk of facial deformity and unreliable ventilatory support during a time of significant neurodevelopment.[6]

Annual, in-hospital physiologic monitoring and assessment of ventilatory needs should take place over a multiday hospitalization under the supervision of trained personnel. This testing should include evaluation of ventilatory needs during all stages of sleep, varying levels of exertion, and with and without mechanical ventilation. Testing should also assess the ventilatory response to physiologic challenges during wakefulness and sleep. At a minimum, continuous recording of respiratory inductance plethysmography, electrocardiography, hemoglobin saturation, pulse waveform, end-tidal carbon dioxide, sleep staging, blood pressure, and core body temperature should accompany the evaluation. The goal of such evaluation is to optimize ventilatory support and oxygenation during activities of daily living, with a focus on safety and positive developmental outcomes.

In cases of untreated LO-CCHS or in patients with insufficient oxygenation despite artificial ventilation, progression to right ventricular dilation, cor pulmonale, and polycythemia may occur. It is important, consequently, to perform annual echocardiograms to check for right ventricular hypertrophy/cor pulmonale and to monitor levels of hemoglobin, hematocrit, and reticulocyte counts to identify any early signs of polycythemia.

Neurocognitive function
It is expected that earlier identification and clinical intervention in CCHS cases, coupled with more standardized patient care, will lead to improved neurocognitive outcomes in CCHS. Neurocognitive testing should be performed annually.

Table 3
Recommended testing to characterize CCHS and ROHHAD phenotypes

	Annual In-Hospital Comprehensive Physiologic Testing (Awake and Asleep), Exogenous and Endogenous Gas Challenges, and Autonomic Testing	Assessment for Hirschsprung Disease	Annual Neurocognitive Assessment	Annual 72-h Holter Recording and Echocardiogram	Annual Imaging to Assess for Tumors of Neural Crest Origin	Hypothalamic/Pituitary Axis Endocrine Testing[a]
CCHS and LO-CCHS						
PHOX2B Mutations PARMs						
20/24–20/25	X			X		
20/26	X	X	X	X		
20/27	X	X	X	X		
20/28–20/33	X	X	X	X	X[b]	
NPARMs	X	X	X	X	X[c]	
ROHHAD	X		X	X	X[b]	X

Abbreviations: NPARM, non–polyalanine repeat expansion mutation; PARM, polyalanine repeat expansion mutation.

[a] Endocrine testing every 3–4 months from time of ROHHAD diagnosis.

[b] Annual chest and abdominal imaging to identify ganglioneuromas and ganglioneuroblastomas.

[c] Chest and abdominal imaging and urine catecholamines every 3 months in first 2 years, then every 6 months until 7 years of age to identify neuroblastomas.

Table 4
Multidisciplinary pediatric specialty care for children with CCHS (including LO-CCHS) and ROHHAD

Specialist	Role in Regard of CCHS Management	Role in Regard of ROHHAD Diagnosis and Management
General pediatrician	Coordination of care Coordination of parental *PHOX2B* genetic testing	Initial recognition of rapid-onset weight gain Coordination of care
Neonatologist	Diagnosis Coordination of proband *PHOX2B* genetic testing	
Geneticist	Coordination of prenatal and parental *PHOX2B* genetic testing	Coordination of *PHOX2B* genetic testing
Emergency care physician	Identifies LO-CCHS cases	Identifies ROHHAD after cardiorespiratory arrest
Intensivist or pulmonologist	Management of home mechanical ventilation Coordination of care	Involved after cardiorespiratory arrest, postoperative care, and with acute respiratory illness
Respiratory physiologist	Comprehensive testing as recommended by 2010 American Thoracic Society (ATS) Statement	Comprehensive testing comparable with 2010 ATS Statement on CCHS Evaluation/management for altered circadian rhythm
Psychologist	Formal neurocognitive testing Diagnosis and management of behavioral issues	Formal neurocognitive testing Diagnosis and management of behavioral issues
Psychiatrist		In severe cases, management of psychosis
Surgeon	Resection of neural crest tumors Surgical treatment of Hirschsprung disease	Resection of neural crest tumors
Cardiologist	Evaluation for sinus pauses and cor pulmonale Holter monitoring	Evaluation for severe bradycardia Holter monitoring
Cardiovascular surgeon	Implantation of cardiac pacemaker	
Oncologist	Identification and management of neural crest tumor if identified	Identification and management of neural crest tumor if identified
Neurologist	Management of seizures	Management of seizures
Ophthalmologist or neuro-ophthalmologist	Evaluation for developing ophthalmologic abnormalities	Evaluation for developing ophthalmologic abnormalities
Otolaryngologist	Tonsillectomy and adenoidectomy Tracheostomy placement Annual bronchoscopy	Tonsillectomy and adenoidectomy if indicated Tracheostomy placement if indicated
Endocrinologist	Evaluation as indicated by symptoms	Investigation for hypothalamic/pituitary axis dysfunction every 3–4 mo

Hirschsprung disease

A rectal biopsy should be performed in all CCHS newborn patients presenting with failure to pass meconium, and barium enema or manometry in older patients with severe constipation, to identify or rule out HSCR. Treatment of HSCR involves surgical removal of the aganglionic segments of the colon, ideally in the first days or weeks of life, and intensive involvement by a team experienced in HSCR management.

Neural crest cell–derived tumors

Screening can include chest radiography or ultrasonography in infants, and chest and abdominal MRI or CT scans for older children and adults. A meta-iodobenzylguanidine scan can identify neuroblastomas in patients who are at highest risk for the development of such tumors (NPARMs). Tumors of neural crest origin are typically surgically resected, but the treatment plan is contingent on the type, size, location, and stage of the tumors.

Cardiac rhythm abnormalities
Patients with sinus pauses of 3 seconds or longer may require implantation of a cardiac pacemaker. Sudden death has been reported in CCHS for those with sinus pauses of 3 seconds or longer who have not received pacemakers.[24]

Autonomic nervous system dysregulation
Improved characterization of ANSD can be achieved through more formal clinical assessment of ANS function including head-up tilt testing with cerebral regional blood flow, heart rate–deep breathing, Valsalva maneuver, thermoregulatory chamber sweat testing, and pupillometry, among other noninvasive tests. Most manifestations of ANSD can be managed on a per-symptom basis, and referred to appropriate specialists when necessary.

ROHHAD

Central hypoventilation
In approximately half of patients, ventilation is only required for use during sleep. Noninvasive positive airway pressure ventilation may be sufficient in such individuals. Another subset of the patient population will develop alveolar hypoventilation necessitating 24-hour mechanical ventilation via tracheostomy. Limited experience with diaphragm pacing in ROHHAD precludes specific recommendations.

Early identification and characterization of the respiratory deficit in individual patients remains a crucial facet of patient care in ROHHAD. In acknowledgment of the variable onset of symptomatic alveolar hypoventilation and the potential for its progressive nature in ROHHAD, routine assessment of ventilatory needs as part of a comprehensive examination of all affected systems is recommended to be provided every 4 to 6 months after initial onset of symptoms, and annually once they have stabilized. Respiratory evaluation should be inclusive of all parameters described herein for CCHS. Annual neurocognitive testing is further recommended to assess the intellectual function as a correlate to the efficacy of the clinical management of ventilatory needs, and provide an early indication of any neurologic decline.

Hypothalamic dysfunction
Obesity in ROHHAD is very difficult to manage, even with diet and exercise. Caution should be used during exercise, as individuals with ROHHAD are often fundamentally unable to meet increased respiratory demands arising from significantly increased levels of exertion. Given the variable presentation of the hypothalamic dysfunction in ROHHAD, care must be provided in conjunction with a pediatric endocrinologist to identify and treat hypothalamic abnormalities on a case-by-case basis and with advancing age. Special attention should be paid to hormonal levels, water balance, urine and plasma osmolarity, and any other issues arising from dysfunction in the hypothalamic/pituitary axis, all with advancing age.

Neural crest cell–derived tumors
Initial screening of patients through chest radiography and abdominal ultrasonography is recommended. Based on these results, more aggressive imaging including CT and MRI can be pursued to accurately identify the presence of ganglioneuromas and ganglioneuroblastomas. Tumors are typically surgically resected.

Autonomic nervous system dysregulation
ANSD within ROHHAD varies greatly as the phenotypic features seem to unfold with advancing age. Seventy-two hour Holter monitoring, electrocardiography, and echocardiography are recommended to check for any rhythm abnormalities or pathologic anatomy. Eye abnormalities such as pupillary dysfunction warrant regular ophthalmologic follow-up. Stool softeners can be used in the treatment of altered gut motility.

Annual testing
Successful management of these disorders requires regular follow-up and clinical assessment of the many manifestations of these diseases (see **Table 3**).

CLINICAL OUTCOMES
CCHS

If untreated, central hypoventilation can result in cardiorespiratory arrest, severe morbidity, and death. Increased recognition and diagnosis of CCHS, introduction of clinical *PHOX2B* testing, and modern techniques for home ventilation and monitoring with pulse oximetry and capnography have significantly improved the prognosis for affected individuals. With early clinical intervention and regular follow-up, individuals with CCHS are expected to achieve a high quality of life and a normal life span. Neonatally identified patients have graduated from high school and college, married, and maintained steady employment. Annual physiologic evaluation and screening for all features of the disease are integral to the success of patients with such disorders. Significant disability has been noted in individuals with CCHS who experienced long-term inconsistent or insufficient management of their condition, stressing the importance of regular evaluation and adjustment of management.

ROHHAD

When undiagnosed or insufficiently managed, individuals with ROHHAD can progress to significant irreversible neurocognitive compromise or death.[32,34] Diagnosis, however, only represents the first step in the ongoing care of affected individuals. Given the evolving nature of the disorder and its variable presentation of symptoms, frequent comprehensive evaluation of individuals with ROHHAD can allow for the anticipatory management of the unfolding phenotype and meet developing needs accordingly. Ongoing evaluation should be performed frequently in the early phases and then every 10 to 12 months thereafter. If treated expediently and adequately, individuals with ROHHAD can maintain a good quality of life with the potential to achieve above-average intellectual ability. The life span of individuals with ROHHAD is unknown, although anecdotal evidence for improved breathing during wakefulness with increasing age is certainly encouraging. Conversely, individuals who have not been identified promptly or who have had suboptimal ventilatory support are at increased risk of premature death.

COMPLICATIONS AND CONCERNS
CCHS

With advancements made in the early identification and improved management of the condition, individuals with CCHS are now surviving well into adulthood, bringing about a set of issues that merit concern and clinical consideration.

Alcohol and drug abuse
Use of depressants such as alcohol or other drugs can have potentially fatal consequences during wakefulness and sleep, particularly in the absence of artificial ventilation. Parents and patients should be counseled on the harms of their use. Similarly, caution should also be applied when administering prescribed medications with a respiratory depressant effect (including sedatives and anesthetics).

Pregnancy
Prenatal *PHOX2B* testing is recommended in any pregnancy in which the mother or father has been diagnosed with CCHS or a somatic mosaicism. Even when termination is not expected, prenatal testing can allow for adequate planning for the immediate care of a CCHS infant. Pregnancy poses specific risks to a mother with CCHS because the increased respiratory demand may exceed the ventilatory support. For women undergoing cesarean section who use diaphragm

pacing, bilevel positive airway pressure ventilation or, potentially, intubation after delivery may be needed, as abdominal incisions may make diaphragm pacing too painful. During delivery and the postpartum period, all women with CCHS should be provided sufficient ventilatory support.

Breath-holding spells
As noted earlier, individuals with CCHS exhibit a loss of or an attenuated responsiveness to hypercarbia and hypoxemia. Concomitant with this loss of chemosensitivity in CCHS is the absence of "air hunger." Consequently, individuals with CCHS must not engage in risk-taking respiratory behaviors, including voluntary extended breath-holding spells[6] or swimming.

ROHHAD

As ROHHAD is extremely rare and patients are only now surviving to adulthood, issues of alcohol or drug abuse and pregnancy have not yet been encountered. However, other psychosocial issues have been identified in the disorder.

Behavioral and mood disorders
Both behavioral and mood disorders have been reported in ROHHAD with mention of frequencies of approximately 31% and 16%, respectively, across 51 literature-reported cases in a recent case report.[40] Increased anxiety, emotional lability, and psychosis have also been reported in a recent ROHHAD case report.[41] Individuals exhibiting psychiatric symptoms should be referred to the appropriate health provider and treated accordingly. From the authors' experience, the issues of behavior and mood were reported most typically in the earliest reports, and in the event of suboptimal artificial ventilation in more recent cases.

Developmental disorders
Developmental issues, as noted by low intelligence quotient (IQ) from neurocognitive testing, are most likely related to inadequate cardiorespiratory arrest intervention, as several patients with ROHHAD have above-average IQ. In addition, suboptimal ventilatory management may result in chronic intermittent hypoxia. Taken together, these risks underscore the value of early identification and clinical intervention to reduce the risk of neurocognitive decline.

Seizures
Seizures have been reported in a subset of individuals with ROHHAD. Seizures can occur secondary to hypoxemia resulting from inadequate ventilatory support, or hyponatremia or hypernatremia attributable to disordered hormonal secretion and the

accompanying electrolyte imbalances. Correction of these underlying causes, when appropriate, can help prevent additional seizures.

SUMMARY

Early clinical identification and intervention, along with regular surveillance of all clinical features as part of ongoing care, are paramount in ensuring that individuals with CCHS and ROHHAD maximize their neurocognitive potential and ability to lead stable, relatively normal lives. With the discovery of a genetic basis and the advent of diagnostic testing, significant strides have been made in the clinical management and understanding of CCHS/LO-CCHS. These advances highlight the potential value of an analogous discovery in ROHHAD, for which efforts are ongoing.

As disorders with phenotypic manifestations that span an array of medical systems and processes, CCHS/LO-CCHS and ROHHAD warrant specialized medical attention. Ideally this care should be provided at centers dedicated specifically to the care of individuals with these unique disorders, with continuous collaboration and coordination with regional providers. Such consolidation of principal care can allow for improved recognition and management of clinical symptoms of these disorders and, accordingly, improve outcomes for affected individuals.

To further aid with these efforts, registries have been established for both CCHS and ROHHAD. These secure online systems aim to consent and enroll all individuals internationally with CCHS and ROHHAD to systematically document their clinical development with advancing age. Such documentation allows for strengthened coordination and dissemination of novel developments related to the evolving understanding of the diagnosis and management of these disorders, and notice of any ongoing clinical or drug intervention trials. Further information on the International CCHS and ROHHAD REDCap Registries can be found on the Center for Autonomic Medicine in Pediatrics (CAMP) at the Ann & Robert H. Lurie Children's Hospital of Chicago Web site (http://www.luriechildrens.org/en-us/care-services/conditions-treatments/autonomic-medicine/Pages/basics/basics.aspx), or by e-mailing CRand@LurieChildrens.org.

REFERENCES

1. Mellins RB, Balfour HH Jr, Turino GM, et al. Failure of automatic control of ventilation (Ondine's curse). Report of an infant born with this syndrome and review of the literature. Medicine (Baltimore) 1970; 49(6):487–504.
2. Weese-Mayer DE, Shannon DC, Keens TG, et al. Idiopathic congenital central hypoventilation syndrome: diagnosis and management. American Thoracic Society. Am J Respir Crit Care Med 1999; 160(1):368–73.
3. Amiel J, Laudier B, Attie-Bitach T, et al. Polyalanine expansion and frameshift mutations of the paired-like homeobox gene PHOX2B in congenital central hypoventilation syndrome. Nat Genet 2003;33(4): 459–61.
4. Weese-Mayer DE, Berry-Kravis EM, Zhou L, et al. Idiopathic congenital central hypoventilation syndrome: analysis of genes pertinent to early autonomic nervous system embryologic development and identification of mutations in PHOX2b. Am J Med Genet A 2003;123A(3):267–78.
5. Pattyn A, Morin X, Cremer H, et al. The homeobox gene Phox2b is essential for the development of autonomic neural crest derivatives. Nature 1999; 399(6734):366–70.
6. Weese-Mayer DE, Berry-Kravis EM, Ceccherini I, et al. An official ATS clinical policy statement: congenital central hypoventilation syndrome: genetic basis, diagnosis, and management. Am J Respir Crit Care Med 2010;181(6):626–44.
7. Trochet D, Hong SJ, Lim JK, et al. Molecular consequences of PHOX2B missense, frameshift and alanine expansion mutations leading to autonomic dysfunction. Hum Mol Genet 2005;14(23): 3697–708.
8. Bachetti T, Matera I, Borghini S, et al. Distinct pathogenetic mechanisms for PHOX2B associated polyalanine expansions and frameshift mutations in congenital central hypoventilation syndrome. Hum Mol Genet 2005;14(13):1815–24.
9. Low KJ, Turnbull AR, Smith KR, et al. A case of congenital central hypoventilation syndrome in a three-generation family with non-polyalanine repeat PHOX2B mutation. Pediatr Pulmonol 2014. [Epub ahead of print].
10. Jennings LJ, Yu M, Rand CM, et al. Variable human phenotype associated with novel deletions of the PHOX2B gene. Pediatr Pulmonol 2012;47(2): 153–61.
11. Fleming PJ, Cade D, Bryan MH, et al. Congenital central hypoventilation and sleep state. Pediatrics 1980;66(3):425–8.
12. Huang J, Colrain IM, Panitch HB, et al. Effect of sleep stage on breathing in children with central hypoventilation. J Appl Physiol 2008;105(1): 44–53.
13. Weese-Mayer DE, Silvestri JM, Menzies LJ, et al. Congenital central hypoventilation syndrome: diagnosis, management, and long-term outcome in thirty-two children. J Pediatr 1992;120(3):381–7.

14. Harper RM, Kumar R, Macey PM, et al. Affective brain areas and sleep-disordered breathing. Prog Brain Res 2014;209:275–93.

15. Oren J, Kelly DH, Shannon DC. Long-term follow-up of children with congenital central hypoventilation syndrome. Pediatrics 1987;80(3):375–80.

16. Marcus CL, Jansen MT, Poulsen MK, et al. Medical and psychosocial outcome of children with congenital central hypoventilation syndrome. J Pediatr 1991;119(6):888–95.

17. Silvestri JM, Weese-Mayer DE, Nelson MN. Neuropsychologic abnormalities in children with congenital central hypoventilation syndrome. J Pediatr 1992;120(3):388–93.

18. Zelko FA, Nelson MN, Leurgans SE, et al. Congenital central hypoventilation syndrome: neurocognitive functioning in school age children. Pediatr Pulmonol 2010;45(1):92–8.

19. Carroll MS, Patwari PP, Kenny AS, et al. Residual chemosensitivity to ventilatory challenges in genotyped congenital central hypoventilation syndrome. J Appl Physiol 2014;116(4):439–50.

20. Nagashimada M, Ohta H, Li C, et al. Autonomic neurocristopathy-associated mutations in PHOX2B dysregulate Sox10 expression. J Clin Invest 2012; 122(9):3145–58.

21. Gorodn SC, Rand CM, Vitez SF, et al. Ganglion cell presence is only part of the story: gastrointestinal symptoms as a measure of enteric autonomic dysfunction in CCHS (congenital central hypoventilation syndrome). Pediatric Academic Societies Annual Research Conference; Pediatr Res E-PAS 2014:3807.178.

22. Berry-Kravis EM, Zhou L, Rand CM, et al. Congenital central hypoventilation syndrome: PHOX2B mutations and phenotype. Am J Respir Crit Care Med 2006;174(10):1139–44.

23. Trochet D, O'Brien LM, Gozal D, et al. PHOX2B genotype allows for prediction of tumor risk in congenital central hypoventilation syndrome. Am J Hum Genet 2005;76(3):421–6.

24. Gronli JO, Santucci BA, Leurgans SE, et al. Congenital central hypoventilation syndrome: PHOX2B genotype determines risk for sudden death. Pediatr Pulmonol 2008;43(1):77–86.

25. Antic NA, Malow BA, Lange N, et al. PHOX2B mutation-confirmed congenital central hypoventilation syndrome: presentation in adulthood. Am J Respir Crit Care Med 2006;174(8):923–7.

26. Goldberg DS, Ludwig IH. Congenital central hypoventilation syndrome: ocular findings in 37 children. J Pediatr Ophthalmol Strabismus 1996;33(3):175–80.

27. Saiyed R, Rand CM, Patwari PP, et al. Altered temperature regulation in respiratory and autonomic disorders of infancy, childhood, and adulthood (RADICA). Am J Respir Crit Care Med 2011; 183(A):6394.

28. Patwari PP, Stewart TM, Rand CM, et al. Pupillometry in congenital central hypoventilation syndrome (CCHS): quantitative evidence of autonomic nervous system dysregulation. Pediatr Res 2012; 71(3):280–5.

29. Rand CM, Yu M, Jennings LJ, et al. Germline mosaicism of PHOX2B mutation accounts for familial recurrence of congenital central hypoventilation syndrome (CCHS). Am J Med Genet A 2012;158A(9): 2297–301.

30. Fishman LS, Samson JH, Sperling DR. Primary alveolar hypoventilation syndrome (Ondine's curse). Am J Dis Child 1965;110:155–61.

31. Katz ES, McGrath S, Marcus CL. Late-onset central hypoventilation with hypothalamic dysfunction: a distinct clinical syndrome. Pediatr Pulmonol 2000; 29(1):62–8.

32. Ize-Ludlow D, Gray JA, Sperling MA, et al. Rapid-onset obesity with hypothalamic dysfunction, hypoventilation, and autonomic dysregulation presenting in childhood. Pediatrics 2007;120(1):e179–88.

33. Ouvrier R, Nunn K, Sprague T, et al. Idiopathic hypothalamic dysfunction: a paraneoplastic syndrome? Lancet 1995;346(8985):1298.

34. Bougneres P, Pantalone L, Linglart A, et al. Endocrine manifestations of the rapid-onset obesity with hypoventilation, hypothalamic, autonomic dysregulation and neural tumor (ROHHADNET) syndrome in early childhood. J Clin Endocrinol Metab 2008; 93(10):3971–80.

35. Paz-Priel I, Cooke DW, Chen AR. Cyclophosphamide for rapid-onset obesity, hypothalamic dysfunction, hypoventilation, and autonomic dysregulation syndrome. J Pediatr 2011;158(2):337–9.

36. Rand CM, Patwari PP, Rodikova EA, et al. Rapid-onset obesity with hypothalamic dysfunction, hypoventilation, and autonomic dysregulation (ROHHAD): analysis of hypothalamic and autonomic candidate genes. Pediatr Res 2011;70(4):375–8.

37. De Pontual L, Trochet D, Caillat-Zucman S, et al. Delineation of late onset hypoventilation associated with hypothalamic dysfunction syndrome. Pediatr Res 2008;64(6):689–94.

38. Patwari PP, Rand CM, Berry-Kravis EM, et al. Monozygotic twins discordant for ROHHAD phenotype. Pediatrics 2011;128(3):e711–5.

39. Chin AC, Shaul DB, Patwari PP, et al. Diaphragmatic pacing in infants and children with congenital central hypoventilation syndrome (CCHS). In: Kheirandish-Gozal L, Gozal D, editors. Sleep disordered breathing in children: a clinical guide. New York: Springer Press; 2012. p. 553–73.

40. Grudnikoff E, Foley C, Poole C, et al. Nocturnal anxiety in a youth with rapid-onset obesity, hypothalamic dysfunction, hypoventilation, and autonomic dysregulation (ROHHAD). J Can Acad Child Adolesc Psychiatry 2013;22(3):235–7.

41. Chew HB, Ngu LH, Keng WT. Rapid-onset obesity with hypothalamic dysfunction, hypoventilation and autonomic dysregulation (ROHHAD): a case with additional features and review of the literature. BMJ Case Rep 2011;2011. pii:bcr0220102706.

42. Jennings LJ, Yu M, Zhou L, et al. Comparison of PHOX2B testing methods in the diagnosis of congenital central hypoventilation syndrome and mosaic carriers. Diagn Mol Pathol 2010;19(4): 224–31.

Sleep Hypoventilation Syndromes and Noninvasive Ventilation in Children

 CrossMark

Rakesh Bhattacharjee, MD[a,b,]*, David Gozal, MD[a,b]

KEYWORDS

- Hypoventilation • Children • Nocturnal noninvasive ventilation • Bilevel positive airway pressure

KEY POINTS

- Current evidence supports the application of noninvasive ventilation devices in most disorders of nocturnal hypoventilation in childhood.
- Technical limitations inherent to noninvasive ventilation devices must be acknowledged before using these devices in children.
- Current evidence supports bilevel positive airway pressure devices in treating childhood nocturnal hypoventilation disorders. Novel devices already established in treating adults with sleep-disordered breathing may represent alternative strategies in treating young children.
- Studies have revealed favorable outcomes regarding adherence to these devices in children.

The wide spectrum of nocturnal hypoventilation in children is attributable largely to the various disturbances of normal ventilation related to a plethora of disease states that can affect either the central ventilatory drive or the ventilatory mechanical apparatus. Our understanding of diseases that lead to hypoventilation during childhood has evolved a great deal over the years. In parallel, any discussion of supportive ventilation including noninvasive ventilation in children would reveal a progression of clinical practice over the past several decades. Classically, invasive mechanical ventilation, typically via a tracheostomy, was the mainstay in managing many disorders of hypoventilation in children, ranging from infectious destruction of anterior horn cells, as is the case in poliomyelitis, to gene-specific disorders such as congenital central hypoventilation syndrome.

However, with advances in noninvasive ventilation in adults its implementation in children was also initiated, but has only recently emerged as an efficacious treatment of disordered breathing in young persons. Furthermore, in the context of conditions under which supportive ventilation is only required at night, whereby the need for a permanent interface such as a tracheostomy can be obviated altogether, the application of noninvasive ventilation becomes highly attractive.

Before a discussion of nocturnal noninvasive ventilation (nNIV) in children, one must acknowledge that clinicians' familiarity with its use stems from the vast experience of these devices in adults with sleep-disordered breathing (SDB). Notwithstanding, the evidence, particularly from studies with large sample sizes, supporting its use in managing SDB in children is sparse. In fact, despite the

[a] Section of Pediatric Sleep Medicine, Department of Pediatrics, Comer Children's Hospital, Pritzker School of Medicine, The University of Chicago, 5841 S Maryland Avenue, MC 4064, Chicago, IL 60637, USA; [b] Section of Pediatric Pulmonology, Department of Pediatrics, Comer Children's Hospital, Pritzker School of Medicine, The University of Chicago, 5841 S Maryland Avenue, MC 4064, Chicago, IL 60637, USA
* Corresponding author. Sections of Pediatric Pulmonary and Pediatric Sleep Medicine, Department of Pediatrics, The University of Chicago, 5841 South Maryland Avenue MC, Chicago, IL 60637.
E-mail address: rbhattac@peds.bsd.uchicago.edu

Sleep Med Clin 9 (2014) 441–453
http://dx.doi.org/10.1016/j.jsmc.2014.05.009
1556-407X/14/$ – see front matter © 2014 Elsevier Inc. All rights reserved.

sleep.theclinics.com

evidence from published studies, nNIV remains to be approved by the Food and Drug Administration (FDA) for use in children weighing less than 30 kg.

In discussing nNIV in treating children with nocturnal hypoventilation disorders, a brief introduction to the pathophysiology of hypoventilation in children is relevant. As hypoventilation disorders in children are discussed elsewhere in this issue by Weese-Meyer and colleagues, herein each of the major categories and conditions of hypoventilation disorders is addressed, including insight into their prevalence and the challenges to diagnosis. The efficacy of current treatment strategies is discussed, including the indications for noninvasive ventilation in children and an analysis of the evidence that describes the unique hurdles that are emerging in the context of adherence among children using noninvasive ventilation. Lastly, evidence is presented suggesting novel modalities that have become recently available and may be applied to children in an off-label manner.

It is crucial to bear in mind that delineation of the specific indications for implementation of nNIV in children has yet to be defined in a formal consensus statement, and there is clearly a pressing need for such guidelines, as illustrated by the beneficial outcomes regarding life expectancy in children and adults with specific hypoventilation syndromes.[1,2]

NOCTURNAL ALVEOLAR HYPOVENTILATION IN CHILDREN

A heterogeneous group of conditions can culminate in nocturnal alveolar hypoventilation in children of variable severity (**Box 1**). Salient conditions include the classic congenital central hypoventilation syndrome (CCHS) but also encompass neuromuscular disorders, metabolic storage diseases including obesity, and musculoskeletal confinement of the thoracic cage, as in the case of scoliosis or thoracic dystrophies. The marked variance in antecedents of nocturnal alveolar hypoventilation is the central hurdle to establishing universal practice parameters for the care of these children, as the progression of disease and overall prognosis differs drastically.

As outlined by *The International Classification of Sleep Disorders* (second edition) (ICSD-2),[3] nocturnal alveolar hypoventilation consists of reduced ventilation secondary to decreased tidal volume, with ensuing hypercapnia and/or hypoxemia. As a manifestation to this variant of sleep-disturbed breathing, there often is accompanying sleep fragmentation related to increases in lighter sleep stage, transient arousals, and/or awakenings. The muscular atonia, a feature of rapid eye

movement (REM) sleep, augments this variant of SDB in most disease states associated with nocturnal hypoventilation with the exception of CCHS, in which non-REM (NREM) stage III sleep accounts for more profound changes in ventilation.

The normative alveolar ventilatory parameters of children during sleep have been only recently defined. In a cross-sectional study of 542 children undergoing nocturnal polysomnography by Montgomery-Downs and colleagues,[4] average nocturnal oxygen saturations, oxygen saturation nadir, and oxygen desaturation indices did not differ by age. Furthermore, end-tidal carbon dioxide (ET_{CO_2}) measurements captured by nocturnal polysomnography did not differ by age, with the average ET_{CO_2} being 40.7 mm Hg. Twenty percent of studied children spent 50% or more of total sleep time with an ET_{CO_2} of at least 45 mm Hg, and 2.2% spent 50% or more of total sleep time with an ET_{CO_2} of at least 50 mm Hg. These findings closely concur with previous smaller-sized studies assessing normative polysomnographic measures in children.[5–7]

The ICSD-2[3] establishes criteria for nocturnal hypoventilation largely based on oxygen saturation (Sp_{O_2}) during polysomnography, such that hypoventilation is defined by an Sp_{O_2} during sleep of less than 90% for more than 5 minutes, with a nadir of at least 85% or more than 30% of total sleep time at an of Sp_{O_2} of less than 90%. A sleeping arterial blood gas level with a partial pressure of CO_2 (P_{CO_2}) that is abnormally high or disproportionately higher than during wakefulness can also define nocturnal hypoventilation. The diagnostic criteria for children are exclusively defined by carbon dioxide monitoring measured during polysomnography. Specifically, the American Academy of Sleep Medicine scoring manual[8] defines alveolar hypoventilation during sleep as greater than 25% of total sleep time spent with a P_{CO_2} greater than 50 mm Hg when measured by either the arterial P_{CO_2} or surrogate. Children, with an overall reduced pulmonary functional residual capacity (FRC), are especially prone to alveolar hypoventilation, which is the premise for routine monitoring of carbon dioxide during pediatric polysomnography.[8]

Although the aforementioned diagnostic criteria for alveolar hypoventilation need to be endorsed by a formal consensus process, there is great variance in opinion regarding the parameters for establishing nNIV in treating disorders associated with nocturnal hypoventilation in children. Recently, a task force put forth guidelines[9] for the treatment of hypoventilation syndromes in adults and children, and largely focused on the

Box 1
Various causes of nocturnal hypoventilation in children

- Central apnea/hypoventilation
  - Congenital central hypoventilation
    - Congenital central hypoventilation syndrome (neonatal/early-onset and late-onset)
    - Rapid-onset obesity, hypoventilation, hypothalamic dysfunction, and autonomic dysregulation (ROHHAD)
    - Secondary to central nervous system (CNS) structural anomalies: Chiari malformation type I and type II, hydrocephalus, syringomyelia
    - Secondary to CNS injury during birth and cerebral palsy (severe asphyxia, CNS hemorrhage/stroke)
    - Other genetic conditions: Prader-Willi syndrome, Rett syndrome, familial dysautonomia, Joubert syndrome
  - Acquired central hypoventilation
    - CNS damage related to trauma, infection, bleeding, seizures, neoplasms, immune and postinfectious diseases, hypoxia/anoxia, storage diseases, metabolic diseases, obesity
- Neuromuscular disorders
  - Congenital neuropathies
    - For example, spinal muscular atrophy types I, II, III
  - Acquired neuropathies
    - Secondary to trauma, infection, immune and postinfectious diseases
    - Metabolic diseases
  - Congenital myopathies
    - Duchenne and Becker muscular dystrophy, acid maltase deficiency, myotonic dystrophy, metabolic diseases
  - Acquired myopathies
- Skeletal or thoracic cage anomalies
  - Severe kyphoscoliosis, Jeune thoracic dystrophy
  - Obesity hypoventilation: Prader-Willi syndrome
- Lung and airway diseases
  - Cystic fibrosis
  - Bronchopulmonary dysplasia
  - Sickle cell disease
  - Acute asthma

titration of bilevel positive airway pressure (BPAP). While these laudable efforts certainly have provided a framework to the clinical practice regarding nNIV titration studies in nocturnal hypoventilation, they also stress the paucity of data concerning the timing of starting therapy, the standard of care for follow-up, and the efficacy of nNIV in treating nocturnal hypoventilation. Before summarizing the treatment of nocturnal hypoventilation, a brief overview the major disorders of hypoventilation in children is presented.

Nocturnal Hypoventilation in Neuromuscular Disorders: Pathophysiology

In the absence of large cross-sectional studies, the exact prevalence of nocturnal hypoventilation has not been established in children with any of the more frequent neuromuscular disorders. For example, there are estimates that 27% to 62% of children with Duchenne muscular dystrophy (DMD) display some form of SDB.[10] However, because there are no longitudinal assessments, such figures may be skewed and represent a later stage of disease, at a time when symptoms prompt referral to pulmonary services. The pathophysiology of SDB[11] in children with neuromuscular disorders depends mostly on the nature and severity of the underlying disorder, but is also affected by the patient's age, particularly if the disorder is progressive, and the type and extent of muscle involvement. Children with neuromuscular disorders have largely preserved central ventilatory drive with the exception of some children with myotonic dystrophy, in whom reduction in respiratory drive may be a component of the disease.[12] However, the overall loss of muscular tone, especially muscles that are integral to the respiratory system, begins an inexorable course that ultimately leads to profound disturbances of ventilation during sleep, even if respiratory muscle training and other rehabilitation approaches may slow down the process.[13] Furthermore, as previously stated, the atonia associated with REM sleep further accentuates the muscular weakness associated with neuromuscular disorders. Therefore in conditions leading to intercostal muscle weakness, the loss of FRC augmented by the supine position of sleep is especially vulnerable during REM sleep, resulting in reduced oxygen reserves and an increased predisposition to carbon dioxide retention.

Neuromuscular disorders that cause tonic deficits of the upper respiratory muscle, such as exist in cerebral palsy, myotonic dystrophy, sensory and motor neuropathies such as Charcot-Marie-Tooth, or poliomyelitis, are likely to contribute to the occurrence of obstructive SDB. Neuromuscular disorders such as DMD and Becker muscular dystrophy (BMD), mitochondrial myopathies, spinal muscular atrophy (SMA) cervical spine injuries, and metabolic and congenital myopathies are all associated with intercostal muscle weakness (sometimes preferentially affecting inspiratory or expiratory intercostals) that contribute to the pathogenesis of hypoventilation. In addition, certain disease states, including DMD and BMD, increase the risk of obesity or of disproportionate adipose tissue distribution in visceral and intramuscular regions even when body mass index is preserved,[14–16] and all children are at risk for adenotonsillar hypertrophy, which further increases the risk for SDB. Taken together, the extent of SDB in children with neuromuscular disorders is largely contingent on the nature of the primary disease, more specifically the degree and nature of muscular insufficiency and the presence of disease-specific comorbidities.[17] In addition, related to intercostal muscular weakness, children with neuromuscular disorders often have an ineffective cough and ineffective airway clearance.

Consequently, pulmonary mucus plugging is a common occurrence in many children, and predisposes children to recurrent pneumonias and atelectasias that secondarily contribute to the onset of pulmonary scarring and respiratory insufficiency. Furthermore, the absence of sufficient muscle tone does not provide the necessary structural support to the rib cage, such that these children are often prone to impaired thoracic cage development manifesting as severe scoliosis, pectus excavatum, flattening of the anteroposterior chest diameter, and a funnel-shaped chest. The consequence of these skeletal changes is a loss of chest wall compliance and subsequent reduction in pulmonary volumes including FRC, paradoxic breathing, and elevated work of breathing, all of which further predispose the child to nocturnal hypoventilation.

Although nNIV and invasive ventilation represent the mainstay modality for treating SDB in these children, it is again emphasized that the diagnosis of nocturnal hypoventilation in these children is not easy to establish and requires a high level of suspicion. Implementing a systematic diagnostic approach is necessary, when possible, while preserving individualized diagnostic and management decisions.

Nocturnal Hypoventilation and Neuromuscular Disorders: Treatment

Most commonly, the initial treatment of hypoventilation in these children consists in the initiation and implementation of nNIV, most commonly BPAP (**Fig. 1**). This approach has been shown to improve most parameters related to SDB, including severity of hypoxemia, the magnitude of carbon dioxide retention, sleep efficiency, arousal index, sleep architecture, overall sleep quality, and reductions in daytime sleepiness. In addition, nNIV leads to significant reduction in the frequency and severity of multiple morbidities, including substantially lower numbers of hospitalizations and pneumonia episodes, while improving the quality of life and potentially prolonging survival.

In a study of 9 infants and young children with SMA, Petrone and colleagues[18] found significant improvements in oxygen desaturation index, mean transcutaneous carbon dioxide, and thoracic abdominal muscular synchrony following just 10 days of BPAP. However, long-term outcomes of nNIV in children with neuromuscular disorders have been investigated in only a few small studies. Bach and colleagues[19] reported improvements in survival and fewer hospitalizations with nNIV in children with SMA. nNIV has been shown to be effective in reducing the frequency of

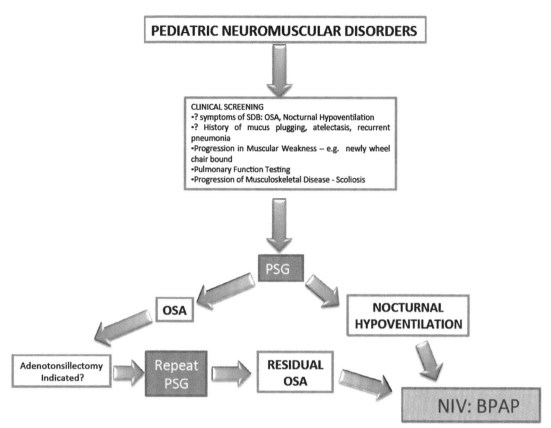

PEDIATRIC NEUROMUSCULAR DISORDERS

CLINICAL SCREENING
•? symptoms of SDB: OSA, Nocturnal Hypoventilation
•? History of mucus plugging, atelectasis, recurrent pneumonia
•Progression in Muscular Weakness – e.g. newly wheel chair bound
•Pulmonary Function Testing
•Progression of Musculoskeletal Disease - Scoliosis

PSG

OSA

NOCTURNAL HYPOVENTILATION

Adenotonsillectomy Indicated?

Repeat PSG

RESIDUAL OSA

NIV: BPAP

Fig. 1. Therapeutic algorithm for the clinical approach to children with neuromuscular disorders. BPAP, bilevel positive airway pressure; NIV, noninvasive ventilation; OSA, obstructive sleep apnea; PSG, polysomnogram; SDB, sleep-disordered breathing.

pneumonia[20] but also in ruling out invasive ventilation, thereby promoting survival.[21] Mellies and colleagues[22] reported the long-term effects of nNIV on both nocturnal and diurnal gas exchange in 30 patients (mean age 12.3 years) with various neuromuscular disorders. This group reported improvements or normalization of nocturnal mean Spo_2 and transcutaneous Pco_2 in addition to improvements in diurnal arterial tension of oxygen and carbon dioxide. In addition, this group reported significant reductions in nocturnal heart rate and improvements in sleep architecture. Improvements in gas exchange, prevention of atelectasis, and reductions in respiratory muscular work have also been described in other long-term studies of children with neuromuscular disorders. Katz and colleagues[23] retrospectively analyzed 15 children with various neuromuscular disorders, and showed that nNIV led to significant reductions in hospitalization episodes, duration of hospitalizations, and admissions to the intensive care unit, in agreement with other similar studies. In addition to improving the overall morbidity associated with neuromuscular disease, nNIV has been shown to be effective in improving overall health quality in

these children. In a retrospective review of 14 patients with various neuromuscular disorders, Young and colleagues[24] reported significant improvements in many symptoms of nocturnal hypoventilation in children aged 1.5 to 16 years using patient and parental questionnaires. There was a resolution of excessive daytime sleepiness in all children, and significant improvements in the frequency of morning headaches. Quality of life was reported to be stable rather than in steady decline as would be anticipated by disease progression. Moreover, there was a significant reduction in hospitalization rates and health care costs following the institution of nNIV. Perez and colleagues[25] further advocated nNIV therapy in 50 children with SMA or muscle myopathy as a method to improve rib-cage development to further enhance pulmonary growth.

The exact timing for nNIV initiation among children with neuromuscular disorders may vary widely; however, the methods used for titration **(Fig. 2)** of nNIV parallel the recommendations as set out by the consensus guidelines.[9] In general, it is not advocated to use oxygen alone in the management of nocturnal hypoventilation, and if

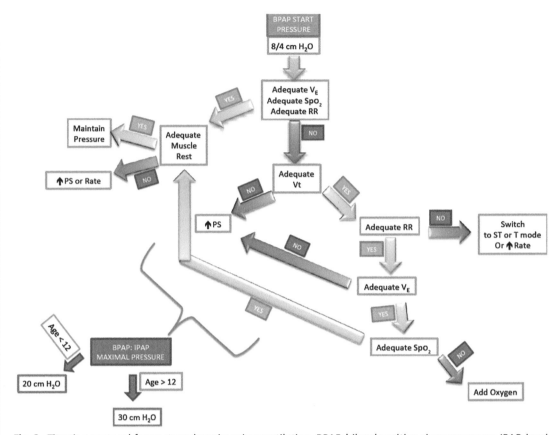

Fig. 2. Titration protocol for nocturnal noninvasive ventilation. BPAP, bilevel positive airway pressure; IPAP, inspiratory positive airway pressure; RR, respiratory rate; Spo$_2$, oxygen saturation; ST, spontaneous timed; T, timed; V$_E$, minute ventilation; Vt, tidal volume. (*Adapted from* Berry RB, Chediak A, Brown LK, et al. Best clinical practice for the sleep center adjustment of noninvasive positive pressure ventilation (NPPV) in stable chronic alveolar hypoventilation syndromes. J Clin Sleep Med 2010;6:496.)

oxygen is added in addition to nNIV, this should be done in carefully performed overnight polysomnography. Technological advances in nNIV have undoubtedly led to advances in the treatment of young children with neuromuscular disorders. Mask sizes now exist for infants as small as 4 kg. There has been enhancement in the triggering sensitivity of several BPAP devices that now allow for more synchronized and less effort-dependent initiation of inspiration and overall ventilation in children. Notwithstanding, triggering and cycling problems do remain significant issues in children using nNIV, particularly when implemented in very young children and infants.

Nocturnal Hypoventilation: Central Hypoventilation Syndromes

Congenital central hypoventilation syndrome
CCHS, a condition best defined as failure of automatic control of breathing, was first described in 1970.[26] Although CCHS was initially believed to

be a life-threatening condition, the discovery of the genetic origin of the disease has revealed a much wider array of severity than originally thought. The primary manifestation is that of sleep-associated respiratory insufficiency and markedly impaired ventilatory response to hypercapnia and/or hypoxemia.[27,28] Unlike the aforementioned neuromuscular disorders of hypoventilation, the pathophysiologic signature of CCHS is hypoventilation that is most profound during quiet stage NREM 3 sleep, a sleep stage associated with the autonomic neural control of sleep. The variability of ventilatory insufficiency in CCHS can range from mild nocturnal hypoventilation to respiratory failure accompanied by sleep-related apneas and hypoventilation observed even during wakefulness.

The putative affected gene underlying CCHS, paired-link homeobox 2B (PHOX2B), has been described by Amiel and colleagues.[29] This gene plays a crucial role in the embryologic development of the autonomic nervous system.[30] Mutations related to polyalanine expansions and nonpolyalanine repeat mutations have been characterized in CCHS,[31,32] and further recent evidence has led to an ability to predict the phenotype, including the severity of impaired ventilatory control with the underlying genotype, specifically the nature and extent of mutations in PHOX2B.

The treatment of CCHS is largely contingent on the underlying severity of ventilatory insufficiency. Despite a paucity of evidence from large studies owing to the exceptionally rare nature of this disease, there have been several published case reports and case series outlining various successful strategies of ventilation. In the context of severe alveolar hypoventilation during both wakefulness and sleep, the mainstay of treatment has been invasive ventilation using a permanent tracheostomy. However, there has been successful transition to nNIV, particularly later in childhood (typically 4–7 years of age) and in children for whom the burden of ventilatory insufficiency is limited to sleep.[27] Furthermore, recent evidence has also suggested successful application of nNIV in early childhood, including young infants with CCHS.[33–40]

Rapid-onset obesity with hypothalamic dysfunction, hypoventilation, and autonomic dysregulation

The condition termed rapid-onset obesity with hypothalamic dysfunction, hypoventilation, and autonomic dysregulation (ROHHAD) is a novel disorder, even though it was first suggested as a separate entity in 1965.[41] ROHHAD is characterized by a period of normal breathing patterns and growth during early life that is then accompanied by the sudden onset of hypothalamic dysfunction leading to hyperphagia, rapid weight gain, and obesity, followed by development of autonomic dysregulation and later alveolar hypoventilation. The timing of alveolar hypoventilation varies, with a median onset during early childhood (6 years of age).[42] Unlike CCHS, there is currently no identified genotype; however, the strong association with neural crest tumors implicates a pathophysiologic mechanism very similar to that of CCHS, even if the gene or genes involved do not include PHOX2B. The multisystem nature of ROHHAD demands a multidisciplinary therapeutic approach, and it is suggested that stabilization of central alveolar hypoventilation is best achieved by a pediatric sleep physician and/or pulmonologist.[43] There are no current longitudinal studies examining the efficacy of nNIV in children with ROHHAD. However, it is apparent that there is a subset of children with ROHHAD who are managed with continuous ventilation, and some

in whom nNIV represents an attractive paradigm, as supportive ventilation is usually indicated only at night.[44,45]

Nocturnal Hypoventilation: Obesity Hypoventilation and Prader-Willi Syndrome

Prader-Willi syndrome (PWS) is a congenital condition whereby most (75%) individuals have a deletion in the paternally derived chromosome 15q11-q13, in some related to a maternal uniparental disomy (20%), and for which approximately 2% to 5% have abnormal methylation of the imprinting center on chromosome 15. This rare genetic disorder affects anywhere from 1 in 10,000 to 1 in 25,000 live births.[46,47] Classic diagnostic characteristics of PWS include developmental delay, hyperphagia, obesity, hypogonadism, and several behavioral abnormalities.[48] Moreover, excessive daytime sleepiness is highly comorbid in children with PWS.[49]

The pathophysiology of nocturnal hypoventilation in PWS is multifactorial. Obesity and an increased risk of scoliosis amount to reduced pulmonary volumes and reduced FRC.[48,50] Underlying reduced global muscular strength leads to respiratory muscular weakness that diminishes chest wall compliance and augments the losses in FRC. Related to abnormalities in peripheral chemoreceptor activity,[51,52] normal adaptive ventilatory responses to hypoxia or hypercapnia are absent or reduced in PWS, predisposing these children to diurnal and nocturnal hypoventilation.

Successful stabilization of hypoventilation has been achieved with nNIV, as reported in several published case reports of small sample sizes.[53–55] However, because of the rarity of this disease there is a paucity of longitudinal studies examining the long-term efficacy of nNIV in both children and adults with PWS.

EQUIPMENT: IMPLICATIONS IN CHILDREN

The application of nNIV in children does not come without several unique challenges. The primary limitation to treating children using nNIV is that these devices were originally intended to treat adults with SDB. Accordingly, modifications must be made to deal with the fairly large prevalence of children in whom nNIV is indicated.

Interface

Selection of the optimal interface is an important step aiming to secure patient compliance and effectiveness of treatment in children with SDB. Of course, the ideal interface should have minimal air leaks, and be very comfortable and easy to wear.[56] Multiple types of interfaces are available in pediatrics, including nasal prongs, nasal masks, nasal pillows, oronasal masks, full-face masks, and helmets. Although mostly unpredictable, clinical factors affecting interface selection are a child's age and neurologic status, and the presence of pulmonary or facial abnormalities. For example, a nasal mask may not be appropriate for very young or uncooperative children, considering the high probability of mouth air leaks. Similarly, the risk of emesis and aspiration in specific high-risk patients should be factored into the decision of implementing a full-face mask.[57] Infants and small children may better be treated with masks that have an appropriately calculated size of dead space. In addition, especially unique to managing pediatric SDB, both mask type and size will have to be adjusted over time to reflect a child's somatic growth.

Circuit and Machine

An open-system (single tubing) or closed-system (double tubing designated for inspiration and expiration) circuit is usually used and depends on the selection of the ventilator (ie, time-cycled-pressure-limited or volume controlled). Volume-cycled ventilators provide the prescribed volume and will adjust the driving pressure as needed unless a high-pressure limit alarm is imposed. The major caveat to these systems is that they do not compensate for air leaks because the machine cannot differentiate between inspired gas and leaked gas, thereby leading to the potential of reduced tidal volume delivery, which can be a significant limitation in ventilating young children in whom the tidal volume is already somewhat diminished. By contrast, pressure-controlled machines compensate for small to medium-sized air leaks. Pressure mode is usually preferred in children because of the relatively large amount of wasted ventilation in the circuit. However, because the current noninvasive ventilators were designed for adults, they are often not triggered by very small or weak children with low inspiratory flow rates or high respiratory rates.

TECHNIQUES OF NONINVASIVE POSITIVE PRESSURE VENTILATION
Continuous Positive Airway Pressure

Continuous positive airway pressure (CPAP) is delivered to the patient by continuous airflow and a pressure valve. Historically this was the first method developed[58] to prevent airway closure throughout the respiratory cycle while improving FRC and reducing the work of breathing. In addition, CPAP normalizes pharyngeal dilator muscle activity during sleep in patients with obstructive sleep apnea.[59] If cessation of breathing effort is a concern, CPAP is inadequate, and a titration study in the sleep laboratory or hospital is required for optimal pressures to be defined.

Automatically Titrated Positive Airway Pressure

For automatically titrated positive airway pressure (APAP), the machine will continuously adjust delivery pressures as needed to eliminate defined respiratory events during sleep. Experience with APAP in children is scarce and has not been critically studied.[60,61]

Bilevel Positive Airway Pressure Ventilation

BPAP is often prescribed in the management of central apnea/chronic hypoventilation in children.[62] Two levels of pressure are delivered to the patient: a lower pressure during expiration and a higher pressure delivered during inspiration (inspiratory positive airway pressure [IPAP]), thereby requiring triggering of the machine (assist, control, or assist-control modes are available with inherent issues pertaining to patient disease) by the patient and synchronization between the spontaneous respiration of the patient and the device. Concerning the latter, the inspiratory ramp slope and expiratory triggering valve setup may require specific adjustments in individualized situations.[9]

Average Volume-Assured Pressure Support

Average volume-assured pressure support (AVAPS) combines volume-controlled and pressure-controlled ventilation, and was specifically developed for conditions during which BPAP with fixed pressure support may not sustain adequate ventilation over time. These recent modalities estimate the expiratory tidal volume and respond by adjusting the IPAP such as to preserve targeted alveolar ventilation.[63] To date only one case of successful use of AVAPS mode has been reported, in a 16-year-old child with CCHS.[64]

Proportional Assisted Ventilation

If the volume or flow that the patient generates during inspiration is measured, the ventilator will deliver inspiratory flow and pressure that closely tracks the child's spontaneous breathing effort.[65] The respiratory pattern is dialed (normal, obstructive, restrictive, or mixed) and all other machine variables are then programmed (CPAP, maximum pressure, maximum tidal volume, and percent assistance). Initial case series of young infants and children with viral bronchiolitis and in premature infants appear promising.[66,67]

Adaptive Servoventilation

Adaptive servoventilation (ASV) was originally developed to treat Cheyne-Stokes central sleep apnea in adult patients with congestive heart failure, but no experience has been reported thus far in children with irregular breathing patterns.[68] Recently ASV was implemented in 2 children with Joubert syndrome who exhibited the characteristic and markedly erratic breathing patterns during sleep and waking.[69,70]

GENERAL CONSIDERATIONS
Air Leaks

A major issue in nNIV is overcoming air leaks that result from mouth breathing or from poor interface selection and placement. Although the ventilators will compensate for leaks by increasing airflow, the presence of significant air leaks may lead to decreases in tidal volume delivery and to problems in triggering the ventilator, potentially compromising the child's respiratory status.

Humidification

High flow of air and unidirectional inspiratory nasal airflow caused by mouth leaks can lead to significant dryness of the nasal mucosa, potentially promoting substantial discomfort while also increasing the airway resistance.[71] Humidification of inspired gas, preferably with heated humidification, is an important consideration in helping to optimize respiratory support, alleviate such nasal complications, and preserve mucociliary function.

Oxygen Supplementation

Supplemental oxygen can be provided to patients receiving nNIV in an effort to correct hypoxemia or when the patient does not tolerate higher pressures required to maintain adequate ventilation. It should be emphasized that the fraction of inspired oxygen (Fio_2) that is generated by admixing oxygen to the circuit is generally unknown and potentially variable. Owing to the uncertainty regarding the actual Fio_2 being provided to the patient, it is advised to use pulse oximetry monitors for children who require supplemental oxygen.

RESPONSE TO TREATMENT: nNIV ADHERENCE

The extent of the cumulative evidence regarding adherence in children is remarkable for its paucity, not surprisingly considering the relatively short experience of such noninvasive ventilatory support

modalities in the pediatric age range. There have been very few studies using objective criteria to evaluate nNIV adherence in children.[72–74] Even when adherence in the hospital appears to be optimal the overall utilization in the home appears to be different, with substantial problems in adherence emerging.[75,76] Here again it must be emphasized that noninvasive ventilatory support is not approved by the FDA for children younger than 7 years or weighing less than 40 lb (18 kg), even if off-label use does not seem to impose any incremental risk even in very young children at home.[77] The 3 major adherence measures used by the authors include the number of hours of actual use as a proportion of the duration of sleep, the number of nights per week using 6 hours or more per night, and the overall total duration of use (months to years).[78] A major problem with adherence estimates is that many studies are based on subjective reports, mostly overestimating actual usage[79] and therefore stressing the importance of objective adherence monitoring in children. Factors affecting adherence to positive airway pressure have included the underlying disease characteristics and severity, psychosocial factors, socioeconomic status and parental education levels, implementation and titration procedures, mask type, pressure discomfort, perceived benefit, nasal and ocular symptoms, and the ability to use the therapy.[73,76,79,80] Indeed, the approach to improving adherence in children is multifactorial and includes educational, technological, and psychosocial facets of using nNIV.[81] Many children requiring nNIV have underlying chronic illnesses or developmental delays that may impose an additional layer of difficulties in optimizing long-term adherence. Many of these children will object to the caregiver efforts, and may develop conditioned anxiety because of poorly fitting equipment and repeated association of the sight, sound, and sensation of nNIV with discomfort from the mask, a struggle, or both.[82] Considering that parental assessment of the use of nNIV markedly overestimates actual use, efforts to improve adherence are more likely to fail in the context of such misperception, particularly among adolescents.[83] The authors and others traditionally implement a period of acclimatization in the home environment as a useful strategy to achieve improved adherence and outcomes. However, as most studies have assessed adherence for only the first 3 to 6 months of treatment, data for long-term adherence are lacking. Nonetheless, identification of adherence, as early as the first week of therapy, is predictive of long-term adherence, thereby implying that compliance therapy should commence as early as possible.[84] In settings of noncompliance, the authors recommend behavioral interventions using child life therapists and biobehavioral psychological techniques.[85] A period of home acclimatization to the equipment is routinely implemented, whereby children are provided with a practice mask and headgear with which to practice; a gradual application of low-pressure therapy (5 cm H_2O) is then used for 2 weeks while awake and then while asleep to help the child habituate to the intervention. Once the child accepts low pressures through the night as indicated by the digital monitoring card in the machine, an overnight laboratory titration study is performed to determine the optimal pressures required. When comparing BPAP with CPAP with regard to adherence data, in a small, randomized, double-blind trial of 56 children, Marcus and colleagues[75] reported no differences in adherence with either technology, further illustrating the multi-dimensional facets of nNIV adherence. Because children continue to grow, the pressure-setting requirements may change and should be therefore periodically ascertained with regular titration polysomnography. Ensuring adequate pressure settings to restore normal breathing during sleep likely contributes to long-term adherence.

SUMMARY

The data reviewed in this article show that although nNIV treatment of nocturnal hypoventilation in many children would be considered off-label, there is certainly a plethora of indications supporting the use of nNIV in children of all ages. The paucity of longitudinal and large-cohort studies remains the central limitation in the field, and precludes the endorsement of an evidence-based approach to care for all children treated with nNIV. In the context of increasing experience in the implementation of nNIV in children with various forms of SDB, the push for universal standards of care will likely require multicenter investigational approaches whereby outcomes of nNIV for nocturnal hypoventilation will need to be carefully examined. Until then, the approach to managing a child with nNIV remains empiric in nature, and is probably most appropriately assumed by experienced pediatric sleep physicians.

REFERENCES

1. Simonds AK, Muntoni F, Heather S, et al. Impact of nasal ventilation on survival in hypercapnic Duchenne muscular dystrophy. Thorax 1998;53: 949–52.
2. Baydur A, Layne E, Aral H, et al. Long term non-invasive ventilation in the community for patients with musculoskeletal disorders: 46 year experience and review. Thorax 2000;55:4–11.
3. American Academy of Sleep Medicine. The international classification of sleep disorders: diagnostic & coding manual. 2nd edition. Westchester (IL): American Academy of Sleep Medicine; 2005.
4. Montgomery-Downs HE, O'Brien LM, Gulliver TE, et al. Polysomnographic characteristics in normal preschool and early school-aged children. Pediatrics 2006;117:741–53.
5. Marcus CL, Omlin KJ, Basinki DJ, et al. Normal polysomnographic values for children and adolescents. Am Rev Respir Dis 1992;146:1235–9.
6. Uliel S, Tauman R, Greenfeld M, et al. Normal polysomnographic respiratory values in children and adolescents. Chest 2004;125:872–8.
7. Traeger N, Schultz B, Pollock AN, et al. Polysomnographic values in children 2-9 years old: additional data and review of the literature. Pediatr Pulmonol 2005;40:22–30.
8. Berry RB, Brooks R, Gamaldo CD, et al. The AASM manual for the scoring of sleep and associated events: rules, terminology and technical specifications, version 2.0.1. Chicago (IL): American Academy of Sleep Medicine; 2013.
9. Berry RB, Chediak A, Brown LK, et al. Best clinical practices for the sleep center adjustment of noninvasive positive pressure ventilation (NPPV) in stable chronic alveolar hypoventilation syndromes. J Clin Sleep Med 2010;6:491–509.
10. Finder JD, Birnkrant D, Carl J, et al. Respiratory care of the patient with Duchenne muscular dystrophy: ATS consensus statement. Am J Respir Crit Care Med 2004;170:456–65.
11. Arens R, Muzumdar H. Sleep, sleep disordered breathing, and nocturnal hypoventilation in children with neuromuscular diseases. Paediatr Respir Rev 2010;11:24–30.
12. Ono S, Takahashi K, Jinnai K, et al. Loss of catecholaminergic neurons in the medullary reticular formation in myotonic dystrophy. Neurology 1998; 51:1121–4.
13. Gozal D, Thiriet P. Respiratory muscle training in neuromuscular disease: long-term effects on strength and load perception. Med Sci Sports Exerc 1999;31:1522–7.
14. Pruna L, Chatelin J, Pascal-Vigneron V, et al. Regional body composition and functional impairment in patients with myotonic dystrophy. Muscle Nerve 2011;44:503–8.
15. Kim HK, Laor T, Horn PS, et al. T2 mapping in Duchenne muscular dystrophy: distribution of disease activity and correlation with clinical assessments. Radiology 2010;255:899–908.
16. Mok E, Letellier G, Cuisset JM, et al. Assessing change in body composition in children with Duchenne muscular dystrophy: anthropometry

and bioelectrical impedance analysis versus dual-energy X-ray absorptiometry. Clin Nutr 2010;29: 633–8.

17. Gozal D. Pulmonary manifestations of neuromuscular disease with special reference to Duchenne muscular dystrophy and spinal muscular atrophy. Pediatr Pulmonol 2000;29:141–50.

18. Petrone A, Pavone M, Testa MB, et al. Noninvasive ventilation in children with spinal muscular atrophy types 1 and 2. Am J Phys Med Rehabil 2007;86: 216–21.

19. Bach JR, Baird JS, Plosky D, et al. Spinal muscular atrophy type 1: management and outcomes. Pediatr Pulmonol 2002;34:16–22.

20. Bach JR, Rajaraman R, Ballanger F, et al. Neuromuscular ventilatory insufficiency: effect of home mechanical ventilator use v oxygen therapy on pneumonia and hospitalization rates. Am J Phys Med Rehabil 1998;77:8–19.

21. Bach JR, Martinez D. Duchenne muscular dystrophy: continuous noninvasive ventilatory support prolongs survival. Respir Care 2011;56:744–50.

22. Mellies U, Ragette R, Dohna Schwake C, et al. Long-term noninvasive ventilation in children and adolescents with neuromuscular disorders. Eur Respir J 2003;22:631–6.

23. Katz S, Selvadurai H, Keilty K, et al. Outcome of non-invasive positive pressure ventilation in paediatric neuromuscular disease. Arch Dis Child 2004; 89(2):121–4.

24. Young HK, Lowe A, Fitzgerald DA, et al. Outcome of noninvasive ventilation in children with neuromuscular disease. Neurology 2007;68:198–201.

25. Perez A, Mulot R, Vardon G, et al. Thoracoabdominal pattern of breathing in neuromuscular disorders. Chest 1996;110:454–61.

26. Mellins RB, Balfour HH Jr, Turino GM, et al. Failure of automatic control of ventilation (Ondine's curse). Report of an infant born with this syndrome and review of the literature. Medicine 1970;49:487–504.

27. Gozal D. Congenital central hypoventilation syndrome: an update. Pediatr Pulmonol 1998;26: 273–82.

28. Deonna T, Arczynska W, Torrado A. Congenital failure of automatic ventilation (Ondine's curse). A case report. J Pediatr 1974;84:710–4.

29. Amiel J, Laudier B, Attie-Bitach T, et al. Polyalanine expansion and frameshift mutations of the paired-like homeobox gene PHOX2B in congenital central hypoventilation syndrome. Nat Genet 2003;33: 459–61.

30. Pattyn A, Morin X, Cremer H, et al. The homeobox gene Phox2b is essential for the development of autonomic neural crest derivatives. Nature 1999; 399:366–70.

31. Weese-Mayer DE, Berry-Kravis EM, Ceccherini I, et al. An official ATS clinical policy statement: congenital central hypoventilation syndrome: genetic basis, diagnosis, and management. Am J Respir Crit Care Med 2010;181:626–44.

32. Weese-Mayer DE, Rand CM, Berry-Kravis EM, et al. Congenital central hypoventilation syndrome from past to future: model for translational and transitional autonomic medicine. Pediatr Pulmonol 2009;44:521–35.

33. Tibballs J, Henning RD. Noninvasive ventilatory strategies in the management of a newborn infant and three children with congenital central hypoventilation syndrome. Pediatr Pulmonol 2003;36:544–8.

34. Migliori C, Cavazza A, Motta M, et al. Early use of nasal-BiPAP in two infants with congenital central hypoventilation syndrome. Acta Paediatr 2003;92: 823–6.

35. Juhl B, Norregaard FO. Congenital central hypoventilation–treated with nocturnal biphasic intermittent respiration via nasal mask. Ugeskr Laeger 1995;157:1683–4 [in Danish].

36. Villa MP, Dotta A, Castello D, et al. Bi-level positive airway pressure (BiPAP) ventilation in an infant with central hypoventilation syndrome. Pediatr Pulmonol 1997;24:66–9.

37. Ramesh P, Boit P, Samuels M. Mask ventilation in the early management of congenital central hypoventilation syndrome. Arch Dis Child Fetal Neonatal Ed 2008;93:F400–3.

38. Schafer T, Schafer C, Schlafke ME. From tracheostomy to non-invasive mask ventilation: a study in children with congenital central hypoventilation syndrome. Med Klin (Munich) 1999;94:66–9 [in German].

39. Nielson DW, Black PG. Mask ventilation in congenital central alveolar hypoventilation syndrome. Pediatr Pulmonol 1990;9:44–5.

40. Kam K, Bjornson C, Mitchell I. Congenital central hypoventilation syndrome; safety of early transition to non-invasive ventilation. Pediatr Pulmonol 2014; 49(4):410–3.

41. Fishman LS, Samson JH, Sperling DR. Primary alveolar hypoventilation syndrome (Ondine's curse). Am J Dis Child 1965;110:155–61.

42. Ize-Ludlow D, Gray JA, Sperling MA, et al. Rapid-onset obesity with hypothalamic dysfunction, hypoventilation, and autonomic dysregulation presenting in childhood. Pediatrics 2007;120: e179–88.

43. Patwari PP, Rand CM, Berry-Kravis EM, et al. Monozygotic twins discordant for ROHHAD phenotype. Pediatrics 2011;128:e711–5.

44. Katz ES, McGrath S, Marcus CL. Late-onset central hypoventilation with hypothalamic dysfunction: a distinct clinical syndrome. Pediatr Pulmonol 2000; 29:62–8.

45. Luccoli L, Ellena M, Esposito I, et al. Noninvasive ventilation in a child with hypothalamic dysfunction,

hypoventilation, and autonomic dysregulation (ROHHAD). Minerva Anestesiol 2012;78:1171–2.

46. Kaplan J, Fredrickson PA, Richardson JW. Sleep and breathing in patients with the Prader-Willi syndrome. Mayo Clin Proc 1991;66:1124–6.

47. Donaldson MD, Chu CE, Cooke A, et al. The Prader-Willi syndrome. Arch Dis Child 1994;70:58–63.

48. Holm VA, Cassidy SB, Butler MG, et al. Prader-Willi syndrome: consensus diagnostic criteria. Pediatrics 1993;91:398–402.

49. Laurance BM, Brito A, Wilkinson J. Prader-Willi syndrome after age 15 years. Arch Dis Child 1981;56:181–6.

50. Mallory GB Jr, Fiser DH, Jackson R. Sleep-associated breathing disorders in morbidly obese children and adolescents. J Pediatr 1989;115:892–7.

51. Arens R, Gozal D, Omlin KJ, et al. Hypoxic and hypercapnic ventilatory responses in Prader-Willi syndrome. J Appl Physiol (1985) 1994;77:2224–30.

52. Gozal D, Arens R, Omlin KJ, et al. Absent peripheral chemosensitivity in Prader-Willi syndrome. J Appl Physiol (1985) 1994;77:2231–6.

53. Smith IE, King MA, Siklos PW, et al. Treatment of ventilatory failure in the Prader-Willi syndrome. Eur Respir J 1998;11:1150–2.

54. Doshi A, Udwadia Z. Prader-Willi syndrome with sleep disordered breathing: effect of two years nocturnal CPAP. Indian J Chest Dis Allied Sci 2001;43:51–3.

55. Clift S, Dahlitz M, Parkes JD. Sleep apnoea in the Prader-Willi syndrome. J Sleep Res 1994;3:121–6.

56. Robert D, Argaud L. Non-invasive positive ventilation in the treatment of sleep-related breathing disorders. Sleep Med 2007;8:441–52.

57. Kirk VG, O'Donnell AR. Continuous positive airway pressure for children: a discussion on how to maximize compliance. Sleep Med Rev 2006;10:119–27.

58. Sullivan CE, Issa FG, Berthon-Jones M, et al. Reversal of obstructive sleep apnoea by continuous positive airway pressure applied through the nares. Lancet 1981;1:862–5.

59. Deegan PC, Nolan P, Carey M, et al. Effects of positive airway pressure on upper airway dilator muscle activity and ventilatory timing. J Appl Phys 1996;81:470–9.

60. Palombini L, Pelayo R, Guilleminault C. Efficacy of automated continuous positive airway pressure in children with sleep-related breathing disorders in an attended setting. Pediatrics 2004;113:e412–7.

61. Marshall MJ, Bucks RS, Hogan AM, et al. Auto-adjusting positive airway pressure in children with sickle cell anemia: results of a phase I randomized controlled trial. Haematologica 2009;94:1006–10.

62. Liner LH, Marcus CL. Ventilatory management of sleep-disordered breathing in children. Current opinion pediatrics 2006;18:272–6.

63. Murphy PB, Davidson C, Hind MD, et al. Volume targeted versus pressure support non-invasive ventilation in patients with super obesity and chronic respiratory failure: a randomised controlled trial. Thorax 2012;67:727–34.

64. Vagiakis E, Koutsourelakis I, Perraki E, et al. Average volume-assured pressure support in a 16-year-old girl with congenital central hypoventilation syndrome. J Clin Sleep Med 2010;6:609–12.

65. Younes M, Puddy A, Roberts D, et al. Proportional assist ventilation. Results of an initial clinical trial. Am Rev Respir Dis 1992;145:121–9.

66. Liet JM, Dejode JM, Joram N, et al. Respiratory support by neurally adjusted ventilatory assist (NAVA) in severe RSV-related bronchiolitis: a case series report. BMC Pediatr 2011;11:92.

67. Alander M, Peltoniemi O, Pokka T, et al. Comparison of pressure-, flow-, and NAVA-triggering in pediatric and neonatal ventilatory care. Pediatr Pulmonol 2012;47:76–83.

68. Teschler H, Dohring J, Wang YM, et al. Adaptive pressure support servo-ventilation: a novel treatment for Cheyne-Stokes respiration in heart failure. Am J Respir Crit Care Med 2001;164:614–9.

69. Fabbri M, Vetrugno R, Provini F, et al. Breathing instability in Joubert syndrome. Mov Disord 2012;27:64.

70. Kamdar BB, Nandkumar P, Krishnan V, et al. Self-reported sleep and breathing disturbances in Joubert syndrome. Pediatr Neurol 2011;45:395–9.

71. Richards GN, Cistulli PA, Ungar RG, et al. Mouth leak with nasal continuous positive airway pressure increases nasal airway resistance. Am J Respir Crit Care Med 1996;154:182–6.

72. Uong EC, Epperson M, Bathon SA, et al. Adherence to nasal positive airway pressure therapy among school-aged children and adolescents with obstructive sleep apnea syndrome. Pediatrics 2007;120:e1203–11.

73. DiFeo N, Meltzer LJ, Beck SE, et al. Predictors of positive airway pressure therapy adherence in children: a prospective study. J Clin Sleep Med 2012;8:279–86.

74. Ramirez A, Khirani S, Aloui S, et al. Continuous positive airway pressure and noninvasive ventilation adherence in children. Sleep Med 2013;14:1290–4.

75. Marcus CL, Rosen G, Ward SL, et al. Adherence to and effectiveness of positive airway pressure therapy in children with obstructive sleep apnea. Pediatrics 2006;117:e442–51.

76. O'Donnell AR, Bjornson CL, Bohn SG, et al. Compliance rates in children using noninvasive continuous positive airway pressure. Sleep 2006;29:651–8.

77. Downey R 3rd, Perkin RM, MacQuarrie J. Nasal continuous positive airway pressure use in children with obstructive sleep apnea younger than 2 years of age. Chest 2000;117:1608–12.

78. Kheirandish-Gozal L, Sans Capdevila O, Kheirandish E, et al. Elevated serum aminotransferase levels in children at risk for obstructive sleep apnea. Chest 2008;133:92–9.

79. Simon SL, Duncan CL, Janicke DM, et al. Barriers to treatment of paediatric obstructive sleep apnoea: development of the adherence barriers to continuous positive airway pressure (CPAP) questionnaire. Sleep Med 2012;13:172–7.

80. Prashad PS, Marcus CL, Maggs J, et al. Investigating reasons for CPAP adherence in adolescents: a qualitative approach. J Clin Sleep Med 2013;9:1303–13.

81. Sawyer AM, Gooneratne NS, Marcus CL, et al. A systematic review of CPAP adherence across age groups: clinical and empiric insights for developing CPAP adherence interventions. Sleep Med Rev 2011;15:343–56.

82. Koontz KL, Slifer KJ, Cataldo MD, et al. Improving pediatric compliance with positive airway pressure therapy: the impact of behavioral intervention. Sleep 2003;26:1010–5.

83. Beebe DW, Byars KC. Adolescents with obstructive sleep apnea adhere poorly to positive airway pressure (PAP), but PAP users show improved attention and school performance. PLoS One 2011;6: e16924.

84. Nixon GM, Mihai R, Verginis N, et al. Patterns of continuous positive airway pressure adherence during the first 3 months of treatment in children. J Pediatr 2011;159:802–7.

85. Rains JC. Treatment of obstructive sleep apnea in pediatric patients. Behavioral intervention for compliance with nasal continuous positive airway pressure. Clin Pediatr (Phila) 1995;34: 535–41.

Index

Note: Page numbers of article titles are in **boldface** type.

Sleep Med Clin 9 (2014) 455–462

http://dx.doi.org/10.1016/S1556-407X(14)00073-3

1556-407X/14/$ – see front matter © 2014 Elsevier Inc. All rights reserved.

Moving?

Make sure your subscription moves with you!

To notify us of your new address, find your **Clinics Account Number** (located on your mailing label above your name), and contact customer service at:

Email: journalscustomerservice-usa@elsevier.com

800-654-2452 (subscribers in the U.S. & Canada)
314-447-8871 (subscribers outside of the U.S. & Canada)

Fax number: 314-447-8029

Elsevier Health Sciences Division
Subscription Customer Service
3251 Riverport Lane
Maryland Heights, MO 63043

*To ensure uninterrupted delivery of your subscription, please notify us at least 4 weeks in advance of move.

ELSEVIER

Printed and bound by CPI Group (UK) Ltd, Croydon, CR0 4YY

03/10/2024

01040382-0019